Everything You Always Wanted to Know About...

Human Anatomy & Physiology

3rd edition

STERLING
Education

Customer Satisfaction Guarantee

Your feedback is important because we strive to provide the highest quality educational materials. Email us comments or suggestions.

info@sterling-prep.com

We reply to emails – check your spam folder

All rights reserved. This publication's content, including the text and graphic images or part thereof, may not be reproduced, downloaded, disseminated, published, converted to electronic media, or distributed by any means without prior written consent from the publisher. Copyright infringement violates federal law and is subject to criminal and civil penalties.

3 2 1

ISBN-13: 979-8-8855731-3-9

Sterling Education materials are available at quantity discounts.
Contact info@sterling–prep.com

Sterling Education
6 Liberty Square #11
Boston, MA 02109

©2025 Sterling Education

Published by Sterling Education

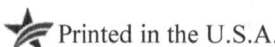 Printed in the U.S.A.

STERLING
Education

From the basic structure of the human body to the complex mechanisms of cellular processes, this comprehensive text is an excellent guide for learning anatomy and physiology. This book provides an essential overview of body structures and functions, elucidating multidimensional concepts of organ systems.

This book is for those who want to develop a better understanding of human anatomy, as well as the relationships between body systems. It uses clear and comprehensible language to explain all essential cellular and physiological processes that affect body functions.

You will learn about cell structure, cell cycle, human body planes and directions, endocrine, nervous, respiratory, circulatory, immune, muscular, skeletal, digestive, excretory, and integumentary systems, reproductive anatomy, and fertilization process.

Created by highly qualified instructors and researchers, this book takes readers on a journey through the fascinating and complex human body. This book educates and empowers readers, regardless of whether they took anatomy and physiology courses or are unfamiliar with the basics.

The editors sincerely hope this guide is a valuable resource for learning human anatomy and physiology.

250411akp

Featured on

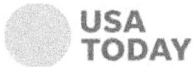 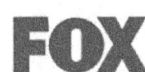 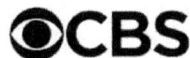 

If you benefited from this book, please leave a review on Amazon so others can learn from your input. Reviews help us understand our customers' needs and experiences while keeping our commitment to quality.

Everything You Always Wanted to Know About…

Chemistry

Physics

Cell & Molecular Biology

Organismal Biology

Human Anatomy & Physiology

American History

American Law

American Government & Politics

Comparative Government & Politics

World History

European History

Psychology

Sociology

Environmental Science

Human Geography

Visit our Amazon store

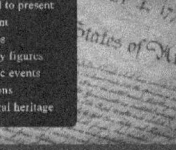

Page intentionally left blank

If you benefited from this book, please leave a review on Amazon so others can learn from your input. Reviews help us understand our customers' needs and experiences while keeping our commitment to quality.

Table of Contents

CHAPTER 1: STRUCTURE & FUNCTION OF EUKARYOTIC CELL 31

Cell Theory 33
- Defining characteristics of cells 33
- History and development 34
- Impact on biology 34

Prokaryotic and Eukaryotic Cells 35
- Nucleus and other defining cellular characteristics 35
- Comparing prokaryotes and eukaryotes 35
- Biochemistry considerations of surface-volume constraints 36
- Nucleus compartmentalizes genetic information 37
- Nucleolus location and function 38
- Nuclear envelope and nuclear pores 38

Membrane-Bound Organelles 41
- Cytoplasm and endomembrane system 41
- Structure of mitochondria 42
- Endosymbiotic theory of evolution 42
- Lysosomes as vesicles containing hydrolytic enzymes 43
- Rough and smooth endoplasmic reticulum 44
- Ribosomes 44
- Smooth endoplasmic reticulum for lipids biosynthesis 45
- Rough endoplasmic reticulum for transmembrane protein biosynthesis 45
- Transmembrane and secreted proteins with signal sequence 45
- Organelles with double-membrane structures 46
- Golgi apparatus modifies, packages and secretes glycoproteins 47
- Peroxisomes 47

Plasma Membrane 49
- Semi-permeable plasma membrane 49
- Phospholipid bilayer with embedded proteins and steroids 49
- Protein components and fluid mosaic model 50
- Fluid mosaic model and associated proteins of membranes 51
- Functional classes of membrane proteins 52
- Semi-permeable membranes produce osmotic pressure 53

Table of Contents (*continued*)

CHAPTER 1: STRUCTURE & FUNCTION OF EUKARYOTIC CELL (*continued*)

Plasma Membrane (*continued*)

Passive transport, diffusion and osmosis	55
ATP needed for primary active transport	56
Energy coupling drives secondary active transport	56
Membrane channels	57
Electrochemical gradient produces a membrane potential	58
Membrane receptors and cell signaling pathway	59
Exocytosis and endocytosis	60
Gap junctions, tight junctions and desmosomes	61

Cytoskeleton **63**

Cytoskeleton for cell support and movement	63
Microfilaments for cleavage and contractility	64
Intermediate filaments for support	64
Microtubules for support and transport	64
Eukaryotic cilia and flagella	65
Centrioles and the microtubule-organizing centers	65

Cell Cycle and Mitosis **67**

Methods for cell division	67
Interphase as the common phase of the cell cycle	67
Four stages of mitosis	68
Cytokinesis divides the cytoplasm to produce two daughter cells	69
Nuclear membrane reorganization during cell division	70
Centrioles, asters and spindles	70
Chromatids, centromeres and kinetochores	70
Mechanisms of chromosome movement	71
Phases of the cell cycle: G_0, G_1, S, G_2, M	71
Sequential phases of the cell cycle	72
Growth arrest	73
Checkpoints during cellular division	73

Table of Contents (*continued*)

CHAPTER 1: STRUCTURE & FUNCTION OF EUKARYOTIC CELL (*continued*)

Cell Cycle Control ... 75
- Cyclin levels regulate cell division ... 75
- Apoptosis as programmed cell death ... 75
- Cancer cells lose cell cycle controls ... 76
- Angiogenesis, oncogenes and tumor suppressor genes ... 77
- Biosignaling ... 78

Tissues Formed by Eukaryotic Cells ... 81
- Simple and stratified epithelium ... 81
- Endothelial cells ... 82
- Connective tissue, loose *vs.* dense fibers and the extracellular matrix ... 82

CHAPTER 2: BASIC HUMAN ANATOMY ... 85

Studying Human Anatomy ... 87
- Categorizing human anatomy ... 87
- Standard anatomical position ... 87

Anatomical Planes and Directional References ... 89
- Anatomical planes ... 89
- Anterior *vs.* posterior relationship ... 90
- Superior *vs.* inferior relationship ... 90
- Medial *vs.* lateral relationship ... 91
- Proximal *vs.* distal relationship ... 91
- Deep *vs.* superficial relationship ... 91
- Ipsilateral *vs.* contralateral relationship ... 91

Body Cavities and Regions ... 93
- Cavities and their associated organs ... 93
- Anatomical terms for body regions ... 94
- Abdominopelvic quadrants and regions ... 94

Table of Contents (*continued*)

CHAPTER 3: ENDOCRINE SYSTEM 97

Hormones and Their Sources 99
- Functions of the endocrine system 99
- Glands secrete direct and trophic hormones 99

Endocrine Glands 101
- Structure and function of major endocrine glands 101
- Anterior pituitary 102
- Thyroid gland 103
- Thyroid disorders and metabolic rates 104
- Adrenal glands for sex hormones and stress responses 105
- Pancreas functions as an exocrine and endocrine gland 106
- Pineal and thymus glands 107

Classifying Hormones 109
- Major classifications of hormones and modes of action 109
- Peptide, steroid and amino acid-derived hormones 110

Hormonal Modes of Action 111
- Insulin regulates blood glucose levels 111
- Peptide hormones' mode of action 111
- Hormones regulate homeostasis 112
- Steroid hormones' mode of action 114
- Androgens and estrogens 115
- Amino acid-derived hormones mode of action 116

Hormone Distribution, Secretion and Effects 119
- Cellular mechanisms of hormone action 119
- Hormone distribution through the blood and lymph fluid 120
- Hypothalamic-hypophyseal and hepatic portal circulation 121
- Target tissue specificity of hormones 121
- Autocrine and paracrine signals 122

Endocrine and Neural Integration 125
- Neuroendocrinology intersects the nervous and endocrine systems 125
- Endocrine integration with the nervous system by feedback control 125
- Regulation by second messengers 126
- Summary table of hormone secretions, targets and effects 128

Table of Contents (*continued*)

CHAPTER 4: NERVOUS SYSTEM 133

- **Vertebrate Nervous System Organization** 135
  - High-level control and integration of body systems 135
  - Central nervous system *vs.* peripheral nervous system 136

- **Nervous System Functions** 137
  - Adaptive capability to external stimuli 137
  - Threshold, all-or-none response 137
  - Efferent control 138
  - Somatic and autonomic nervous systems 138
  - Negative feedback to achieve homeostasis 139
  - Sensory input by the peripheral nervous system 139
  - Limbic system's structures and purpose 140
  - Memory and learning 141

- **Sympathetic and Parasympathetic Nervous Systems** 143
  - Sensory and motor branches of the nervous system 143
  - Sympathetic division of the autonomic nervous system 144
  - Parasympathetic division of the autonomic nervous system 145

- **Reflexes and Feedback Mechanisms** 147
  - Reflex arcs as a survival mechanism 147
  - Feedback loops affect flexor and extensor muscles 147
  - Reflex arc 148

- **Spinal Cord Anatomy** 149
  - Spinal cord function and meninges 149
  - Dorsal and ventral horns for information propagation 150
  - Gray and white matter of the brain and spinal cord 151
  - Descending and ascending tracts connect the brain and spinal cord 151

- **Endocrine System Integration** 153
  - Hormones acting on nervous system 153

- **Neurons** 155
  - Neuron structure and function 155
  - Cell body as the site of nucleus and organelles 156
  - Dendrite and axon structure and function 156
  - Axon: structure and function 156

Table of Contents (*continued*)

CHAPTER 4: NERVOUS SYSTEM (*continued*)

Nerve Structures ... 157
- Neuroglia, glial cells and astrocytes ... 157
- Myelin sheath, Schwann cells, oligodendrocytes ... 157
- Nodes of Ranvier ... 158

Synapses and Neurotransmitters ... 159
- Impulse propagation between cells ... 159
- Classifying electrical and chemical synapses ... 160
- Synaptic propagation between cells without signal loss ... 161
- Neurotransmitters, presynaptic and postsynaptic membranes ... 162
- Postsynaptic neurons and graded potentials ... 163
- Classifying neurotransmitters ... 163

Impulse Propagation ... 165
- Electrochemical gradients ... 165
- Resting potential ... 166
- All-or-none action potentials, depolarization and repolarization ... 166

Excitatory and inhibitory nerve fibers and summation ... 171
- Membrane potentials ... 171
- Excitatory and inhibitory chemical synapses ... 171
- Integration ... 172

Interneurons, Sensory and Efferent Neurons ... 173
- Interneurons integrate and transmit signals ... 173
- Sensory and efferent neurons ... 173

CHAPTER 5: SENSORY RECEPTION & PROCESSING ... 175

Perception of Sensations ... 177
- Psychophysics and experimental psychology ... 177
- Threshold and detecting stimuli ... 177
- Weber's law of just noticeable differences ... 178
- Signal detection theory ... 179
- Sensory adaptation ... 179

Table of Contents (*continued*)

CHAPTER 5: SENSORY RECEPTION & PROCESSING (*continued*)

Sensory Receptors of the Nervous System 181
    Four aspects of stimulus 181
    Sensory receptors 181
    Sensory pathways in the brain and spinal column 183

Sound Perception and Processing 185
    Ear structure and function 185
    Inner ear 186
    Hearing process 187
    Measuring sound and auditory pathways in the brain 188

Vision Perception and Processing 191
    Eye structure and function 191
    Visual acuity and image perception 192
    Cones and rods for light and color perception 193
    Visual image processing 194
    Integration of signals by ganglion cells 195
    Optic nerve 196
    Parallel processing 197
    Feature detection 197

Senses of Touch, Taste, Smell and Balance 199
    Sensation of touch 199
    Taste bud anatomy and function 199
    Olfactory cells detect smells 200
    Pheromones influence behavior 201
    Olfactory pathways in the brain 202
    Kinesthetic and vestibular sense 202
    Dynamic and static equilibrium 203

Perception Processing 205
    Bottom-up and top-down processing 205
    Perceptual organization: depth, form, motion, and constancy 206
    Gestalt principles 207

Table of Contents (*continued*)

CHAPTER 6: RESPIRATORY SYSTEM 209

- **Respiratory System Structure and Function** 211
  - Gas exchange 211
  - Airways enter the lungs 212
  - Protection against disease and particulate matter 213
  - Respiratory ailments 214

- **Lungs and Alveoli** 217
  - Lung structure 217
  - Alveoli as the site of gas exchange 217

- **Mechanisms of Breathing** 219
  - Measuring respiration rates and lung capacity 219
  - Diaphragm and rib cage 219
  - Pressure differences facilitate breathing 221
  - Resiliency and surface tension effects 221
  - Thermoregulation 222

- **Alveolar Gas Exchange** 223
  - Diffusion 223
  - Differential partial pressures of O_2 and CO_2 223
  - Henry's Law 225

- **pH and Neural Regulation** 227
  - pH control 227
  - Henderson-Hasselbalch equation 227
  - Nervous system control 228
  - CO_2 sensitivity 229

CHAPTER 7: CIRCULATORY SYSTEM 231

- **Circulatory System Structure** 233
  - Network for transporting gases, nutrients and hormones 233
  - Role in thermoregulation 233
  - Four-chambered heart structure and function 233
  - Atria and ventricles 234
  - Tricuspid and semilunar valves 235
  - Endothelial cells in heart and blood vessels 236

Table of Contents (*continued*)

CHAPTER 7: CIRCULATORY SYSTEM (*continued*)

Blood Pressure and Cardiac Cycle.. 237
    Systolic and diastolic blood pressure.. 237
    Cardiac cycle.. 238
    Pulse rate... 239
    Cardiac control of heart rate... 239
    EKG and fibrillation.. 240
    Neural and hormonal control of heart rate... 242
    Chemoreceptors and baroreceptors.. 243

Circulation Pathways.. 245
    Pulmonary and systemic circulation... 245
    Blood flow... 246
    Fetal blood pathway.. 246

Arterial and Venous Systems... 249
    Arteries, capillaries and veins... 249
    Structural and functional differences.. 250
    Artery types... 251
    Capillaries as the site of diffusion.. 251
    Venules and veins return blood to the heart...................................... 253

Arterial and Venous Regulation.. 255
    Cardiac output... 255
    Valves regulate blood flow in veins... 256
    Blood volume and pressure.. 257

Oxygen and Carbon Dioxide Transport... 259
    Hemoglobin and hematocrit.. 259
    Sickle cell anemia... 259
    Oxygen content of blood.. 259
    Oxygen affinity and dissociation curves.. 260
    Bohr effects on the oxygen dissociation curves................................ 262
    Oxygen loads in the lungs and dissociates at the tissue.................... 263
    Carbon monoxide binds hemoglobin with high affinity.................... 263
    Carbon dioxide levels and transport by the blood............................. 264

Table of Contents (*continued*)

CHAPTER 7: CIRCULATORY SYSTEM (*continued*)

Exchange Mechanisms 265
    Gas and solute exchange mechanisms 265
    Heat exchange mechanisms 266
    Peripheral resistance impedes blood flow 267
    Vasoconstriction and vasodilation 267

Blood 269
    Blood composition 269
    Leukocytes and cells of the immune system 269
    Lymphocytes and platelets 270
    Erythrocytes, spleen and bone marrow 270
    Regulation of plasma volume 272
    Clotting factors and wound healing 273

Cardiovascular Diseases 277
    Heart failure 277
    Hypertension 277
    Blood clots, myocardial infarction and stroke 278

CHAPTER 8: LYMPHATIC AND IMMUNE SYSTEM 281

Lymphatic System 283
    Lymph nodes, lymphatic vessels and capillaries 283
    Lymphatic system equalizes fluid distribution 283
    Transport of proteins and large glycerides 284
    Lymph returns substances to the blood 284

Lymphatic Fluid 285
    Composition of lymph 285
    The similarity to blood plasma 285
    Lymph transports substances 285
    Diffusion of lymph from capillaries by differential pressure 285

Table of Contents (*continued*)

CHAPTER 8: LYMPHATIC AND IMMUNE SYSTEM (*continued*)

Lymph Nodes **287**
    Lymph nodes anatomy and function 287
    Afferent and efferent lymphatic vessels 288
    Lymph nodes and lymphocytes 288
    Activation of lymphocytes 289

Non-Specific and Specific Immunity **291**
    Active and passive immunity 291
    Vaccination and antibody titer 291
    Major histocompatibility complex 293
    Recognition of self *vs.* non-self 293
    Autoimmune disease 294

Innate Immune System **295**
    Nonspecific immune responses 295
    Complement proteins 296
    Lymphocytes produce antibodies 296
    Macrophages digest foreign material 297
    Phagocytes 298
    Neutrophils 298
    Plasma cells secrete antibodies 299
    Inflammatory response to infection 299
    Allergies 300
    Natural killer cells use cell-to-cell contact 300

Adaptive Immune System **303**
    Specific immune responses 303
    Clonal selection initiated by specific antigens 304
    T lymphocytes, interleukins and cytokines 304
    Roles of B cells and T cells in immunity 307
    Interferons 309

Table of Contents (*continued*)

CHAPTER 8: LYMPHATIC AND IMMUNE SYSTEM (*continued*)

Immune System Tissues and Organs ... 311
- Lymphocytes originate from lymphoid tissue ... 311
- Bone marrow and blood cell production ... 311
- Spleen filters the blood ... 312
- Thymus produces T cells ... 313

Antigen and Antibody ... 315
- Antigen-antibody complex ... 315
- Structure of the antibody molecule ... 315
- Five classes of immunoglobulins ... 316
- Anaphylactic shock ... 317
- Monoclonal antibodies ... 317
- Antigen presentation stimulates antibodies ... 317

Blood Types and Rh Factor ... 319
- Rh factor antigen on red blood cells ... 319
- Blood types and transfusions ... 319

CHAPTER 9: DIGESTIVE SYSTEM ... 323

Digestive System Overview ... 325
- Six processes of the digestive tract ... 325
- Four macromolecules in the digestive tract ... 325
- Gastrointestinal structures ... 326

Ingestion ... 327
- Saliva and digestive enzymes ... 327
- Pharynx, epiglottis and peristalsis ... 328
- Epiglottal action ... 328

Stomach ... 329
- Stomach anatomy and function ... 329
- Mechanical digestion, storage and churning of chyme ... 330
- Mucus, low pH and gastric juice ... 330
- Ulcers ... 331
- Production of digestive enzymes and site of digestion ... 331
- Cardiac and pyloric sphincters of the stomach ... 332

Table of Contents (*continued*)

CHAPTER 9: DIGESTIVE SYSTEM (*continued*)

Liver... 333
    Glandular organ 333
    Nutrient metabolism and vitamin storage 333
    Blood glucose regulation and cellular detoxification 334

Bile.. 337
    Bile production 337
    Gallbladder stores bile 337
    Bile emulsifies fats during digestion 337
    Gallstones and jaundice 338

Pancreas... 339
    Endocrine and exocrine functions 339
    Pancreas produces enzymes and bicarbonate 339
    Transport of enzymes to the small intestine 341

Small Intestine.. 343
    Site of complete digestion and absorption of monomers 343
    Absorption of digested food molecules 343
    Function and structure of villi 344
    Lacteals 345
    Enzyme production and site of digestion 346
    Peptidase and maltase 347
    Pancreatic juices neutralize stomach acid 347
    Anatomical subdivisions of the small intestine 347
    Tissue stratification of the small intestine 348

Large Intestine... 351
    Structure of large intestine 351
    Water absorption by the large intestine 352
    Rectum stores and eliminates waste 352

Muscular Control.. 353
    Sphincter muscles 353
    Peristalsis 353
    Segmentation by the small intestine mixes chyme 354

Table of Contents (continued)

CHAPTER 9: DIGESTIVE SYSTEM (continued)

Gastrointestinal Tract Summary ... **355**
- Anatomy and function of the gastrointestinal (GI) tract ... 355
- Summary of the digestive system ... 355
- Amylase, protease and lipase ... 356

Endocrine Control ... **357**
- Digestive glands and associated hormones ... 357
- Islets of Langerhans, gastrin, histamine and HCl secretions ... 358
- Vitamin D and calcium ... 359
- Receptor regulation and gastrin ... 359

Neural Control by Enteric Nervous System ... **361**
- Neural regulation of the GI tract ... 361
- Unidirectional movement of food ... 362
- Vomit reflex as a survival mechanism ... 362
- Three phases of gastrointestinal control ... 362

Human Nutrition ... **365**
- Macronutrients ... 365
- Carbohydrates ... 365
- Proteins ... 366
- Lipids ... 367
- Absorptive and post-absorptive states ... 368
- Vitamins ... 368
- Minerals ... 370

CHAPTER 10: EXCRETORY SYSTEM ... 373

General Anatomy of Excretory System ... **375**
- Excretory system and kidneys ... 375
- Urinary bladder and urethra ... 375
- Kidneys regulate fluid volume ... 376
- Anatomy of the kidney ... 376

Table of Contents (*continued*)

CHAPTER 10: EXCRETORY SYSTEM (*continued*)

Nephron Structure and Function 377
- Nephron as the functional unit of the kidney 377
- Glomerulus as a capillary bed blood filtration 377
- Bowman's capsule 378
- Proximal tubule 378
- Loop of Henle structure 379
- Loop of Henle reabsorbs salts and water 379
- Distal tubule regulates calcium levels 380
- Collecting ducts and the antidiuretic hormone (ADH) 381

Kidneys and Homeostasis 383
- Kidneys' role in blood pressure regulation 383
- Juxtaglomerular cells 383
- Aldosterone regulates sodium ion reabsorption 383
- Kidneys' role in osmoregulation 384
- Aldosterone regulates blood osmolarity 386
- ADH increases the permeability of collecting ducts 386
- Acid-base balance 387
- Kidneys' role in removing soluble nitrogenous waste 388
- Osmoregulation: reabsorption of H_2O, glucose, ions 389

Urine Formation 391
- Afferent and efferent arterioles at the glomerulus 391
- Tubular reabsorption 391
- Nephron regions and the passage of substances 392
- Location and mechanism for secretion and reabsorption of solutes 394
- Tubular secretions and reabsorption 394
- Proximal convoluted tubules reabsorb salts 395
- Concentration of urine 396
- Countercurrent multiplier mechanism 397

Urine Storage and Elimination 399
- Urinary bladder structure and function 399
- Renal clearance rate 399
- Neural control of the bladder 400

Table of Contents (continued)

CHAPTER 11: MUSCULAR SYSTEM 403

Muscular System Functions 405
- Support and mobility 405
- Assisting peripheral circulation 405
- Thermoregulation 405

Structural Characteristics of Muscles 407
- Skeletal, cardiac and smooth muscle comparison 407
- Voluntary control of skeletal muscle 407
- Cardiac muscle comprises the heart 408
- Involuntary control of smooth muscle 409
- Single-unit and multiunit smooth muscle 410

Muscle Contraction Mechanism 413
- Actin and myosin filaments 413
- Troponin and tropomyosin in muscle contraction 414
- Cross bridges 415
- Sliding filament theory for muscle contractions 416
- Calcium in sarcoplasmic reticulum for muscle contraction 417
- Temporal and spatial response to force 418
- Muscle tension responds to force applied 419
- Muscle contraction types 420

Muscle Regulation 423
- Contractile velocity of different muscle types 423
- Regulation of cardiac muscle contraction 424
- Cardiac muscle contraction pathways 425
- Oxygen debt and muscle fatigue 425

Neural Control of Muscular System 427
- Motor and sensory neurons 427
- Alpha and gamma motor neurons and reflex response 428
- Neuromuscular junctions and motor end plates 428
- Sympathetic and parasympathetic innervation 429
- Voluntary and involuntary muscles 429

Table of Contents (*continued*)

CHAPTER 11: MUSCULAR SYSTEM (*continued*)

Muscle Cell 431
    Muscle cell structure and function 431
    Transverse tubules and calcium 432
    Sarcoplasmic reticulum stores calcium for contractions 432
    Sarcomere anatomy and function for muscle contractions 433
    Muscle fiber types and functions 435
    Myosin ATPase activity 435
    Abundant mitochondria in red muscle cells as ATP source 436
    Muscle types and their properties 437

CHAPTER 12: SKELETAL SYSTEM 441

Skeletal System Functions 443
    Endoskeleton *vs.* exoskeleton 443
    Structural rigidity and support 443
    Storage of calcium under hormonal influence 443
    Physical protection 444
    Skeletal tissues 444

Axial Skeleton Structures 445
    Cranium bones 445
    Facial bones 446
    Vertebral column 446

Appendicular Skeleton Structures 449
    Pectoral and pelvic girdles 449
    Upper limbs 450
    Lower limbs 450

Bone Characteristics 453
    Bone shapes 453
    Bone structure and function 454

Table of Contents (*continued*)

CHAPTER 12: SKELETAL SYSTEM (*continued*)

Cartilage and Joints 457
    Cartilage structure and function 457
    Fibrocartilage 458
    Joint structure and function 459
    Hierarchical structure of ligaments and tendons 461
    Anatomy and functions of ligaments and tendons 462
    Mechanical properties of ligaments and tendons 463
    Stress *vs.* strain for tendons and ligaments 463

Bone Composition 465
    Chemical composition of bone 465
    Four types of bone matrix cells 465
    Compact and spongy bones 466
    Calcium–protein matrix of bones 467

Bone Growth and Remodeling 469
    Bone ossification, formation and growth 469
    Dynamic bone remodeling by osteoblasts and osteoclasts ... 472

Endocrine Control of Skeletal System 473
    Osteoblasts and osteoclasts 473
    Minerals and vitamins for bone deposition and remodeling ... 473
    Hormones of bone remodeling 474
    Bone remodeling for calcium homeostasis 474
    PTH, vitamin D and calcitonin 475

CHAPTER 13: SKIN SYSTEM 477

Skin Structure and Functions 479
    Integument 479
    Essential functions of skin 480
    Layer differentiation, cell types, and tissue 480
    Epidermal layers' structure and function 481
    Dermal layers' structure and function 483
    Skin receptor structure and functions 483
    Skin pigmentation and melanocytes 485
    Relative impermeability to water 485

Table of Contents (*continued*)

CHAPTER 13: SKIN SYSTEM (*continued*)

Thermoregulation Function of Skin 487
    Osmoregulation 487
    Thermoreceptors in skin 487
    Hair and erectile musculature of skin 488
    Adipose tissue layer for energy reserves and insulation 488
    Merocrine and apocrine sweat glands 488
    Vasoconstriction and vasodilation of surface capillaries 489
    Regulation beyond the thermoneutral zone 489

Physical Protection by Skin 493
    Skin functions as the first barrier of defense 493
    Protection against abrasion and pathogens 493
    Nail anatomy 494

Hair Structure 495
    Keratin structure 495
    Hair anatomy and texture 495
    Hair life cycle 496

Skin Tissue Damage 494
    Tissue damage by burns 497
    Wound healing 498
    Skin cancer classification 498

Hormonal Influences 499
    Hormone modulations of skin and fluid balance 499
    Hormones regulate blood flow during thermoregulation 499

CHAPTER 14: REPRODUCTIVE SYSTEM 503

Female Reproductive Structures and Functions 505
    Genitalia of the reproductive system 505
    Female genitalia 505
    Vagina 506
    Uterus 506
    Fallopian tubes 507
    Gonad anatomy and functions 507
    Ovarian anatomy 507

Table of Contents (*continued*)

Male Reproductive Structures and Functions **509**
    Male genitalia 509
    Penis 509
    Blood supply 510
    Scrotum 510
    Spermatic ducts 510
    Gonads 511
    Gonad anatomy and function 511
    Blood supply and innervation 512
    Accessory glands 512
    Semen 513
    Accessory muscles 513
    Sperm pathway 514

Gametogenesis **515**
    Gonads produce gametes 515
    Gamete formation 515
    Gamete development 515
    Meiosis 516
    Diploid zygote 516

Meiosis **517**
    Two stages of meiosis 517
    Phases of meiosis I 517
    Meiosis I: reduction phase from diploid to haploid 518
    Meiosis II: 1N → 1N 519
    Fertilization restores diploid number 520
    Haploid gametes fuse during fertilization 520
    Meiosis *vs.* mitosis summary 521

Oogenesis **523**
    Ovarian cycle 523
    Oogenesis *vs.* spermatogenesis 523
    Oocytes 524
    Polar bodies 524
    Ovum development 525
    Ovulation 525

Table of Contents (*continued*)

CHAPTER 14: REPRODUCTIVE SYSTEM (*continued*)

Spermatogenesis **527**
    Sperm formation 527
    Primary and secondary spermatocytes 527
    Spermatid formation 527
    Spermatogonium 528
    Meiosis II 528
    Sertoli cells 528
    Leydig cells and epididymides 529

Gametes' Structure and Functions **531**
    Female *vs.* male gametes 531
    Egg morphology 532
    Granulosa cell 532
    Sperm morphology and mechanisms 533
    Spermatozoa 533
    Egg and sperm contributions during fertilization 533
    Cytoplasmic nutrients and biomolecules 534

Sexual Development **535**
    Male and female sexual maturity 535
    Reproductive organs mature during puberty 535
    Secondary male characteristics 536
    Secondary female characteristics 536
    Female breast development 537
    Female hormone fluctuations 537
    Male reproductive cycle 538
    Sperm production rate 538
    Neural control of sexual arousal 538
    Sexual excitation 538
    Ejaculation 539
    Orgasm 539

Table of Contents (*continued*)

CHAPTER 14: REPRODUCTIVE SYSTEM (*continued*)

Hormonal Control of Ovarian Cycle **541**
    Female ovarian cycle 541
    Menstrual cycle 541
    Menstrual phase 542
    Menses 542
    LH surge 542
    Endometrium formation 543

Hormonal Control of Female Reproductive Cycle **545**
    Ovulation 545
    Pregnancy maintains endometrium 545
    Hormonal response to fertilization 545
    Female and male infertility 546
    Viviparity 546

Hormonal Control of Gestation and Birthing **547**
    Pregnancy 547
    Corpus luteum 547
    Parturition 547
    Labor 547
    Delivery 548
    Breast development during pregnancy 548
    Lactation 548

APPENDIX **551**

    Glossary of Anatomy & Physiology Terms **553**

Page intentionally left blank

Page intentionally left blank

Chapter 1

Structure & Function of Eukaryotic Cell

Cell Theory

Prokaryotic and Eukaryotic Cells

Membrane-Bound Organelles

Plasma Membrane

Cytoskeleton

Cell Cycle and Mitosis

Cell Cycle Control

Tissues Formed by Eukaryotic Cells

Page intentionally left blank

Cell Theory

Defining characteristics of cells

Cell theory, the scientific theory which describes the morphological and biochemical properties of cells, is a fundamental doctrine of biology.

Classical cell theory includes three fundamental tenets derived from the research of early biologists:

1. *All living organisms are composed of one or more cells.*

    Multicellular organisms are composed of many cells.

    Unicellular organisms (e.g., bacteria) are composed of one cell.

2. *Cells are the smallest, basic units of life.*

    Cells are the smallest units of life because they are the smallest structures capable of carrying out the fundamental metabolic process (e.g., reproduce and divide, extract energy from their environment).

3. *Cells arise from pre-existing cells and cannot be created from non-living material.*

    Creating new cells is cellular division and used in sexual and asexual reproduction.

As the modern understanding of biology evolved, so did the tenets of cell theory.

Modern cell theory adds the following concepts to classical cell theory:

4. *Cells pass on the genetic material during replication in the form of DNA.*
5. *The cells of organisms are chemically similar.*
6. *Cells are responsible for energy flow and metabolism.*

The tenets of cell theory are somewhat dynamic, and as such, some scientists may omit some tenets or include others not mentioned here.

History and development

Robert Hooke first observed the small structural units, which he called "cells," under the light microscope in 1665. However, it was not until nearly 200 years later that significant progress was made in understanding these cells. In the 1830s, botanist Matthias Schleiden discovered cells in the tissues of plants and declared that cells are the building blocks of plants. Simultaneously, Theodor Schwann published his work on cell theory, generalizing it to plants and animals. Shortly after that, Rudolf Virchow overturned the predominating belief that cells were spontaneously generated from non-living matter. He proclaimed that all cells must arise from other living cells.

Cell biology was consistently advanced by new findings in membrane physiology, mitosis, and other cellular and molecular processes.

In the 1950s, James Watson and Francis Crick published their discovery of the molecular structure of DNA, which revolutionized the entire field of biology. Other researchers, including Rosalind Franklin, went uncredited for their seminal work on this monumental discovery.

Impact on biology

Cell theory is an important unifying concept that provides biologists with a common understanding from which they can make further discoveries. Once the foundation of cell theory was laid, along with advances in laboratory techniques and instrumentation, scientific progress in the field of biology rapidly accelerated. The relatively slow progress of biology before the mid-1800s demonstrates the difficulties of advancing in a field where the framework is not understood.

By understanding the basics of a single cell, researchers could add context to life sciences. This is because cells represent the building blocks of all organisms. Multicellular organisms exhibit *emergent properties*, meaning the whole is greater than the sum of its parts. Cells form tissues, tissues form organs, organs form organ systems, and organ systems form multicellular organisms. For example, the individual cells in the lungs are not of much use by themselves, but when combined as a working unit, they create a highly sophisticated set of lungs essential for the organism's survival.

Prokaryotic and Eukaryotic Cells

Nucleus and other defining cellular characteristics

Cells are divided into two taxa: *Eukarya* and *Prokarya*.

Prokaryotes are divided into the domains of Bacteria and Archaea.

Prokaryotes and eukaryotes' salient difference is that prokaryotes lack a nucleus and membrane-bound organelles. A prokaryotic cell's main intracellular components are its single double-stranded circular DNA molecule, ribosomes, and cytoplasm.

Prokaryotic cells include a phospholipid plasma membrane and an outer peptidoglycan cell wall. They are usually smaller than eukaryotic cells with smaller ribosomes (30S and 50S subunits; 70S as assembled).

Eukaryotic cells have linear DNA enclosed in a membrane-bound nucleus and membrane-bound organelles.

Eukaryotic cells replicate via mitosis or meiosis, while prokaryotes replicate via *binary fission*, a form of asexual reproduction.

Many similarities exist between the two cell types.

Prokaryotes and eukaryotes contain cytoplasm, ribosomes, and DNA, and are unicellular or multicellular, although multicellular prokaryotes are rare.

Some eukaryotes are capable of asexual reproduction, albeit differently from prokaryotes.

Plants and fungi (eukaryotes) have cell walls like prokaryotes.

Comparing prokaryotes and eukaryotes

Prokaryotes	Eukaryotes
Domains: Bacteria and Archaea	Domain: Eukarya
Cell wall present in all prokaryotes	Cell wall in fungi, plants, and some protists
No nucleus, circular strand of dsDNA	Membrane-bound nucleus housing dsDNA
Ribosomes (subunits = 30S and 50S; 70S)	Ribosomes (subunits = 40S and 60S; 80S)
No membrane-bound organelles	Membrane-bound organelles

Biochemistry considerations of surface-volume constraints

The cell's metabolic activity describes the biochemical reactions within the cell.

Substances need to be taken into the cell to fuel these reactions, while the reactions' waste products need to be removed.

When the cell increases in size, so do its metabolic activity.

The cell's surface area is vital because it affects the rate particles can enter and exit, with a larger surface area resulting in a higher uptake and excretion rate.

The volume affects the rate at which biochemical materials are made (or consumed) within the cell; the chemical activity per unit of time.

As the volume (and associated chemical activity) of the cell increases, so does the surface area, but not to the same extent. When the cell gets bigger, its surface area-to-volume ratio gets smaller.

If the surface area-to-volume ratio decreases, substances cannot enter the cell fast enough to fuel reactions.

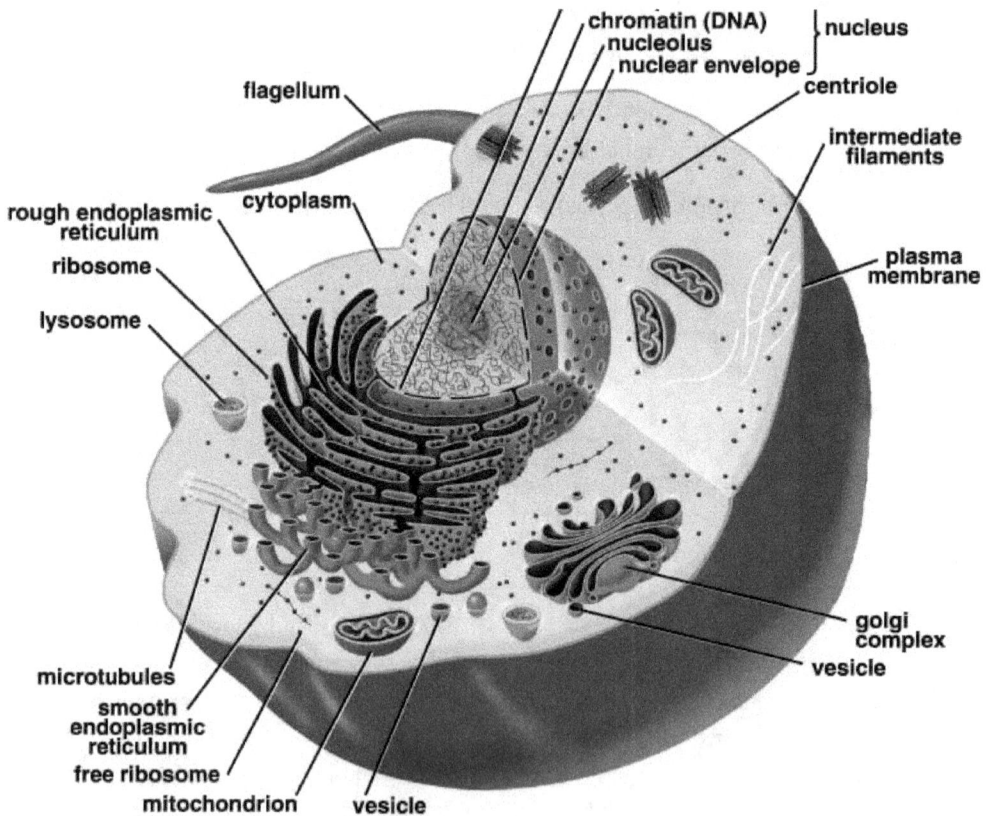

A eukaryotic animal cell with no cell wall or chloroplasts as in eukaryotic plant cells

Waste products are produced faster than they can be excreted, accumulating inside the cell. Cells are not able to lose heat fast enough and may overheat.

The surface-area-to-volume ratio is important for a cell. The physical limitation of the area-to-volume ratio limits the size of cells.

Nucleus compartmentalizes genetic information

The *nucleus* is the largest membrane-bound organelle in the center of most eukaryotic cells. It contains the cell's genetic code—its DNA. The nucleus's function is to direct the cell by storing and transmitting genetic information.

Cells contain multiple nuclei (e.g., skeletal muscle cells), one, or rarely, none (e.g., red blood cells).

Inside the nucleus is the *nuclear lamina*, a dense network of filamentous and membranous proteins associated with the nuclear envelope and its pores.

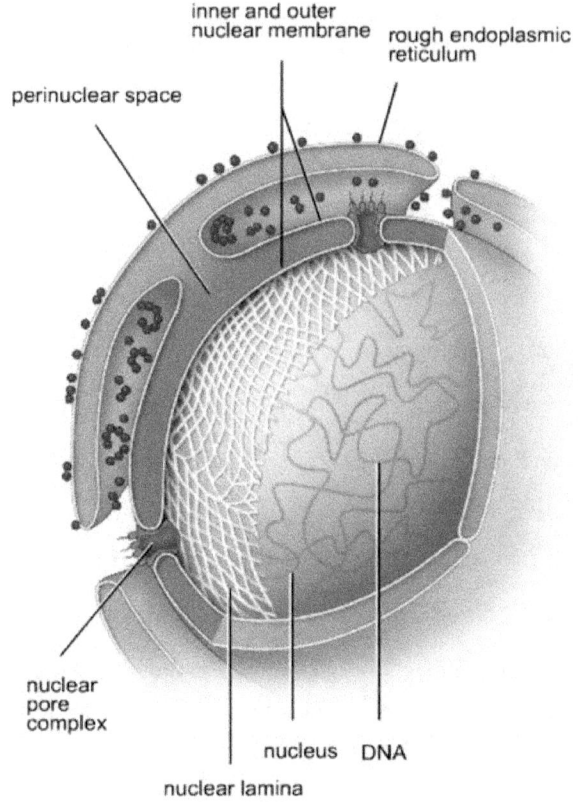

A double membrane surrounds the nucleus of the cell with nuclear pores for select transport of a substance in and out of the nucleus

The lamina provides mechanical support and is involved in crucial cell functions, including DNA replication, cell division, and chromatin organization.

The *nucleoplasm* is the nucleus's semifluid medium, analogous to the cell's cytoplasm. In the nucleoplasm, DNA and proteins interact to form *chromatin*.

Nucleolus location and function

The *nucleolus* is a nonmembrane-bound region in the nucleus where ribosomal RNA (rRNA) is transcribed subunits assembled.

Chromosomal loci of the ribosomal RNA (rRNA) genes are known as nucleolar organizing regions (NORs). rRNA is essential for ribosome formation during protein synthesis (i.e., translation).

The rRNA subunits are exported from the nucleolus to the cytoplasm for assembly into ribosomes to translate mRNA into proteins. The nucleolus is the site of transcription and processing of rRNA subunits.

Thus, it has DNA, RNA, and ribosomal proteins, including RNA polymerases, imported from the cytosol. Under the light microscope, the nucleolus is prominent in cells with high protein production.

Nuclear envelope and nuclear pores

Nuclear envelope (or *nuclear membrane*) is a double membrane system composed of an outer and inner membrane.

The nuclear envelope is analogous to the plasma membrane surrounding the cell.

Perinuclear space is between the two layers of the nuclear membrane.

Nuclear pores punctuate the nuclear double membrane for selective passage of specific biomolecules entering the nucleus.

Cell processes and communications require the segregation of biomolecules.

The number of nuclear pores is not static but changes based on the cell's needs.

Through the pores, signal molecules, nucleoplasm proteins, nuclear membrane proteins, lipids, and transcription factors can enter the nucleus, while mRNA, rRNA, and ribosomal proteins exit into the cytoplasm.

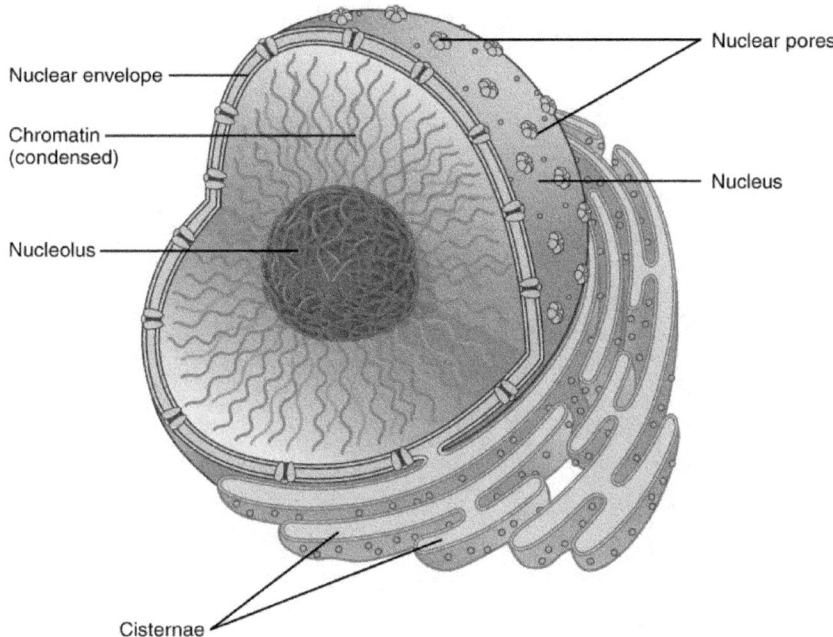

The nucleolus is within the nucleus and assembles ribosomal subunits in eukaryotic cells

Notes for active learning

Membrane-Bound Organelles

Cytoplasm and endomembrane system

The cytoplasm is the cellular material outside the nucleus and within the cell's plasma membrane. It includes the *cytosol*, the cell's fluid medium, and the *organelles*, small, usually membrane-bound subunits with specialized functions (ribosomes are not membrane-bound). Among other functions, organelles structurally support the cell, facilitate cell movement, store and transfer energy, and exchange products in transport vesicles. Mitochondria in animal cells and chloroplasts in plant cells are organelles with genetic material and replicate independently of the nucleus.

The *endomembrane system* is a series of intracellular membranes that compartmentalize the cell. Vesicles bud from the endomembrane system as transport molecules within the cell. Products synthesized in the cell pass through at least some portion of the endomembrane system.

A typical pathway through the endomembrane system is:

1. Proteins produced in rough ER (endoplasmic reticulum) and lipids from smooth ER are carried in vesicles to the Golgi apparatus.

2. The Golgi apparatus modifies these products and sorts and packages them into vesicles transported to various cell destinations (e.g., organelles or exported from the cell).

3. Secretory vesicles transport products to organelles or the plasma membrane, secreted via exocytosis.

Aside from the Golgi apparatus, smooth and rough ER, and secretory vesicles, the endomembrane system includes the membranes of lysosomes, peroxisomes, and other organelles within the cell.

While most cells have the same organelles, their distribution may differ depending on the cell's function. For example, cells that require much energy for locomotion (e.g., sperm cells) have many mitochondria; cells involved in secretion (e.g., pancreatic islet cells) have many Golgi apparatuses; and cells that primarily serve a transport function (e.g., red blood cells) lack organelles.

Structure of mitochondria

Mitochondria (singular, *mitochondrion*) are responsible for aerobic respiration, converting chemical energy into ATP (adenosine triphosphate) using oxygen. ATP is used as the primary energy source within cells. Mitochondria vary in shape; they may be long and thin or short and broad. Mitochondria can be fixed in one location or form long, moving chains. They have a double membrane, with the outer membrane separating the mitochondria from the cytoplasm.

The inner membrane has folds as *cristae*, which project into the inner fluid, the *matrix* (analogous to the cytoplasm of the cell). Between the outer and inner membrane is the intermembrane space. This region is high in protons, creating a proton gradient, which drives ATP synthesis.

The cristae are dotted with *ATP synthase* protein complexes, powered by the proton gradient (used in the electron transport chain) to transform ADP into ATP. This process is essential to producing the energy that organisms require for metabolic functions. Thus, cells with higher energy needs require more mitochondria.

Endosymbiotic theory of evolution

Mitochondria are unique because they have their genome, distinct from the genome within the nucleus. They have circular DNA, inherited exclusively from the mother, containing genes for synthesizing some mitochondrial proteins.

Mitochondria can replicate their DNA independently from the nucleus. They have ribosomes independent from the host cell's ribosomes in sequence and structure.

The unique characteristics of mitochondria support the *endosymbiosis theory* for the origin of eukaryotic cells. The endosymbiosis theory states that mitochondria were once free-living aerobic prokaryotes consumed by another cell about 1.5 billion years ago.

The prokaryote (likely a proteobacterium) became an endosymbiont within the cell, providing the anaerobic host cell with ATP via aerobic respiration. In return, the host cell provided the endosymbiont with a stable environment and nutrients.

Over time, the endosymbiont transferred most of its genes to the host nucleus, to the point that it became obligate (i.e., could no longer survive outside the host cell) and evolved into a mitochondrion.

Biologists largely accept the endosymbiosis theory. One of the most compelling evidence is that mitochondrial DNA does not encode its proteins.

Many of its genes are in the nuclear DNA; therefore, proteins must be imported into the mitochondria.

Mitochondrial DNA, ribosomes, and enzymes are similar to bacterial forms, and mitochondria replicate by a process similar to binary fission.

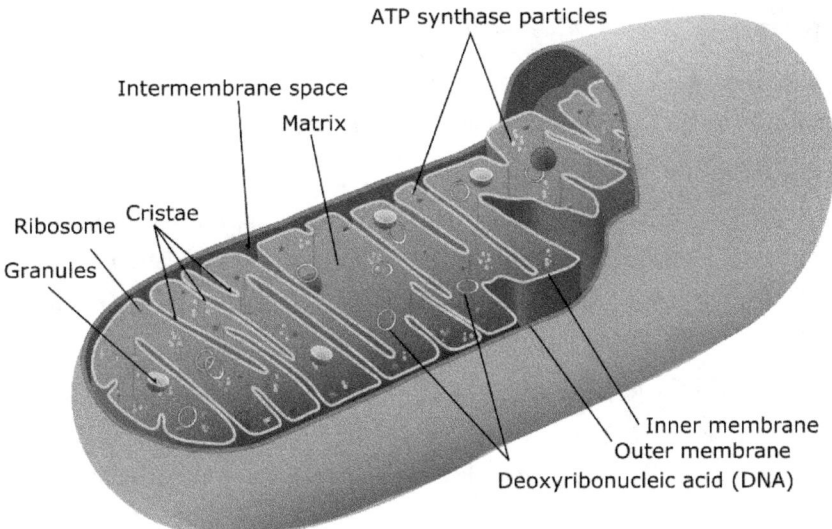

Mitochondria have double membrane enclosure with ATPase embedded in the inner membrane

Additionally, some of the proteins within the mitochondria's plasma membrane are like prokaryotes, different from proteins in the eukaryotic plasma membrane.

Chloroplasts, the organelles that conduct photosynthesis, exhibit strong evidence of an endosymbiotic origin, although they are hypothesized to have descended from cyanobacteria rather than proteobacteria. Chloroplasts and other plastids can undergo secondary and even tertiary endosymbiosis, causing the development of other membranes.

Lysosomes as vesicles containing hydrolytic enzymes

Lysosomes, only in animal cells, are membrane-bound vesicles produced by the Golgi apparatus. These small organelles contain hydrolytic enzymes (low pH) to digest macromolecules: proteins, nucleic acids, carbohydrates, and lipids. These macromolecules may originate from food, from the waste products of cells, or foreign agents, such as viruses and bacteria. After these particles enter a cell in vesicles, lysosomes fuse with vesicles and digest their contents by hydrolyzing the macromolecules into their monomers.

Lysosomes are especially important in specialized immune cells. For example, white blood cells that engulf foreign agents use lysosomes to digest the invaders.

Autodigestion is when lysosomes digest parts of the body's cells due to disease or trauma or for immune purposes (e.g., programmed cell death).

Mutations in the genes that encode lysosomal enzymes cause *lysosomal storage disorders*. When a mutation renders certain lysosomal enzymes inefficient (or inoperable), waste products accumulate in the cells and cause severe, often incurable complications.

Rough and smooth endoplasmic reticulum

Endoplasmic reticulum (ER) is a system of membrane channels (or *cisternae*) continuous with the outer membrane of the nuclear envelope. The space enclosed within the cisternae, the *lumen*, is thus continuous with the perinuclear space.

The rough ER, so-called because of its rough appearance, is studded with ribosomes on the cytoplasmic side. Here, proteins are synthesized and enter the ER interior for processing and modification. Modifications may include folding the protein or combining multiple polypeptide chains to form proteins with several subunits.

The smooth ER is usually interconnected with the rough ER but lacks ribosomes, hence its smooth appearance. It is the site of various synthesis, detoxification, and storage processes, such as synthesizing lipids and steroids and the metabolism of carbohydrates and other molecules.

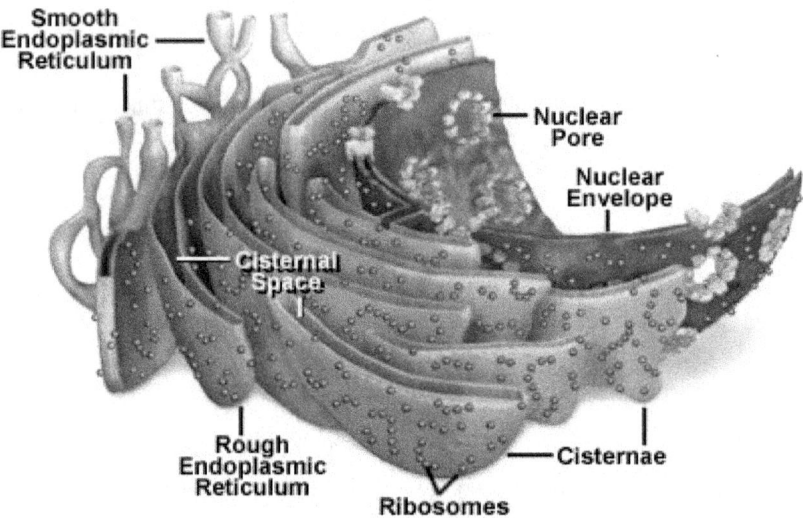

The ER forms transport vesicles for trafficking particles to the Golgi apparatus

Ribosomes

Ribosomes are organelles composed of proteins and ribosomal RNA (rRNA). They are either floating free in the cytoplasm, attached to the rough ER's surface, or within mitochondria and chloroplasts.

Ribosomes translate messenger RNA (mRNA) to coordinate the assembly of amino acids into polypeptide chains, which fold into functional proteins.

Ribosomes of eukaryotic cells are 20 to 30 nm in diameter, while those in prokaryotic cells are slightly smaller. They are composed of one large and one small subunit; each with its mix of proteins and rRNA. *Polyribosomes* are several ribosomes simultaneously synthesizing the same protein; they may be attached to ER or floating freely in the cytosol.

Smooth endoplasmic reticulum for lipids biosynthesis

The smooth ER and rough ER synthesize key membrane components. The smooth ER synthesizes the major lipids of a membrane: phospholipids, glycolipids, and steroids.

Some lipid products are already in the correct form for incorporation into a membrane once secreted by the smooth ER. Other lipids require modification by the Golgi apparatus.

Lipids synthesized in the smooth ER must pass through the Golgi apparatus before heading to their destination at the plasma membrane or membrane-bound organelles.

Rough endoplasmic reticulum for transmembrane protein biosynthesis

The rough ER synthesizes the protein components of cell membranes. This includes the plasma membrane, the membranes of the ER, Golgi apparatus, lysosomes, and other organelles.

Membrane proteins are divided into several classes (discussed later), but some of their functions include membrane transport, cell-to-cell adhesion, cell signaling, and catalysis.

Like lipids synthesized on the smooth ER, proteins synthesized on the rough ER follow a set pathway through the Golgi apparatus towards their destinations.

Transmembrane and secreted proteins with signal sequence

Proteins destined for the plasma membrane, Golgi apparatus membrane, ER membrane, or lysosomal membranes are inserted into the ER membrane immediately after synthesis on the cytosolic side of the rough ER membrane. These proteins are transported as membrane components rather than soluble proteins.

ER membrane proteins end their journey here, but the others proceed to the Golgi apparatus.

Upon post-translational processing, Golgi membrane proteins remain in the Golgi apparatus. The remaining proteins (secretory pathway) travel to the lysosome, the plasma membrane or undergo exocytosis to leave the cell.

Secretory proteins and proteins destined for the *lumen* of the ER or Golgi apparatus are released into the ER lumen following ER synthesis. ER lumen proteins remain in the ER lumen.

Golgi lumen proteins travel to the Golgi lumen, and secretory proteins travel to the Golgi and then the plasma membrane or are secreted by the cell.

Not all protein synthesis takes place on the rough ER. Free-floating ribosomes synthesize proteins designated for use in the cytosol and some organelles (e.g., nucleus, mitochondria, chloroplasts, peroxisomes) in the cytosol. After synthesis, cytosolic proteins are released directly into the cytosol.

Nuclear, mitochondrial, chloroplastic, and peroxisomal proteins are escorted to their destinations by receptor molecules.

Protein synthesis begins on free ribosomes. Therefore, proteins that need to be synthesized in the ER must be translocated there.

Posttranslational translocation to the ER occurs after a free-floating ribosome synthesizes a polypeptide.

Cotranslational translocation (common in mammalian cells) occurs as the polypeptide is synthesized.

Cotranslational translocation is facilitated by a *signal sequence* on the growing polypeptide chain. This sequence is a short chain of amino acids, mostly hydrophobic. As soon as the signal sequence emerges on the polypeptide from the ribosome, a protein-RNA complex called a *signal recognition particle* (SRP) recognizes and binds to the signal sequence and ribosome, halting translation. The SRP then targets the ribosome and polypeptide chain to the rough ER membrane, where the SRP binds to an SRP receptor.

Binding to the SRP receptor releases the SRP from the ribosome and polypeptide, allowing the ribosome itself to bind to a protein translocation complex next to the SRP receptor called *Sec61*. After binding, the signal sequence is inserted into the Sec61 membrane channel (part of the translocation complex), and polypeptide synthesis resumes.

As it grows, the polypeptide chain is translocated through the membrane channel. A *signal peptidase* enzyme cleaves the signal sequence from the rest of the polypeptide, allowing the finished polypeptide to be released into the lumen, where it undergoes folding and modification.

If the polypeptide is a membrane protein that must enter the ER membrane and not the lumen, it is inserted into the ER membrane in a variety of ways. For example, transmembrane proteins may contain a *stop-transfer sequence*, which anchors the polypeptide in the ER membrane partway through synthesis so that the polypeptide is anchored to the ER membrane rather than located in the ER lumen.

Organelles with double-membrane structures

While most organelles of the eukaryotic cell are composed of a single bilayer membrane, three key organelles have a double membrane: mitochondria, chloroplasts, and the nucleus.

Mitochondria have a double membrane structure due to their proposed evolution from an endosymbiotic prokaryote. The intermembrane space is high in proton concentration, while the matrix (like cytosol) within the mitochondria is relatively low in proton concentration.

This double membrane is crucial for creating the proton gradient that drives ATP synthesis. This proton gradient powers ATP synthases, with cytochrome proteins dotting the inner membrane's cristae, combining ADP with Pi and O_2 forming ATP by oxidative phosphorylation.

Chloroplasts, the sites of photosynthesis and ATP synthesis in plant cells, have a double membrane of endosymbiotic origin, the *chloroplast envelope*. The two membranes regulate the passage of particles into and out of the chloroplast. The outer membrane is permeable to ions and metabolites, while the inner membrane is specific to transport proteins.

Unlike mitochondria, chloroplasts contain *thylakoids* as additional membrane-bound structures. The thylakoid membranes are analogous to mitochondrial inner membranes, and the spaces within the thylakoids (lumen) are analogous to the mitochondrial intermembrane space. The high proton concentration in the lumen creates the proton gradient that drives ATP synthesis on the thylakoid membranes.

A sophisticated, double-membrane nuclear envelope surrounds the nucleus. The highly selective nuclear protein pores dotting the envelope regulate gene expression by controlling the passage of transcription factors, biomolecules, and mRNA into and out of the nucleus. Since the outer membrane is continuous with the rough ER, no vesicle transport is required to transport ER proteins into the nucleus. As a result, the cell's energy requirements are lower than if transport were required.

Golgi apparatus modifies, packages and secretes glycoproteins

The *Golgi apparatus*, named for the Italian 1906 Noble laureate Camillo Golgi, consists of a stack of flattened sacs. It acts as an intermediary in the secretion of biomolecules. The Golgi apparatus receives transport vesicles from the ER and may modify their contents before packaging the protein or lipid in vesicles for transport to their destination.

Glycosylation affects a protein's structure and function and protects it from degradation. Glycosylation is when the Golgi apparatus modifies a protein by adding carbohydrates. The Golgi apparatus glycosylates proteins (i.e., add sugar residues to a protein) and modifies existing glycosylations. The finished glycosylation product is a *glycoprotein* protein with attached sugars or carbohydrates.

Peroxisomes

Peroxisomes are membrane-bound vesicles containing enzymes for a variety of metabolic reactions. They are involved in the catabolism (i.e., degradation) and anabolism (i.e., synthesis) of macromolecules, including fatty acids, proteins, and carbohydrates. When peroxisomes were first discovered, they were defined as organelles that produce hydrogen peroxide through oxidation reactions. Peroxisomes use catalase (enzymes end with *~ase*) to degrade the produced hydrogen peroxide into water and oxygen or oxidize compounds.

Peroxisomes are abundant in the liver, where they are notable for producing bile salts from cholesterol and metabolizing alcohol. They participate in lipid biosynthesis. Peroxisomes' functions are vast and varied, making them a vital part of eukaryotic cells.

Notes for active learning

Plasma Membrane

Semi-permeable plasma membrane

The *semi-permeable plasma membrane* separates cell contents from the extracellular environment and regulates the passage of materials into and out of the cell. The plasma membrane surrounds the cell, providing support, protection, and a boundary from the outside environment. It is primarily composed of lipids and proteins, forming a dynamic bilayer of lipids with membrane proteins. The function and composition of the two layers of a plasma membrane differ; therefore, the membrane is asymmetric.

Phospholipid bilayer with embedded proteins and steroids

Lipids are a large group of naturally occurring hydrophobic molecules. They are vital components of the plasma membrane. Lipids in the plasma membrane include phospholipids, steroids, and glycolipids. The foundation of the plasma membrane is the *phospholipid bilayer*. Phospholipids are molecules with a phosphate head and two long hydrocarbon tails. The head is hydrophilic and attracts water and other polar molecules, while the hydrocarbon tails are hydrophobic and repel water molecules.

The special dual nature of phospholipids, called *amphipathic*, allows them to align into a bilayer when placed in water spontaneously. In the bilayer, the hydrophilic phosphate heads point out towards the aqueous solution, while the hydrophobic tails point inward towards one another. Thus, the plasma membrane's extracellular and intracellular surfaces are hydrophilic, while the membrane's interior is hydrophobic. Hydrophobic interactions in the interior of the membrane hold the entire structure together.

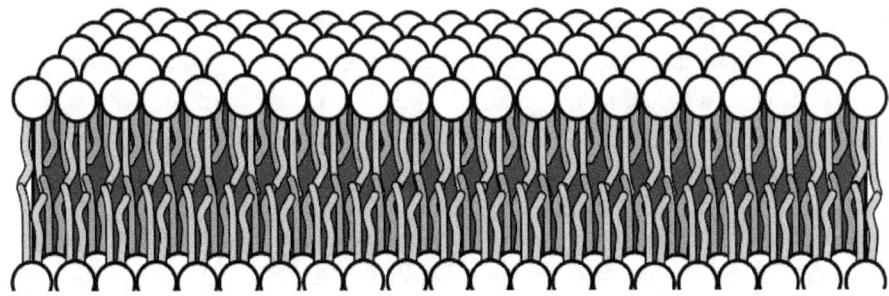

Phospholipid bilayer (absent in the schematic are embedded proteins)

The bilayer provides the plasma membrane with stability and with extraordinary flexibility. Lipids exhibit free lateral diffusion about the bilayer, resulting in varying lipid compositions across the membrane sections. Generally, cell membranes have a consistency like that of olive oil at room temperature.

Increasing the concentration of lipids with unsaturated hydrocarbon tails increases membrane fluidity; the addition of saturated hydrocarbon tails makes the membrane rigid.

Cells regulate membrane fluidity by lengthening phospholipid tails, altering the cytoskeleton, changing their protein composition, and adding steroids (e.g., cholesterol).

Steroids are a class of lipids that regulate membrane fluidity by hindering phospholipid movement. Cholesterol, a steroid in animal plasma membranes, plays a crucial role in maintaining membrane fluidity despite temperature fluctuation. At high temperatures, membranes become dangerously fluid and permeable unless cholesterol interferes with extreme phospholipid movement.

At low temperatures, membranes may freeze unless cholesterol prevents phospholipids from becoming stationary due to strong hydrophobic interactions.

Cholesterol molecules facilitate cell signaling and vesicle formation.

Glycolipids are lipids modified with a carbohydrate. In the plasma membrane, they assist in various functions and anchor the plasma membrane to the *glycocalyx*, a layer of polysaccharides linked to the membrane lipids and proteins.

Essentially, the glycocalyx is a carbohydrate coat present on the extracellular surface of the plasma membrane and the extracellular surface of the cell walls of some bacteria. The glycocalyx's carbohydrate chains face outwards, providing markers for cell recognition and adhesive capabilities to the cell.

Protein components and the fluid mosaic model

In the early 1900s, researchers noted that lipid-soluble molecules entered cells more readily than water-soluble molecules, suggesting that lipids are a component of the plasma membrane. Chemical analysis later revealed that the membrane indeed contained phospholipids. The amount of phospholipid extracted from a red blood cell was just enough to form one bilayer. The analysis suggested that the nonpolar tails were directed inward and polar heads outward. To account for the permeability of the membrane to non-lipid substances, researchers initially proposed a *sandwich model*, describing a phospholipid bilayer in between two layers of protein.

After investigation with an electron microscope, the *unit membrane model* was proposed, which was based on the "trilaminar" appearance of two dark outer lines and a light inner region visible under the electron microscope. The dark outer lines were believed to be protein monolayers, while the inner region was thought to be a phospholipid bilayer. The unit membrane model was essentially in agreement with the sandwich model. However, both of these models failed to explain permeability satisfactorily.

Fluid mosaic model and associated proteins of membranes

In 1972, Garth L. Nicholson and Seymour J. Singer published the currently accepted *fluid-mosaic model*, which describes a plasma membrane as a phospholipid bilayer embedded with proteins. Electron micrographs of the freeze-fractured membrane (and other evidence) supported the fluid-mosaic model. The lipid portion of the plasma membrane gives it its "fluid" characteristic. Thus, fluidity describes the lipids that diffuse freely throughout the membrane and regulate consistency.

The membrane's protein components contribute to the "mosaic." Protein composition in the plasma membrane depends on the function of the cell. Some proteins are held in place by cytoskeletal filaments, but most migrate within the fluid bilayer.

The proteins embedded in a membrane are grouped into two classes by location.

Peripheral membrane proteins are on the membrane surface, mainly the intracellular side, interacting with cytoskeletal elements to influence cell shape and motility.

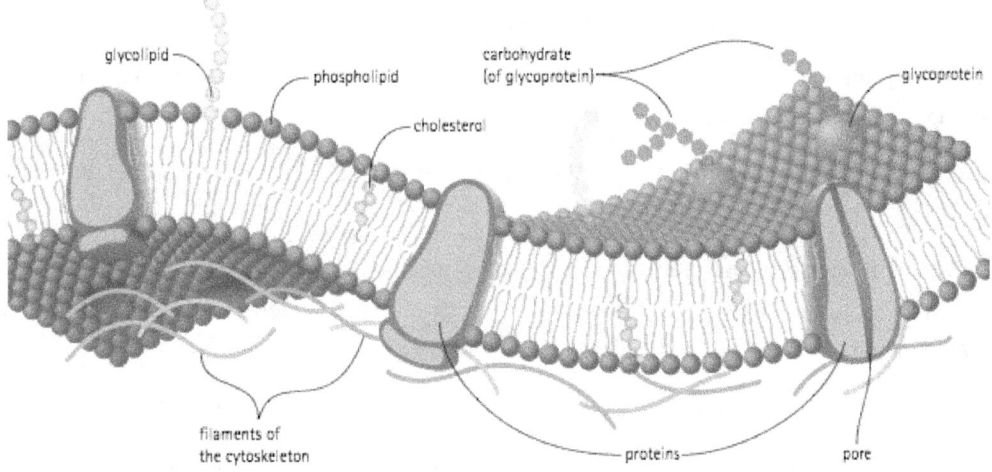

Phospholipid bilayer with cholesterol between hydrophobic lipid tails and embedded proteins

These proteins are not amphipathic; they interact with the membrane's hydrophilic heads.

Peripheral membrane proteins are removed from the membrane with relative ease using high salt or high pH, and therefore are not permanently attached to the membrane.

Integral membrane proteins are permanently attached to the membrane and cannot be removed without disrupting the lipid bilayer. They possess hydrophobic domains anchored to hydrophobic lipids.

Most integral membrane proteins are *transmembrane* proteins, spanning the entire membrane.

Membrane proteins participate in cell signaling, cell-to-cell adhesion, transport through the membrane, enzymatic activity, and other biochemical activities.

Functional classes of membrane proteins

When divided by function, several key classes of membrane proteins emerge.

Receptor proteins provide a binding site for hormones, neurotransmitters, and other signaling molecules. Receptor proteins are usually specific in that they bind to a single molecule or class of molecule. The binding of the signal molecule to the receptor triggers a cellular response corresponding to a specific biochemical pathway.

Adhesion proteins attach cells to neighboring cells for cell-to-cell communication and tissue structure. These proteins generally attach to one cell's cytoskeleton and extend through the plasma membrane to the extracellular environment, where they bind and interact with the adhesion proteins of another cell.

Transport proteins move materials into and out of the cell.

These include *channel proteins* and *carrier proteins*.

Channel proteins provide a passageway for large, polar, or charged molecules that cannot pass through the lipid bilayer without assistance.

The channel proteins facilitate the passive transport of molecules; they do not require ATP to operate.

However, carrier proteins may facilitate passive and active (energy-requiring) transport of molecules. They bind to specific molecules on one side of the cell membrane and changes conformation to release the molecule on the other side of the membrane.

Enzymatic membrane proteins carry out metabolic reactions at the cell membrane.

For example, enzymatic membrane proteins help digest membrane components for recycling. The mitochondrial membrane contains enzymatic proteins (e.g., protein complexes of the electron transport chain in aerobic cellular respiration).

Recognition proteins are glycoproteins that identify a cell to the body's immune system. They allow immune cells to recognize a substance as belonging to the body or as an invasive foreign agent to be destroyed.

Antigens are the basis for A, B, and O blood groups in humans.

Immune cells recognize the sugars attached to these proteins and attack any red blood cells with foreign sugars, so patients of blood groups cannot donate blood or receive blood from people with other blood groups.

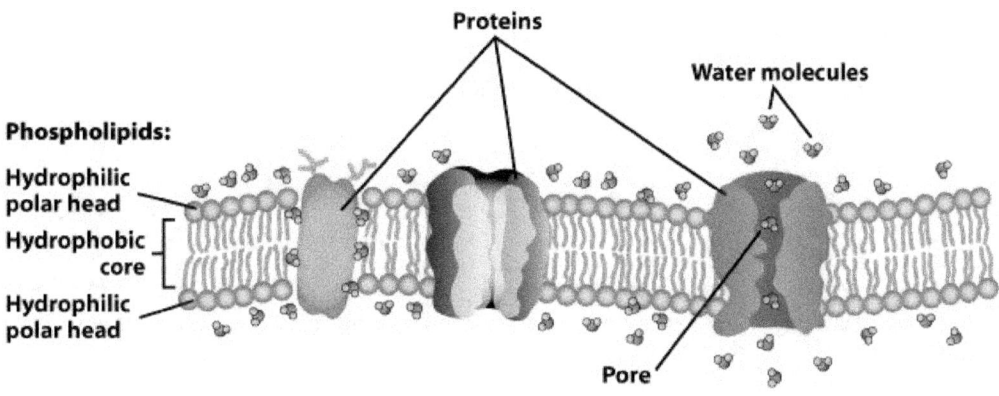

Semi-permeable membranes produce osmotic pressure

All fluids of the body are *solutions*: they contain dissolved substances (solutes) and a fluid (water) in which the substances dissolve (solvent).

Diffusion is the movement of solutes from an area with a higher to an area with a lower concentration.

Osmosis is the diffusion of water from a low solute concentration to an area of high solute concentration. Solutes diffuse to an area of lower solute concentration, while water (a solvent) diffuses to an area of higher solute concentration. The solute and solvent offset unequal solute concentration and restore equilibrium.

The natural inclination of solutes is to diffuse until they are evenly distributed. However, areas of the cell/tissue/organ/body require different solute concentrations. Separation areas are accomplished via the complex system of membrane compartmentalization in organs, tissues, and cells.

The body must prevent body compartments from reaching equilibrium but must allow the passage of certain atoms, ions, and molecules through membranes to the areas needed. Membranes are highly selective and tightly regulated.

Colligative properties of solutions depend on the concentration of a solute in the solution. They do not depend on the chemical nature of the solutes. The most important colligative property for the regulation of body fluids is *osmotic pressure*, the pressure that must be applied to prevent the net flow of water into a solution separated by a membrane (i.e., a measure of water's tendency to flow from one solution to another). This property is related to several other key terms in osmoregulation (the regulation of osmotic pressure).

Osmolarity is the total solute concentration of a solution measured in *osmoles*. Osmolarity considers penetrating and non-penetrating solutes and describes a single solution or compares different solutions.

A *hyperosmotic* solution has a higher osmolarity.

A *hypoosmotic* solution has a relatively low osmolarity.

Isosmotic solutions have the same osmotic pressure.

Tonicity describes the relative concentration of two solutions separated by a selectively permeable membrane and explains how diffusion occurs between them (e.g., between intracellular and extracellular fluid). Unlike osmolarity, tonicity refers to non-penetrating solutes (solutes that cannot cross a membrane) and describes how one solution compares to another.

A *hypertonic* solution has a relatively higher concentration of solute. Conversely, a *hypotonic* solution has a relatively lower concentration of solute. Therefore, a cell with a lower concentration of solute than the extracellular fluid is hypotonic to the fluid, while the extracellular fluid is hypertonic to the cell.

The reverse is true for a cell with a higher concentration of solute than the extracellular fluid.

A cell placed in a hypertonic solution shrinks through a process of *crenation* (i.e., shrinking of the cell) as water diffuses out of the cell to offset the high concentration of the outside solution. Conversely, a cell in a hypotonic solution swells as water rushes into the cell, causing *cytolysis* (i.e., bursting of a cell due to osmotic imbalance caused by excess water entering the cell.

Too much water can enter the cell, resulting in *lysis* (breakage of the cell).

An *isotonic* solution has an equal solute concentration to the solution it is being compared to. In this situation, there is no net water movement.

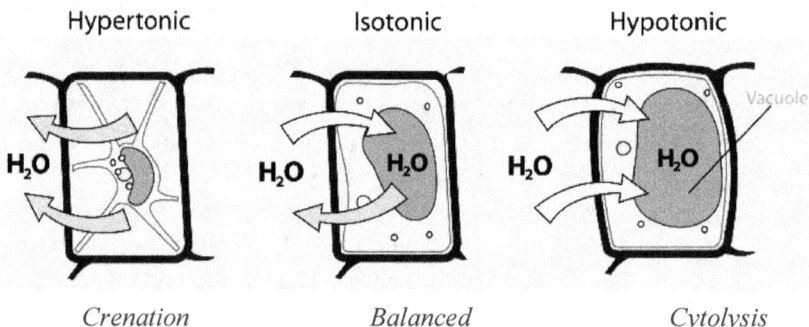

Crenation   *Balanced*   *Cytolysis*

Passive transport, diffusion and osmosis

The plasma membrane is selectively permeable; specific molecules can pass through. A molecule's ability to diffuse through the plasma membrane depends on the molecule's size, charge, and polarity. The greater the diffusing particle's lipid solubility, the easier it passes through the membrane.

Generally, smaller particles diffuse more rapidly than larger ones, and hydrophobic solutes diffuse faster than hydrophilic solutes.

Many particles cannot diffuse through the plasma membrane without assistance. Small, non-charged, or non-polar molecules pass through the membrane freely. Large, charged, or polar molecules usually require assistance to pass through the membrane.

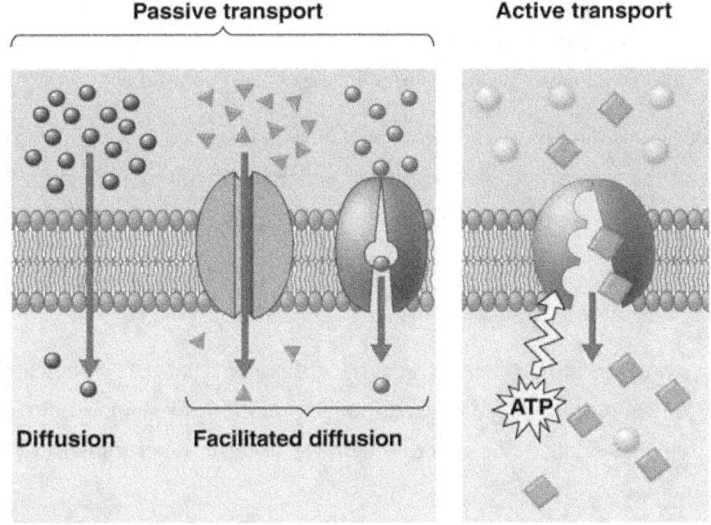

Passive transport includes diffusion and facilitated diffusion with the expenditure of energy as molecules move down the concentration gradient

Passive transport enables the movement of molecules across a membrane without energy expenditure by the cell. The methods include simple diffusion, osmosis, and facilitated diffusion. Passive transport utilizes a *concentration gradient*, whereby particles diffuse from an area of higher to an area of lower solute concentration.

Simple diffusion is the process for smaller, lipid-soluble molecules to diffuse through the phospholipid bilayer. For example, oxygen and carbon dioxide pass through the membrane via simple diffusion.

While water is a polar molecule, it is small enough to diffuse freely across a plasma membrane. *Osmosis* is the passive diffusion of water molecules.

Osmosis occurs when water moves from a region of lower solute concentration to a higher solute concentration region and is facilitated by *aquaporins* as channel proteins. Osmosis is classified as simple diffusion, despite requiring transport proteins like facilitated diffusion.

Facilitated diffusion allows larger, lipid-insoluble molecules that cannot freely pass through the phospholipid bilayer (e.g., sugars, ions, and amino acids) to get transported down their concentration gradient with the assistance of a carrier protein or channel proteins, often as a *uniporter*.

ATP needed for primary active transport

Active transport requires cellular energy to move solutes against their concentration gradient. Unlike passive transport, which exploits molecules' natural inclination to move down their concentration gradient, active transport requires energy expenditure to resist this opposing force. Carrier proteins are the transmembrane proteins that mediate molecules' movement too polar or too large to move across a membrane by diffusion, thereby governing active transport.

During this process, a solute (molecule to be transported) binds to a specific site on a transporter on one surface of the membrane. The transporter changes shape to expose the bound solute to the opposite side of the membrane. The solute dissociates from the transporter and is on the opposite side from which it started.

There are two types of active transport: primary and secondary.

Primary active transport utilizes energy generated directly from ATP. The carrier proteins for primary active transport are pumps. An example is a sodium-potassium pump, which works by moving 3 Na^+ ions out and 2 K^+ ions into a cell, resulting in a net transfer of positive charge outside the membrane.

For a cell at rest, intracellular K^+ concentration is high, and Na^+ concentration is low, while extracellular K^+ concentration is low and Na^+ concentration is high. These concentration gradients facilitate transport across the plasma membrane and help the cell manage its *membrane potential*, the difference in electrical charge between the outside and inside the cell.

Cellular sodium and potassium concentrations are maintained via active transport by the sodium-potassium pump (Na^+ / K^+ ATPase). When the intracellular Na^+ concentration is too high, and K^+ concentration is too low, the sodium-potassium pump must pump Na^+ out of the cell and K^+ into the cell to restore the appropriate concentration gradients.

Energy coupling drives secondary active transport

The energy for *secondary active transport* comes from an electrochemical gradient established by primary active transport. Secondary active transporters work via a mechanism of *cotransport*.

Cotransport occurs when one molecule moves with (down) its concentration gradient, while another molecule moves against (up) its concentration gradient.

The energetically favorable movement of the molecule moving with its concentration gradient powers the other molecule's movement against its concentration gradient.

Antiporters (e.g., sodium-calcium exchanger) move molecules in opposite directions, i.e., one is transported out while the other is transported into the cell.

Symporters move both molecules in the same direction.

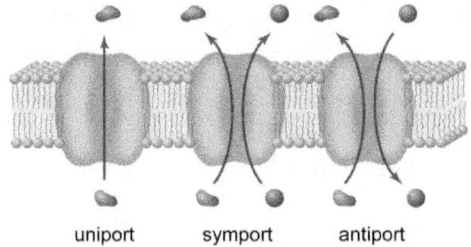

One example of a symporter is the sodium-glucose linked transporter (SGLT), which transports sodium *with* its concentration gradient from the exoplasmic space to the cytoplasmic space, and transports glucose *against* its concentration gradient from the exoplasmic space to the cytoplasmic space. These movements are energetically coupled. Note that while both molecules are moving in the same *physical* direction in a symporter, the molecules are moving in opposite directions but are energetically favorable with one process driving the other.

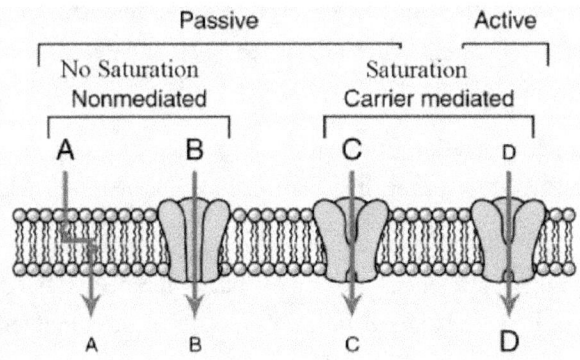

Comparison of passive and active transport: A is diffusion with movement unaided by a protein, B is passive transport down the concentration gradient through a channel (no saturation), C is passive transport through a carrier protein (saturation), D is active transport up a concentration gradient (saturation possible and energy needed)

Membrane channels

Membrane channels are transmembrane proteins that allow ions to diffuse across the membrane via passive transport.

Individual cells have different permeabilities, depending on their membrane channels.

The channel's diameter and the polar groups on the protein subunits forming channel walls determine the permeability of the channels for various ions and molecules.

Porins are channel proteins less chemically specific than many other channel proteins; generally, if a molecule can fit through the porin, it can pass through it.

Ion channels allow for the passage of ions.

Channel gating is the opening and closing of ion channels to the molecules they transport.

Changes in membrane potential modulate voltage-gated channels.

Ligand-gated channels are modulated by allosteric or covalent binding of ligands to the channel protein.

Ligands are small molecules that bind to a protein or receptor, usually to trigger a signal.

Mechanically gated channels are modulated by mechanical stimuli such as stretching, pressure, or temperature.

Several factors influence a single channel, and the same ion may pass through several channels.

Electrochemical gradient produces a membrane potential

The membrane potential is the electrical potential difference between the intracellular and extracellular environments. Nearly all eukaryotic cells maintain a non-zero membrane potential. The membrane potential is mediated by channels and pumps, altering electrochemical gradients as needed by the cell.

Whenever there is a net separation of electric charges across a cell membrane; a membrane potential exists for all cells. However, it is often the focus of neurons and depolarization with action potentials.

The concentration gradient influences molecules, but differences influence ions, creating the resting membrane potential. The *electrochemical gradient* is the combined forces of membrane potential and concentration gradient. These forces may oppose one another, work independently, or work in conjunction.

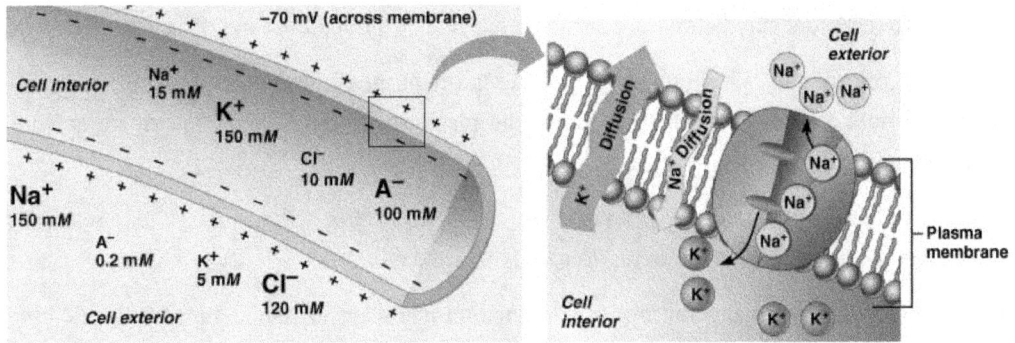

The differences in ion concentrations maintain membrane potential (i.e., voltage)

Nearly all eukaryotic cells maintain a non-zero membrane potential. In animal cells, this value ranges from −40 mV to −80 mV; thus, with respect to the extracellular environment, the inside of the cell has a negative voltage. Membrane potential is especially important for neurons, which have a *resting membrane potential* of about −70 mV. Changes in this resting potential allow for the electrical communications of neurons.

Membrane receptors and cell signaling pathway

Cells must communicate with their neighbors as well as their environment.

Cell signaling is the system by which cells receive, integrate, and send signals to communicate information.

Signals are sent through the *extracellular matrix*, a collection of polysaccharides and proteins secreted by cells in multicellular organisms.

This matrix fills the space between cells, providing structure, facilitating cell signaling, and allowing cells to move and change their shape.

The composition of the extracellular matrix is highly variable depending on tissue type, as different tissues have different functions. For example, the extracellular matrix of bone is highly calcified, while the extracellular matrix of blood is fluid, containing dissolved proteins and other molecules. The most extensive extracellular matrices are of connective tissues, which are found throughout the body and include bone and blood. Connective tissues are largely composed of their extracellular matrix and are only sparsely populated with cells.

A typical connective tissue extracellular matrix includes fibrous proteins and *proteoglycans*, glycoproteins that form a packing gel around the fibrous proteins. The primary fibrous proteins are *collagen* and *elastin*, which provide structure and flexibility, along with *fibronectin* and *laminin*, which assist in adhesion and cell migration. Transmembrane proteins such as *integrins* bind to specific proteins in the extracellular matrix and membrane proteins on adjacent cells. Integrins help organize cells into tissues. They are responsible for transmitting signals from the extracellular matrix to the cell interior.

Membrane receptors may be on the plasma membrane or intracellular membranes.

Not all signal molecules bind to membrane receptors at the plasma membrane. For example, steroid hormones and gases diffuse across the plasma membrane and bind to intracellular receptors.

Other signal molecules enter the cell via endocytosis. In addition to hormones and gases, signal molecules include neurotransmitters, proteins, and lipids.

Membrane receptors are crucial in the cell-signaling pathways. When a signal molecule binds to a membrane receptor, it may initiate a metabolic response, change the membrane potential or alter gene expression.

Signal transduction is when one signaling molecule triggers a multi-step chain reaction, which indirectly transmits the initial signal to its destination. *Second messengers* are the molecules that relay the signal.

At steps in the signal transduction pathway, second messengers can greatly amplify the strength of the original signal by increasing the number of molecules they activate. For example, one signal molecule at the membrane receptor may produce 10 second messengers, and these 10 second messengers may each produce another 10 second messengers, and so on, amplifying the signal significantly.

Cell signaling is a complex process but can be divided into four general categories. *Endocrine signaling* is when a cell secretes a signal that travels to a distant target cell. *Paracrine signaling* is when the target cell is nearby, but not in direct contact. *Juxtacrine signaling* is the signaling of a target cell in direct contact with the secreting cell. *Autocrine signaling* targets the same cell that secreted the signal.

Exocytosis and endocytosis

The plasma membrane's fluidity allows it to change shape, pinch off, and reform. This fluidity enables substances to exit the cell via *exocytosis* and enter the cell via *endocytosis*.

Both processes require cellular energy and are therefore a form of active transport.

During exocytosis, membrane-bound vesicles in the cytoplasm fuse with the plasma membrane, and their contents are released outside the cell. The vesicle assimilates into the plasma membrane, replenishing portions of the membrane that would otherwise be lost.

The exocytosis process is triggered by stimuli, leading to an increase in cytosolic calcium concentration, which activates proteins required for the vesicle membrane to fuse with the plasma membrane. Exocytosis provides a route for releasing synthesized proteins as either extracellular secretions or proteins and lipids destined for the plasma membrane.

Endocytosis is essentially the opposite process of exocytosis. During endocytosis, extracellular molecules destined for the plasma membrane or the cytoplasm are imported into the cell.

In preparation for endocytosis, a region of the outer side of the plasma membrane invaginates to enclose the imported material. This indentation folds and pinches into a membrane-bound vesicle inside the cell.

Pinocytosis ("cell-drinking" or fluid endocytosis) is a form of endocytosis that cells use to import small amounts of extracellular fluid containing molecules absorbed by the cell. The process of pinocytosis may be non-specific or mediated by receptors on the plasma membrane.

A few types of specialized cells perform phagocytosis. Phagocytosis (or *cell-eating*) involves importing larger particulate matter than imported by pinocytosis.

The particulate matter must be degraded before it is absorbed by the cell. As such, phagocytes digest bacteria, viruses, and cell debris as a function of our immune system.

Some unicellular eukaryotes, such as amoeba, rely on phagocytosis for nutrient intake.

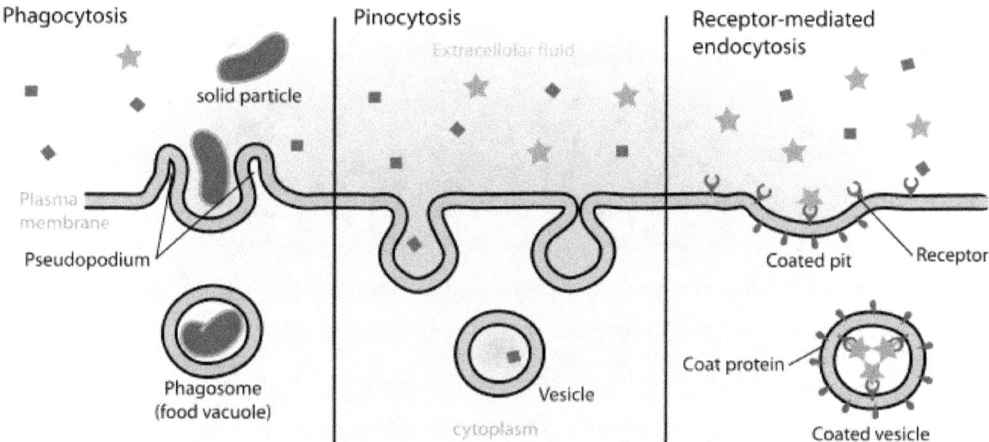

Types of endocytosis with substrates taken into the cell

Gap junctions, tight junctions and desmosomes

Cell junctions are points of contact that physically link neighboring cells.

Animal cells have three intercellular junctions: gap junctions, tight junctions, and anchoring junctions.

Gap junctions are protein channels that link the cytoplasms of adjacent cells. Gap junctions are communicating junctions because they allow for rapid cell-to-cell communication. They form by joining two membrane channels on adjacent cells, allowing small molecules and ions between cells while still preventing their cytoplasms from mixing.

Gap junctions are essential in cardiac muscle tissues, where electrical impulses must be transmitted through cells exceptionally rapidly so that the muscle fibers contract as a single unit.

The *tight junction* has plasma membrane proteins attach in zipper-like fastenings, holding cells so tightly that the tissues become barriers to molecules.

Tight junctions are formed by the physical joining of the extracellular surfaces of two adjacent plasma membranes, producing a seal that prevents the passage of materials between cells.

Materials must enter the cells by passive or active transport to pass through the tissue.

Tight junctions are essential in areas where more control over tissue processes is needed. For example, the epithelial cells in the intestine involved in nutrient absorption.

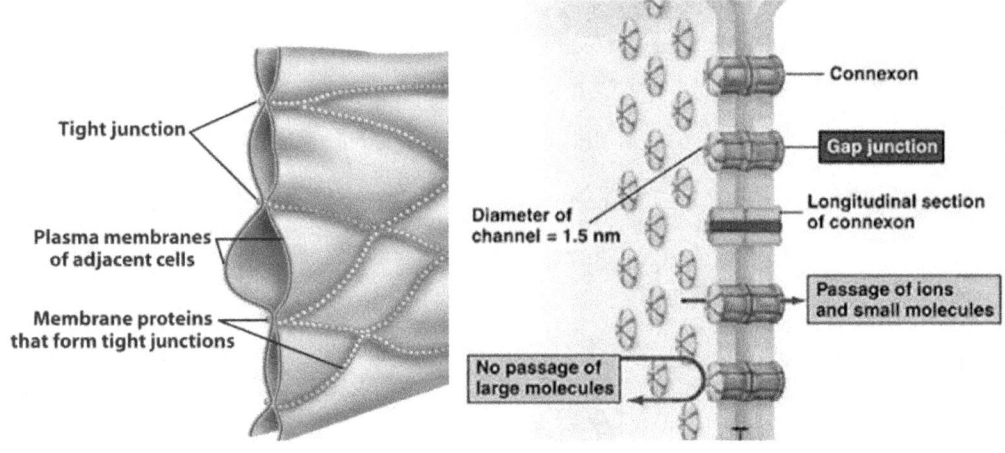

Tight junctions　　　*Gap junctions*

Anchoring junctions use proteins extended through one cell's plasma membrane and attached to another cell. Anchoring junctions are firm but still allow for spaces between adjacent cells.

Desmosomes, an anchoring junction, are created by dense protein patches on the plasma membranes of two cells. Internally, proteins anchor to the cell's cytoplasm, while the proteins adhere to one another.

The purpose and function of desmosomes are to hold adjacent cells firmly in place in tissue areas subject to stretching (e.g., bladder, skin, stomach).

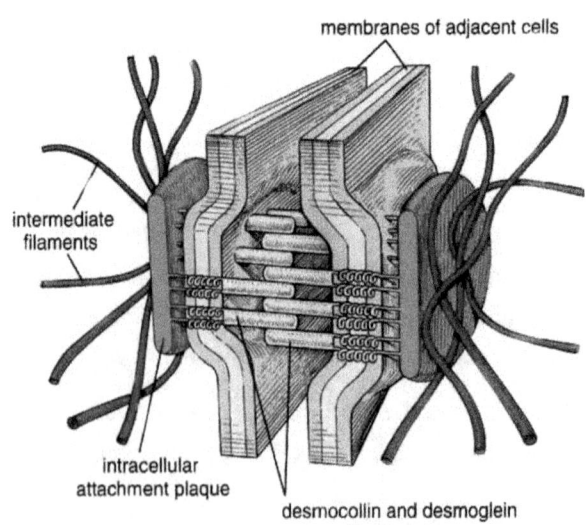

Desmosome

Cytoskeleton

Cytoskeleton for cell support and movement

The *cytoskeleton* is a scaffold of flexible, tubular protein fibers extending between the nucleus to the plasma membrane in eukaryotes. This vast network of fibers maintains the shape of the cell, provides support, and facilitates vesicular transport.

The cytoskeleton is the cellular analogy to an animal's bones and muscles. It anchors organelles and enzymes to cell regions to keep them organized in the cytosol.

The cytoskeleton changes shape to facilitate contractility and movement, allowing the cell to divide, migrate or undergo endocytosis and exocytosis.

During cell division, the cytoskeletal elements rapidly assemble and disassemble, forming spindles for chromosomes' organization and cleaving the cell into two daughter cells.

The cytoskeleton's long fibers serve for intracellular transport, upon which vesicles and organelles move via motor proteins (e.g., dynein and kinesin).

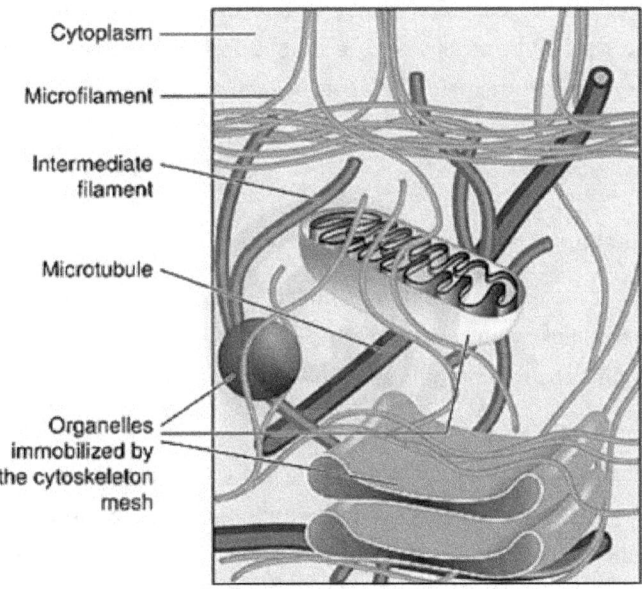

The cytoskeleton is a network of tubular proteins to provide shape and facilitate the transport of vesicles

Microfilaments for cleavage and contractility

Microfilaments (i.e., actin filaments) are the thinnest and abundant of the cytoskeleton proteins. They are contractile protein *actin* composed of long, thin fibers, about 7 nm in diameter, in bundles or mesh-like networks. Microfilament consists of two globular actin subunits chains twisted to form a helix.

Microfilaments assemble and disassemble quickly according to the needs of the cell. They are involved in cell motility functions, such as muscle cells' contraction, the formation of amoeba pseudopodia, and cleavage of the cell during cytokinesis. While flexible, microfilaments are strong and prevent deformation of the cell by their tensile strength.

Microfilaments provide tracks for the movement of myosin. Myosin attaches to vesicles (or organelles) and pulls them to their destination along the microfilament track. Additionally, the interaction between microfilaments and myosin is crucial to the cell's function.

Intermediate filaments for support

Intermediate filaments are thicker than microfilaments but thinner than microtubules. Typically, they are 8 to 11 nm in diameter. These rope-like assemblies of fibrous polypeptides are found extensively in regions of cells subjected to stress. Most intermediate filaments are in the cytoplasm, supporting the plasma membrane and forming a cell-to-cell junction. However, *lamins* are a class of intermediate filaments responsible for structural support within the nucleus. Unlike microfilaments and microtubules, intermediate filaments cannot rapidly disassemble once assembled.

Microtubules for support and transport

Microtubules (tubulin) are hollow protein cylinders about 25 nm in diameter and 0.2–25 μm in length. They are the thickest and most rigid of filaments. Microtubules are globular proteins of *tubulin* and β tubulin. The microtubule assembly combines these as dimers, and the dimers are arranged in rows.

Microtubule strength and rigidity make them ideal for resisting the compression of the cell. However, these fibers serve functions similar to microfilaments. Microtubules act as tracks for intracellular transport, but they interact primarily with *kinesin* and *dynein* motor proteins rather than myosin.

Microtubules' transport function is crucial for trafficking neurotransmitters throughout nerve cells. Like microfilaments, microtubules are rapidly assembled or disassembled. Regulation of microtubule assembly is under the control of a *microtubule-organizing center* (MTOC). Microtubules radiate from the MTOC and extend throughout the cytoplasm. During cell division, the centrosome generates the microtubule spindle fibers necessary for chromosome separation.

Eukaryotic cilia and flagella

Cilia and *flagella* are two microtubule complexes that protrude from the cell body and serve cell motility and sensory functions. Eukaryotes are membrane-bounded cylinders that enclose a matrix of nine pairs of microtubules encircling two single microtubules, a *9 + 2 pattern*. Movement occurs when these microtubules slide past one another. A basal body anchors the cilium (or flagellum) to the cell body at the plasma membrane. The basal body is derived from a centriole formed by nine pairs of microtubules without central microtubules, the *9 + 0 patterns*. Eukaryotic cilia and flagella grow by polymerizing (adding) tubulin to their tips.

Cilia are short, hair-like projections. Nearly every human cell has at least one cilium, *non-motile,* and functions as a sensory antenna important in cell signaling pathways. Non-motile cilia lack the 2 central microtubules and have a 9 + 0 pattern.

Many cells are covered with *motile* cilia, which undulates to transport particles across the cell surface. For example, motile cilia in the respiratory tract push mucus and irritants out of the lungs, trachea, and nose.

Eukaryotic flagella are structurally like eukaryotic cilia, so distinctions are often not drawn between them. Like cilia, they have sensory and motility functions. However, eukaryotic flagella tend to be longer and move with a whip-like motion. An example of a eukaryotic flagellum is the tail of a sperm cell.

Prokaryotic flagella are notably different from their prokaryotic cilia counterparts. Prokaryotic flagella are noted for their long, whip shape and functional differences from cilia.

Centrioles and the microtubule-organizing centers

The *centrosome* is the main microtubule-organizing center at the poles during mitosis and meiosis.

Centrosomes contain a pair of barrel-shaped organelles of *centrioles.*

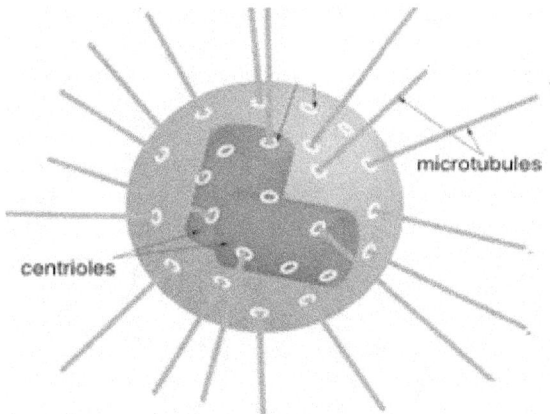

Centrosome is the microtubule organizing center with microtubules attached to the centrioles

The centrosome has a crucial role in mitosis when it divides into two centrosomes, interacting with chromosomes via microtubules to form the mitotic spindle

Centrioles are components of the centrosome. Microtubules radiate from these barrel-shaped structures, made of microtubules themselves. They are short cylinders with a ring pattern (9 + 0) of microtubule triplets.

In animal cells and most protists, a centrosome contains two centrioles oriented at right angles.

In mitosis, the terms centrioles and centrosomes are often used interchangeably because centrioles form the crucial parts of a centrosome.

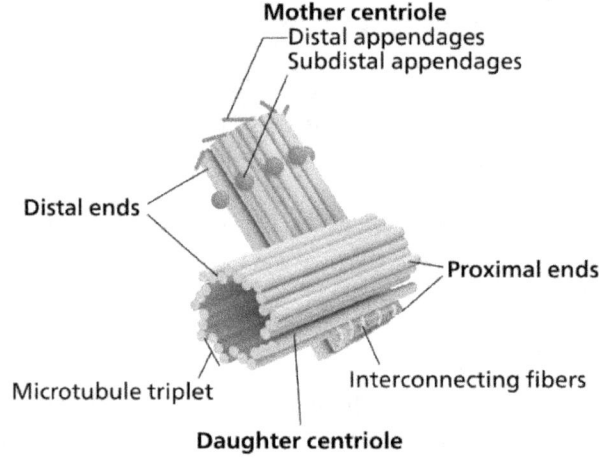

Centrosome contains two centrioles oriented at right angles

Cell Cycle and Mitosis

Methods for cell division

The cell cycle describes a cell's lifetime, detailing the life stages from creating a cell to its division into two daughter cells.

Most of an organism's cells divide throughout their lifetime (i.e., an exception is nerve cells), as cell division is the process by which organisms grow, repair tissues, and reproduce.

Mitosis and meiosis are two types of cell division.

Mitosis is cell division when new *somatic* (or *body*) cells are added to multicellular organisms as they grow and when tissues are repaired or replaced.

As a cell prepares for mitosis, it grows larger, the number of organelles doubles, and the DNA replicates.

Meiosis produces gametes (reproductive cells of egg and sperm) by organisms that reproduce sexually. Meiosis is discussed separately. .

Mitosis does not introduce genetic variations.

A daughter cell is identical in chromosome number and genetic makeup to the parent cell.

Mitosis distributes identical genetic material to two daughter cells.

What is remarkable is the fidelity with which the DNA is passed along, without dilution or error, between generations.

Eukaryotes divide by mitosis, but prokaryotes undergo *binary fission*, a form of asexual reproduction.

Binary fission is a simpler process wherein the parent cell replicates its DNA and then divides. Since prokaryotes have a single and circular DNA without a nucleus, there are no complex steps of chromosome formation and separation by mitosis with microtubules between the centromere and centrioles as in eukaryotic cells.

Interphase as the common phase of the cell cycle

Interphase is the stage before mitosis and represents most of the cell's life. This is not a static state but rather a progression towards mitosis.

However, in some cases, a cell halts its progress through interphase, either temporarily or permanently.

This may be because it is a non-dividing cell (e.g., nerve cell) or not healthy enough to perform growth and replicate interphase functions.

During interphase ($G_1 \rightarrow S \rightarrow G_2$), the cell prepares to divide by growing, replicating DNA and organelles, and synthesizing mRNA and proteins.

When it has completed interphase functions, the cell exits interphase and enters mitosis.

Four stages of mitosis

The four phases of mitosis: prophase, metaphase, anaphase, and telophase (PMAT).

1. Prophase = *Prepare*: cell *prepares* for mitosis
2. Metaphase = *Middle*: chromosomes align in the *middle* of the cell
3. Anaphase = *Apart*: centromere splits

    The sister chromatids pull *apart* by microtubules to the opposite poles
4. Telophase = *Two*: two daughter nuclei reform with separate nuclei

Prophase, the first phase of mitosis, involves chromatin condensation, nucleolus dissolution, nuclear membrane fragmentation, and centrosome movement. *Chromatin condensation* is the process by which loose euchromatin condenses into chromosomes. Currently, the chromosomes have no fixed orientation in the cell.

Upon chromatin condensation, the nucleolus dissolves, and the nuclear membrane begins to fragment, exposing the chromosomes to the cytoplasm of the cell. Simultaneously, centrosomes begin to migrate to opposite sides of the cell. Microtubules start to extend from the centrosomes, forming the *spindle apparatus.*

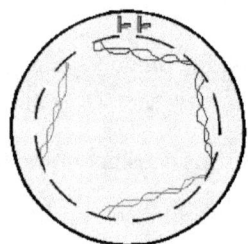

Prophase

Metaphase follows prophase when nuclear fragmentation completes, and the centrosomes are at opposite poles of the cell. Microtubules emerge from the centrosomes and attach to the chromosomes.

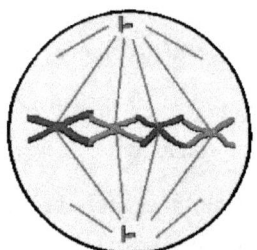

Metaphase

Microtubules align chromosomes along an imaginary line in the center of the cell, the *metaphase plate* (or *equatorial plate*) completing the formation of the spindle apparatus. Chromosomes must be attached and aligned at the metaphase plate before the cell proceeds dividing.

During *anaphase, sister chromatids* (i.e., chromatin strands replicated during the S phase of interphase but attached at the centromere) are pulled apart to opposite poles of the cell.

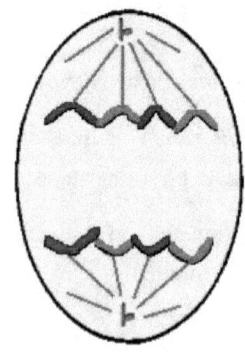

Anaphase

The sister chromatids separate at their centromere and travel towards opposite centrosomes by the spindle microtubules. By the end of anaphase, equal numbers of sister chromatids are stationed by both centrosomes.

Telophase is the cell reverse action of prophase as it prepares to divide.

The spindle apparatus disassembles, and two daughter nuclei reform.

As spindle microtubules disassemble, two regions of identical chromatids are present.

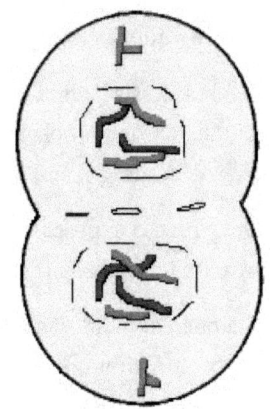

Telophase

A nuclear envelope develops around each region, forming two daughter nuclei.

Within the nuclei, chromosomal DNA uncoils into chromatin, and nucleoli form. The cell contains two identical daughter nuclei, and cell division proceeds.

Cytokinesis divides the cytoplasm to produce two daughter cells

Cytokinesis is the division of the cytoplasm to create two daughter cells. This usually coincides with the end of telophase but is *not* a phase of mitosis. Instead, it is a separate event that does not always occur.

When mitosis occurs but cytokinesis does not, multinucleated cell form; (often in plants, but in skeletal muscle cells of animals).

In animal cells, cytokinesis occurs by the process of *cleavage*.

First, a *cleavage furrow*, a shallow groove between the two daughter nuclei, appears. The cleavage furrow deepens as a microfilament band; the *contractile ring* constricts between the two daughter cells. A narrow bridge exists between daughter cells during telophase until constriction separates the cytoplasms.

The result is two daughter cells enclosed in their plasma membrane and their identical nuclei. Recall that the parent cell replicated its organelles before mitosis; thus, daughter cells contain a complete set of organelles smaller than the parent's cell size.

Cytokinesis in plant cells is different because plant cells have rigid cellulose cell walls which do not permit cytokinesis by furrowing. In plants, vesicles containing cellulose move to the middle of the cell. Additional vesicles arrive and coalesce, building a *cell plate* of cellulose (cell wall). When the cell plate is complete, the parent has divided into two separate daughter cells.

Nuclear membrane reorganization during cell division

Before mitosis begins, the cell's DNA is contained inside the nucleus, inaccessible to the mitotic spindle. During prophase and metaphase, the nucleolus disintegrates, chromatin condenses (i.e., heterochromatin), and the nuclear membrane breaks down.

This process exposes chromosomal DNA to the cell's cytoplasm and allows mitosis to divide the parental (original) cell into two identical daughter (new) cells.

The nuclear membrane does not reform until telophase, when the two daughter nuclei are each enclosed within nuclear membranes from fragments of the parental cell's nuclear membrane. Chromosomes then uncoil into relaxed chromatin (i.e., euchromatin), and the nucleoli reform, making nuclear reorganization complete.

Centrioles, asters and spindles

As discussed, centrioles are the microtubule-organizing centers of the cell. Centrioles replicate during interphase in preparation for mitosis.

During prophase, *polar microtubules* emerge from pairs of centrioles and centrosomes and push against each other and move the centrosomes to opposite sides of the cell. *Astral microtubules* extend from the centrioles to assist in orienting the mitotic spindle apparatus.

At the end of prophase, kinetochore microtubules originate from the centrioles and attach to the chromosomes' kinetochores.

The spindle apparatus consists of two centrosomes (composed of two centrioles each), polar microtubules, astral microtubules (asters), and *kinetochore microtubules* (k-fibers) attached to the kinetochores on chromosomes.

Like animal cells, plant cells have a spindle apparatus, but many do not have centrioles or astral microtubules. Centrioles are not strictly necessary for mitosis, even in animal cells.

Chromatids, centromeres and kinetochores

As the cell enters metaphase, kinetochore microtubules extend from the centrosomes and attach to *kinetochores* on the chromosomes. Kinetochores are assembled on the *centromere*, the chromosome region linking two sister chromatids.

There are two sections of the kinetochore: the inner kinetochore, which associates with the DNA of the centromere, and the outer kinetochore, which interacts with the kinetochore microtubules attached to the centriole.

During metaphase, microtubules pull on the chromosomes with tension, eventually aligning them at the metaphase plate. After successful attachment of chromosomes to the spindle via the kinetochore and microtubules, proteins are released from the kinetochore, which signals the end of metaphase and the beginning of anaphase.

Mechanisms of chromosome movement

In anaphase, the centromere holding the sister chromatids (S phase of interphase when the chromosome replicated to form two sister chromatids) dissolves, and the sister chromatids are released from their attachment point. The chromosomes are pulled to opposite sides of the cell by the shortening of kinetochore microtubules.

Shortening occurs when the motor protein attached to a kinetochore "walks" along the kinetochore-microtubule, dissembling the microtubule into tubulin subunits as it passes.

Polar microtubules assist the separation of chromosomes by lengthening the spindle. Wherever the ends of two polar microtubules from opposite poles overlap, motor proteins interact between the fibers and push them in opposite directions, thus pushing the entire spindle apart.

Phases of the cell cycle: G_0, G_1, S, G_2, M

Interphase is divided into three phases: G_1, S, and G_2.

G_0 is another resting phase when the cell is not dividing nor preparing to divide. G_0 is the static state in which cells remain permanently (e.g., nerve cells) and others temporarily.

A cell exits G_0 and reenter the active cell cycle upon receipt of signals from *growth factor* proteins.

Under a microscope, a cell is recognized as being in interphase by the lack of visible chromosomes because the DNA is uncoiled as loose chromatin (i.e., euchromatin).

During the *G_1 phase* (*Gap phase 1*), the cell continues normal function as it grows larger and replicates its organelles, including ribosomes, mitochondria, and chloroplasts (if a plant cell).

The mitochondria generate sufficient storage of energy for the functions of mitosis.

In G_1, the cell synthesizes mRNA and proteins in preparation for the *S phase*.

In the S (*Synthesis*) phase, the cell replicates DNA and produces two sister chromatids attached at the centromere. During the S phase, DNA nucleotide damage must be detected and fixed before the cell proceeds.

G_2 phase (*Gap phase 2*) is where the cell grows and synthesizes proteins needed for mitosis.

Completing G_2 marks the end of interphase and the beginning of mitosis, abbreviated as M.

Sequential phases of the cell cycle

The sequential phases of the cell cycle are:

G_0 = no DNA replication or cell division

G_1 = making of organelles, increase in cell size (growth)

S = DNA replication, complete duplication of chromosomes (sister chromatids)

G_2 = making of organelles, increase in cell size (growth), cell committed to mitosis

M = mitosis (PMAT); prophase, metaphase, anaphase, and telophase

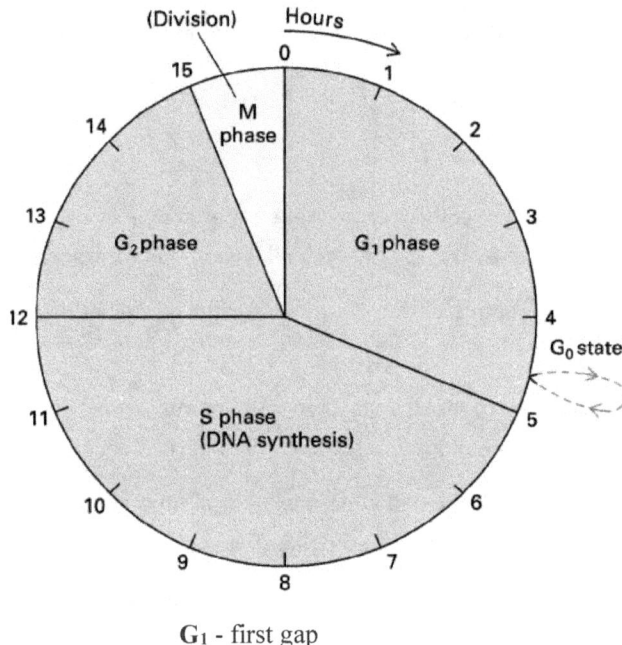

G_1 - first gap

S - DNA synthesis (replication)

G_2 - second gap

M - mitosis

The cell cycle divided between interphase and mitosis

Growth arrest

Cell growth is *cell proliferation* (for populations of cells) or an individual cell's growth, whereby biomolecules are synthesized.

Cell proliferation is the goal of unicellular organisms.

However, in multicellular organisms, cell proliferation must be carefully monitored to prevent tumor formation and invasion into nearby tissues.

Contact inhibition, the tendency for cells to cease dividing when they come into physical contact with their neighbors, regulates this. Therefore, lack of free space signals growth arrest.

The growth of the individual cells regulates cell populations.

For individual cell development, growth arrest is *cellular quiescence* or *cell cycle arrest*.

During the cell cycle, the cell encounters checkpoints where the cell cycle is halted before proceeding.

Checkpoints during cellular division

1. **The G_1 Checkpoint** – *Restriction Point*

    Partway through G_1, the cell reaches the restriction point.

    The cell checks for biomolecules, nutrients, and growth factors.

    If the cell is not sufficiently prepared for mitosis, the cycle halts, and the cell returns to G_0.

    Additionally, if DNA damage is detected, this triggers *apoptosis* (cell death) if the DNA is not repaired.

    If there are no inhibitory signals, the cell clears the checkpoint and proceeds toward DNA replication (S phase).

    G_1 is the checkpoint mediated by extracellular signals.

    After this point, intracellular signals direct the cell cycle to proceed or halt progress.

2. **The G_2 Checkpoint** – *DNA Damage Checkpoint*

    At the end of G_2, there is another checkpoint before the cell proceeds with mitosis.

    The cell checks for size and proper DNA replication.

    If the DNA has not finished replicating or damaged and requiring repair, it remains in G_2 until these issues are resolved.

3. **The M Checkpoint** – *Mitotic Spindle Checkpoint*

   After the cell has entered mitosis and has reached metaphase, a final checkpoint occurs.

   The M checkpoint ensures that the correct number of chromosomes are aligned at the mitotic plate and secured to the mitotic spindle.

   Errors during chromosome segregation (e.g., nondisjunction) can cause defects resulting in genetic conditions (e.g., Down syndrome).

   The M checkpoint reduces defects by arresting the cell in metaphase until the chromosomes are correctly attached to the spindle apparatus and aligned for anaphase.

Cell Cycle Control

Cyclin levels regulate cell division

The cell cycle is controlled by intracellular and extracellular signals that stimulate or inhibit metabolic events. Extracellular stimulatory signal molecules are growth factors; these are proteins or hormones that promote cell growth and differentiation.

Extracellular inhibitory signal molecules are growth suppressors or *tumor suppressors* because they prevent cancer cells' rampant growth.

Tumor suppressors inhibit growth by halting the cell cycle or directing the cell for apoptosis (i.e., cell death).

Intracellular signaling directs the cell cycle and involves the activation and inactivation of proteins; *cyclin-dependent kinases* (CDKs).

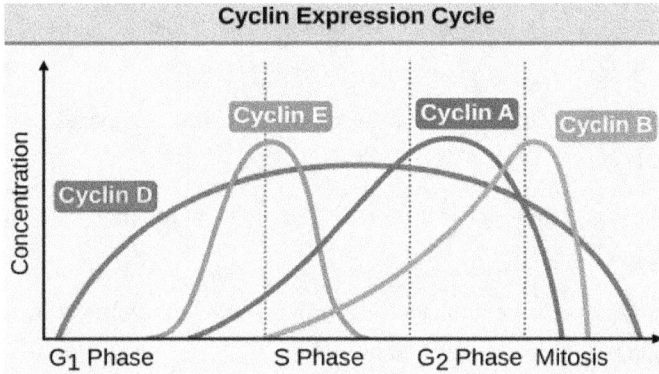

Relative concentrations of cyclin proteins during phases of the cell cycle

Apoptosis as programmed cell death

Apoptosis is the programmed cell death that occurs in multicellular organisms. It occurs in developing tissue (e.g., embryonic development where parts of tissues are no longer needed) and adult tissue (i.e., cell death balances cell division).

Apoptosis destroys cells that threaten the organism, such as infected cells, cells with DNA damage, cancerous cells, and immune system cells no longer needed and are unnecessarily attacking other body cells.

While paradoxical, apoptosis is essential for growth. For example, cells must die to create spaces in the webbed hands of a fetus for the formation of separate digits.

Some internal or external pathways and signals cause cell death, but the morphological changes during apoptosis are consistent whatever the cause.

These changes include shrinkage and *blebbing* (bulging) of the plasma membrane and nuclear envelope and DNA fragmentation.

Engulfment by nearby phagocytic cells occurs as a result.

Apoptotic cells release signals which attract phagocytic cells.

The engulfment of the dying cell's fragments prevents viruses or other dangerous cell contents from spilling out of the damaged cell.

Cancer cells lose cell cycle controls

Cancer cells are abnormal cells with various dangerous properties, making them a serious threat to the body. They invade and destroy normal tissue, causing serious illness and death.

Cancerous cells do not normally respond to the body's control mechanism. They no longer respond to inhibitory growth factors and do not require as many stimulatory growth factors.

Cancer cells may produce the required external growth factor (or override factors) or possess abnormal signal transduction sequences that falsely convey growth signals, thereby bypassing normal growth checks.

Due to their irregular growth cycles, if cancer cells' growth does occur, it does so at random points of the cell cycle.

Cancer can kill the organism because these cells can divide indefinitely (i.e., immortalized cells) if given a continual supply of nutrients.

DNA segments of *telomeres* form the ends of chromosomes and shorten with each cell division, eventually signaling the cell to stop dividing.

However, cancer cells produce telomerase (enzymes end with ~*ase*), which keeps telomeres long and allows cells to continue dividing as "*immortal*."

Unlike normal cells, which differentiate, cancer cells are non-specialized.

Cancer cells do not exhibit contact inhibition; they do not avoid crowding neighboring cells but rather pile up and grow on one another. This behavior creates the characteristic tissue mass as a tumor.

Not all tumors are dangerous.

A *benign tumor* is encapsulated and does not invade adjacent tissue.

However, benign tumors can still compress and damage nearby tissue, and some benign tumors have the potential to become *malignant* (cancerous).

Malignancy occurs when new tumors are spread to areas distant from the primary tumor by *metastasis*.

Angiogenesis, oncogenes and tumor suppressor genes

Angiogenesis, the formation of new blood vessels, is a process required for metastasis. Angiogenesis is triggered when cancer cells release a growth factor that causes nearby blood vessels to grow and transport nutrients and oxygen to the tumor.

Because of angiogenesis in metastasis, angiogenesis inhibitors are an important class of cancer drugs.

Cancer cells have abnormal nuclei that may be enlarged and have an abnormal number of chromosomes, as some chromosomes are mutated, duplicated, or deleted.

When the DNA repair system fails to correct mutations during DNA replication, damage to crucial genes may occur.

Oncogenes encode growth factor proteins such as Ras, which stimulates the cell cycle (analogous to a *gas pedal* in a car).

In contrast, *tumor-suppressor genes* encode proteins such as p53 that inhibit the cell cycle (analogous to the *brake pedal* in a car).

Mutations of oncogenes or tumor suppressors can cause cancer.

Mutation of *proto-oncogenes* may convert them into *oncogenes*, which are cancer-causing genes.

An oncogene can cause cancer by coding for a faulty receptor in the stimulatory pathway, for an abnormal protein, or for abnormally high levels of a normal product that stimulates the cell cycle.

More than 100 oncogenes have been identified; the *ras* gene family includes variants associated with lung cancer, colon cancer, pancreatic cancer, leukemia, and thyroid cancers.

Mutation of tumor-suppressor genes results in unregulated cell growth.

For example, the *p53* tumor-suppressor gene is frequently mutated in human cancers than other known genes; it usually functions to trigger cell cycle inhibitors and stimulate apoptosis.

However, if it malfunctions due to mutation, cell growth is not suppressed, and cancer may result.

Editor's note: Nomenclature in molecular biology uses an italicized lower-case abbreviation for the gene (e.g., p53), while the protein (e.g., Ras*) begins with a capital letter but is not italicized.*

Biosignaling

Rhythmic fluctuations in the abundance and activity of cell-cycle control molecules pace the events of the cell cycle. One example of these control molecules are *kinases*, proteins which activate or deactivate other proteins by phosphorylation. They are responsible for a procession through the G_1 and G_2 checkpoints.

To give the signal, the kinases themselves must be activated by a *cyclin* protein. Because of this requirement, these kinases are called cyclin-dependent kinases (CDKs). Cyclins, named for their cycling concentration in the cell, accumulate during the G_1, S, and G_2 phases of the cell cycle.

By the G_2 checkpoint, enough cyclin is available to form a complex of cyclin and CDK called the *maturation-promoting factor* (MPF), or the M-Phase-promoting factor. MPF initiates progression from the G_2 to the M phase by phosphorylating key proteins involved in mitosis.

Later in mitosis, MPF switches itself off by initiating a process which leads to the destruction of cyclin. Cdk, the non-cyclin component of MPF, persists in the cell in an inactive form until it associates with the new cyclin molecules synthesized during interphase of the next round of the cell cycle.

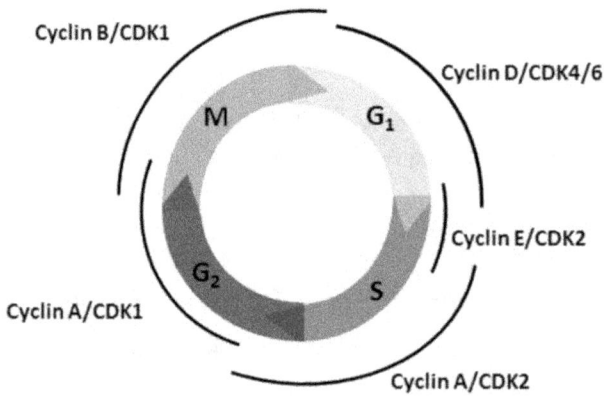

Cyclin-dependent kinases (CDK) and cyclin relationship to regulate the cell cycle

Platelet-derived growth factor (PDGF) is another protein that regulates cell growth and division. PDGF is required for the division of *fibroblasts*, connective tissue cells essential in wound healing. When an injury occurs, platelet blood cells release PDGF, which then binds to fibroblast receptors and activates a signal-transduction pathway that leads to a proliferation of fibroblasts and healing of the wound.

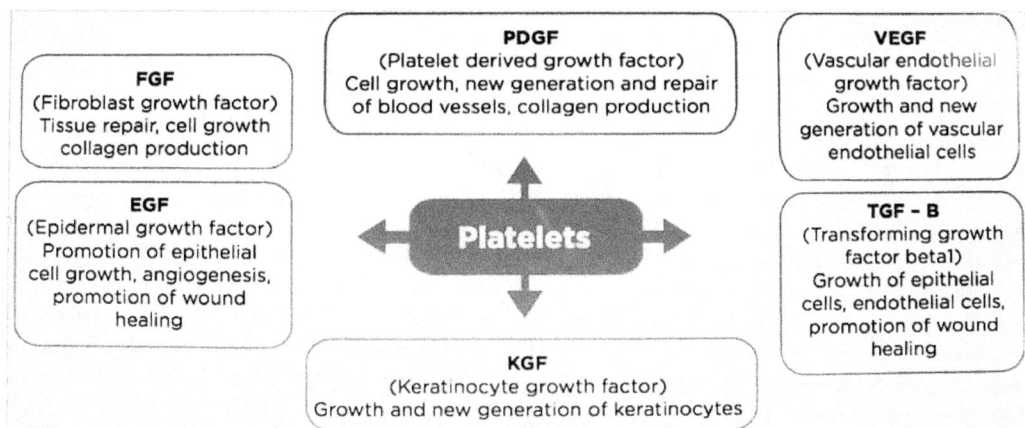

Growth factors released by platelets in wound healing

The extracellular environment has a direct effect on cell division. Cells grown in culture rapidly divide until a single layer of cells is spread over the area of the petri dish. However, if cells are removed, those bordering the open space begin dividing again and continue to do so until the gap is filled.

This propensity to avoid division when in contact with neighboring cells is known as density-dependent inhibition of growth. When a cell population reaches a critical density, the amount of required growth factors and nutrients available to each cell becomes insufficient to allow continued cell growth.

Anchorage is another extracellular factor that controls cell division. For most animal cells to divide, they must be anchored to a substratum, such as the extracellular matrix of a tissue or the inside of a culture plate. Anchorage is signaled via pathways involving membrane proteins and the cytoskeleton.

Notes for active learning

Tissues Formed by Eukaryotic Cells

Simple and stratified epithelium

Epithelial cells comprise epithelial tissues, which line body structures, particularly organs and blood vessels. Several types of epithelial cells perform a variety of functions.

Squamous epithelial cells appear flat, *cuboidal epithelial cells* are cube-shaped, and *columnar epithelial cells* are column-shaped.

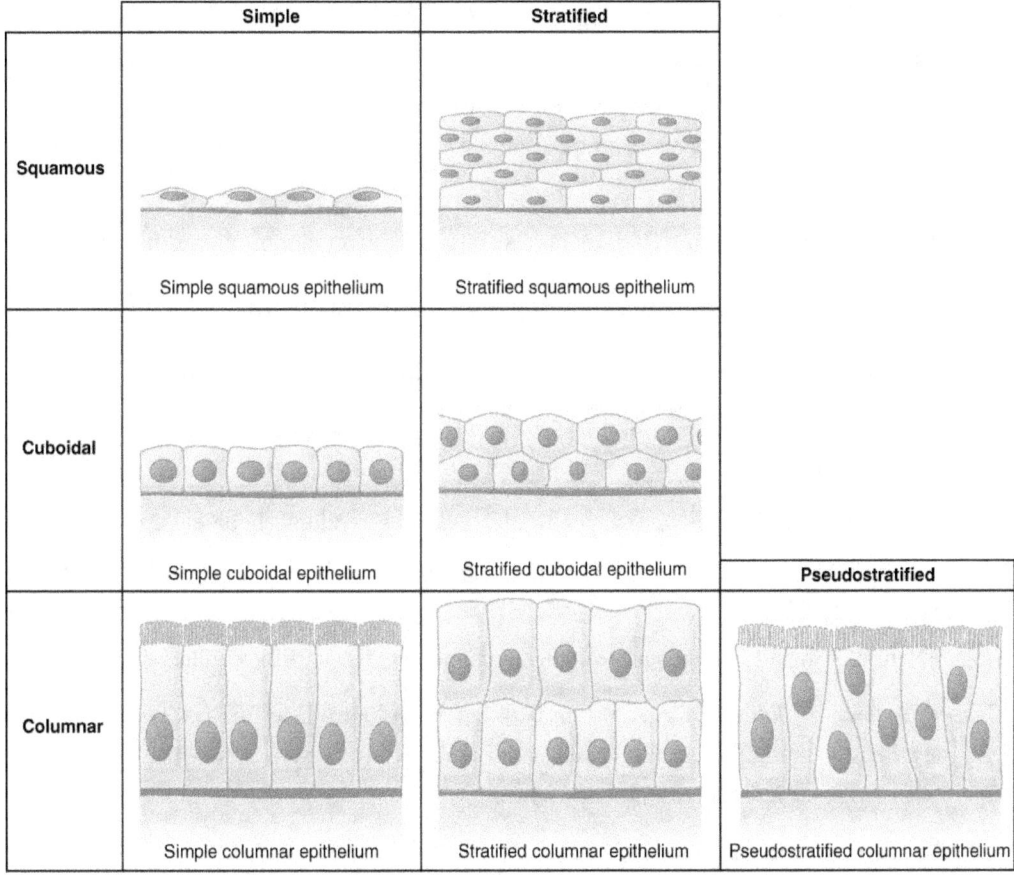

Simple epithelium is a single layer of epithelial cells connected by tight junctions, and its function highly depends on the types of epithelial cells involved.

Simple squamous layers often involve passive diffusion, lining surfaces such as the alveoli during oxygen exchange.

Simple cuboidal layers secrete and absorb (e.g., gland ducts and kidney tubules).

Simple columnar epithelial layers form a protective layer in the stomach and gut.

Stratified epithelium layers protect and facilitate complex functions. For example, stratified columnar epithelium lines the *vas deferens*, protecting the glands and assisting in secretion.

Stratified columnar and cuboidal epithelium are rare in human anatomy; stratified squamous epithelium covers the body as skin.

Endothelial cells

Endothelium is a layer of simple squamous cells forming the interior lining of lymphatic vessels and blood vessels. It is a semi-selective barrier that controls the passage of materials.

Lymphatic endothelial cells are in direct contact with lymph.

Vascular endothelial cells directly contact blood and line every part of the circulatory system, from the tiniest capillaries to larger arteries, veins, and the heart. These endothelial cells have many functions, including blood clotting, forming new blood vessels, blood pressure control, and inflammation control.

Endothelial cells have a strong cell division capacity and movement, proliferating quickly.

Connective tissue, loose *vs.* dense fibers and the extracellular matrix

Connective tissue holds body structures. It consists of specialized cells, ground substances, and fibers. Connective tissue secretes the extracellular matrix held by ground substances.

Fibers, made of collagen, give the matrix its strength.

Several connective tissue cells exist, including bone, fat, tendons, ligaments, cartilage, and blood. For example, chondroblasts make cartilage; fibroblasts make collagen, and hematopoietic stem cells make blood.

Nomenclature of the numerous types of cells in connective tissue differentiates their function.

Cells with the suffix *blast* describe a stem cell that actively produces matrix, while the suffix *cyte* describes a mature cell. For example, osteoblasts (*osteo-* for bone) are specialized connective tissue cells that build the bone matrix.

Osteocytes are mature, immobile osteoblasts involved in bone maintenance.

Various types of fibers make up connective tissue.

The most common protein fiber is collagen or *collagenous fibers*. These coiled fibers give collagen its rigidity.

Many collagenous fibers, including elastic fibers, give connective tissue flexibility, while *reticular fibers* mainly join one connective tissue to an adjacent organ or blood vessel.

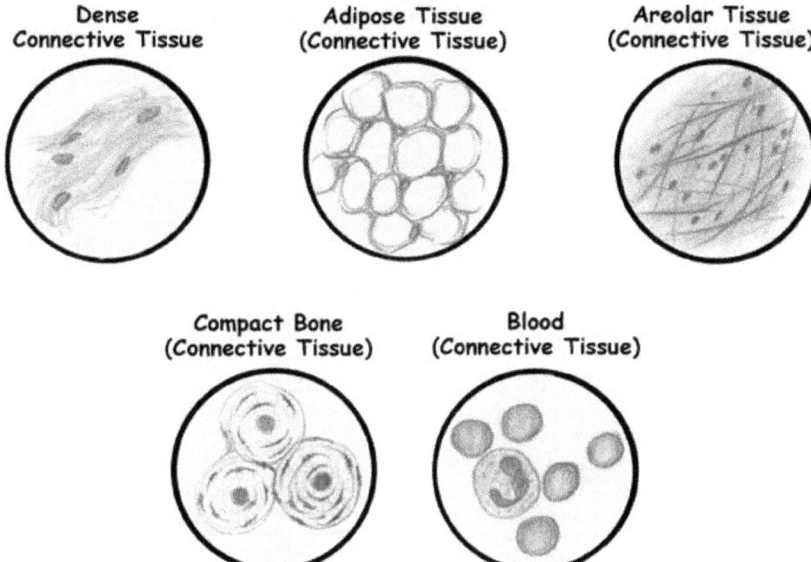

Connective tissue is "loose" or "dense."

Loose connective tissue has a higher concentration of ground substance and cells and fewer fibers. It provides protective padding around the internal organs, as well as fat.

Dense connective tissue has a higher concentration of collagenous fibers than loose connective tissue and is needed in anatomical structures that require great strength (e.g., ligaments and tendons).

Cartilage is a connective tissue that is produced and maintained by chondrocytes.

Cartilage absorbs shock and is on the ends of bones and spinal disks. Since it is more flexible than bone, cartilage is advantageous for structures that do not require much protection, such as the nose or ears.

Extracellular matrix (ECM) exists outside of cells. Cells secrete molecules that make up the matrix, including proteins and polysaccharides.

ECM gives surrounding cells a physical and chemical support system in connective tissue.

Notes for active learning

CHAPTER 2

Basic Human Anatomy

Studying Human Anatomy

Anatomical Planes and Directional References

Body Cavities and Regions

Studying Human Anatomy

Categorizing human anatomy

Human anatomy is the study of the human body and includes gross anatomy and microscopic anatomy.

Physiology is the study of the functions of the body.

Gross anatomy studies the structures of the body that can be seen with the naked eye.

Microscopic anatomy studies those structures of the body that require a microscope.

Microscopic anatomy includes *histology* (i.e., the study of tissues) and *cytology* (i.e., the study of cells).

From the smallest to the largest part of the human anatomy, the sequence is:

$$\text{cells} \rightarrow \text{tissues} \rightarrow \text{organs} \rightarrow \text{systems}$$

Standard anatomical position

The anatomical position is the frame of reference for other terms relating to anatomy, structures, and directions. The anatomical position consists of a standing upright person facing forward with the person's arms on their sides next to the body and feet together.

The anatomical position is different from a normal standing position because the palms of the hands are unnaturally facing forward rather than naturally facing the legs.

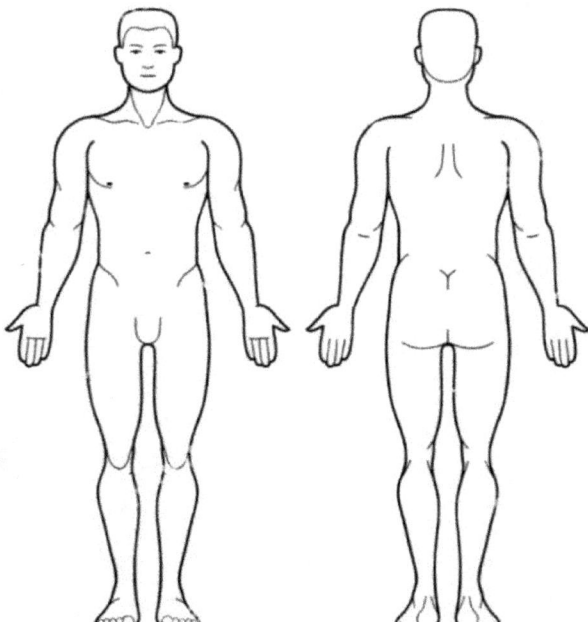

Standard anatomical position: anterior (left) and posterior view (right)

Notes for active learning

Anatomical Planes and Directional References

Anatomical planes

The *anatomical planes* are imaginary lines going through the body and referenced in anatomy.

The *coronal plane* (or *frontal plane*) is the imaginary line separating the front from the back of the body.

The *ventral surface* is a term for the front of the body.

The *dorsal surface* is a term for the back of the body.

The *sagittal plane* (or *medial plane*) is the imaginary line separating the right from the left side of the body.

The *transverse plane* (or *cross-sectional plane*) is the imaginary line separating the upper portion at the waist from the bottom of the body.

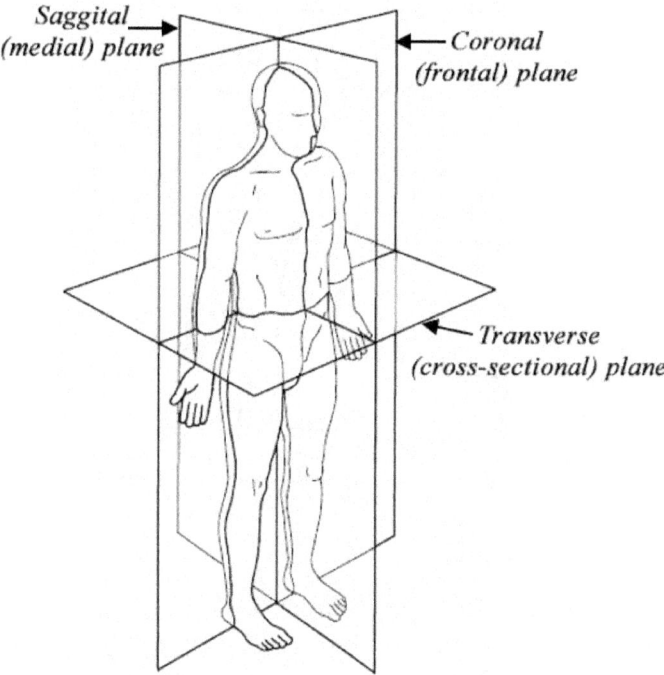

Anatomical planes of the human body

Anterior vs. posterior relationship

Anterior (or *ventral*) is a relative and comparative directional term describing a body part or anatomical structure closer to the front of the body than another body part or anatomical structure. For example, the sternum is anterior to the esophagus.

Posterior (or *dorsal*) is a relative and comparative directional term describing a body part or anatomical structure behind another body part or anatomical structure. For example, the heart is posterior to the ribs.

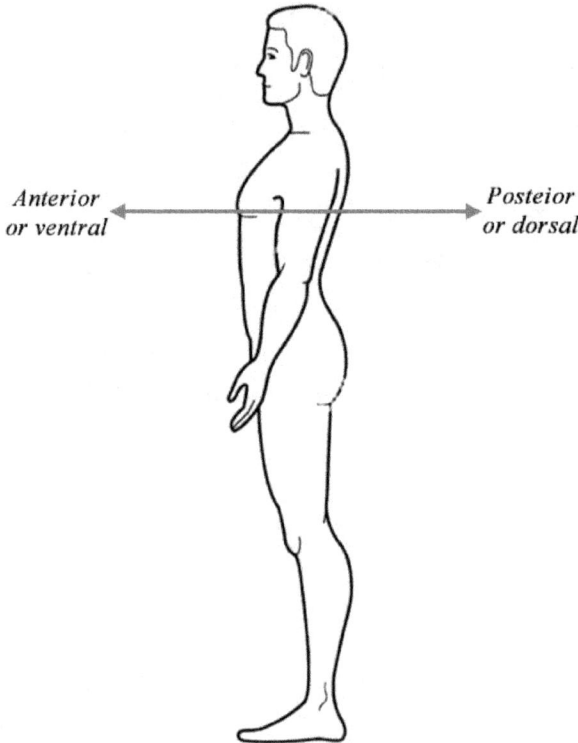

Lateral view of the body with the anterior–posterior directional relationship noted

Superior vs. inferior relationship

Superior (or *cranial*) is a relative and comparative directional term describing a body part or anatomical structure above another body part or anatomical structure. For example, the knee is superior to the ankle in the anatomical position.

Inferior (or *caudal*) is a relative and comparative directional term for a body part or anatomical structure below another part or structure. For example, the ankle is inferior to the knee in the anatomical position.

Medial *vs.* lateral relationship

Medial is a relative and comparative directional term describing a body part or anatomical structure towards the center of the body, compared to another body part or anatomical structure. For example, the nipple is medial to the shoulder.

Lateral is a relative and comparative directional term for a body part or anatomical structure away from the center of the body compared to another part or structure. For example, the nipple is lateral to the sternum.

Proximal *vs.* distal relationship

Proximal is a relative and comparative directional term describing an anatomical structure (or body part) closer to the body core than another. For example, the hip is proximal to the knee.

Distal is a relative and comparative directional term for a body part or anatomical structure further from the body's core than another part or structure. For example, the ankle is distal to the knee.

Deep *vs.* superficial relationship

Deep is a term describing a body part or anatomical structure further from the surface of the body than another body part or structure. For example, muscle is deeper than the skin.

Superficial is a term for a body part or anatomical structure closer to the surface of the body than another part or structure. For example, the skin is the most superficial organ of the body.

Ipsilateral *vs.* contralateral relationship

Ipsilateral describes that two structures are on the same side of the body. For example, the spleen and descending colon are ipsilateral.

Contralateral describes that two structures are on the opposite side of the body. For example, the spleen and gallbladder are contralateral.

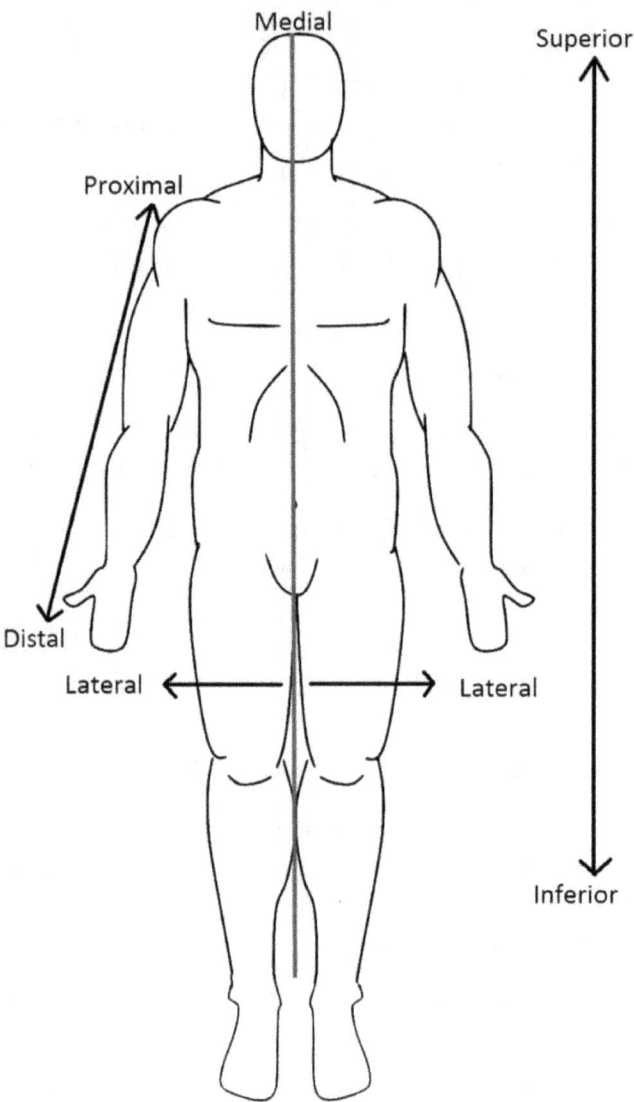

Directional references of the human body

Body Cavities and Regions

Cavities and their associated organs

Body cavities are hollow spaces within the body that contain internal organs and structures.

The *dorsal cavity* is located toward the back of the body.

It is divided into the *cranial cavity*, which holds the brain and the *vertebral* (or *spinal*) *cavity*, which holds the spinal cord.

The *ventral cavity* is located toward the front of the body and is divided by the diaphragm into the abdominopelvic and thoracic cavities.

The *abdominopelvic cavity* is subdivided into the *abdominal cavity* (holding the stomach, pancreas, spleen, kidneys, liver, gallbladder, small and large intestines) and the *pelvic cavity* (holding the urinary bladder and reproductive organs).

The *thoracic cavity* is subdivided into the *pleural cavity*, which holds the lungs.

The *pericardial cavity* holds the heart.

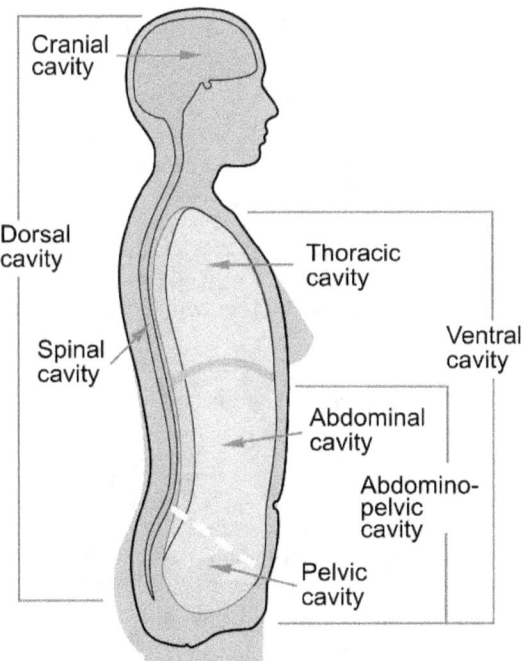

Cavities of the human body

Anatomical terms for body regions

Some common anatomical terms to describe a region of the body.

Abdominal – region between thorax and pelvis   *Cervical* – the neck

Antebrachial – the forearm   *Costal* – the ribs

Antecubital – the front of elbow   *Cubital* – the elbow

Axillary – the armpit   *Femoral* – the thigh

Brachial – the upper arm   *Gluteal* – the buttock

Celiac – the abdomen   *Lumbar* – the lower back

Cephalic – the head   *Pedal* – the foot

Abdominopelvic quadrants and regions

The abdominopelvic area is divided into four quadrants and nine regions.

This division allows the localization of pain or other symptoms for diagnosis and treatment.

The quadrants are the *left lower, left upper, right upper,* and *right lower quadrant.*

The nine regions are smaller areas than quadrants, as shown below.

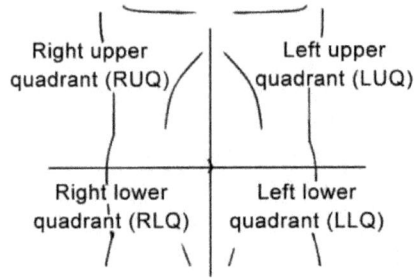

Four abdominopelvic quadrants

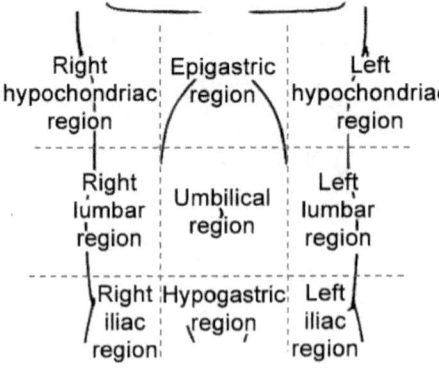

Nine abdominopelvic regions

Notes for active learning

Notes for active learning

CHAPTER 3

Endocrine System

Hormones and Their Sources

Endocrine Glands

Classifying Hormones

Hormonal Modes of Action

Hormone Distribution, Secretion and Effects

Endocrine and Neural Integration

Page intentionally left blank

Hormones and Their Sources

Functions of the endocrine system

Endocrine system synthesizes and secretes hormones into the bloodstream (*endo* means "within"). The target cell of a hormone has a receptor, allowing it to respond to the stimulus.

Exocrine system secretions travel through ducts to external environments. Several glands in the body create hormones of the endocrine system, such as sudoriferous (i.e., sweat), sebaceous (i.e., oily), mucous, digestion, and mammary glands.

A few glands, such as the pancreas, have endocrine and exocrine functions.

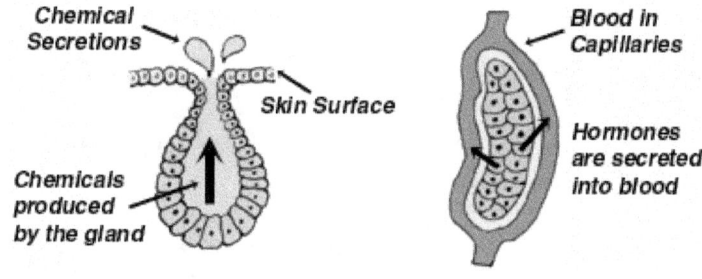

Exocrine Gland *Endocrine Gland*

Glands secrete direct and trophic hormones

Hormones are molecules created by glands that affect distant organs through the circulatory system. Hormones regulate metabolism and other functions of cells. Tiny amounts of the hormone may have a widespread effect.

Hormones are divided into two categories based on their target: *direct hormones* (or *non-tropic hormones*) directly stimulate target hormones, and *tropic hormones* stimulate endocrine glands.

Endocrine glands are ductless glands in the endocrine system that secrete hormones into the bloodstream, affecting target cells. A single gland may produce several hormones.

Multiple glands may produce the same hormone. Principal human endocrine glands include the hypothalamus, pineal, and pituitary glands in the brain; the thyroid and parathyroid glands (located in the neck); the ovaries (located in the abdomen); the testes (in the scrotum); and the thymus (in the thorax).

The chemical demands of an organism vary by daily function and life cycle. When a cellular demand is recognized, genes (located on DNA) are transcribed (mRNA production) and translated (making proteins). This process secretes the hormone into the bloodstream and affects the target cells (with hormone receptors).

In general, hormones instruct cells in tissues to devote their resources to protein production. For example, human adolescents require gonadotropic hormones, which target the sex organs during puberty. Adolescent changes include the ability to produce functional gametes for reproduction and growth and develop secondary sex characteristics.

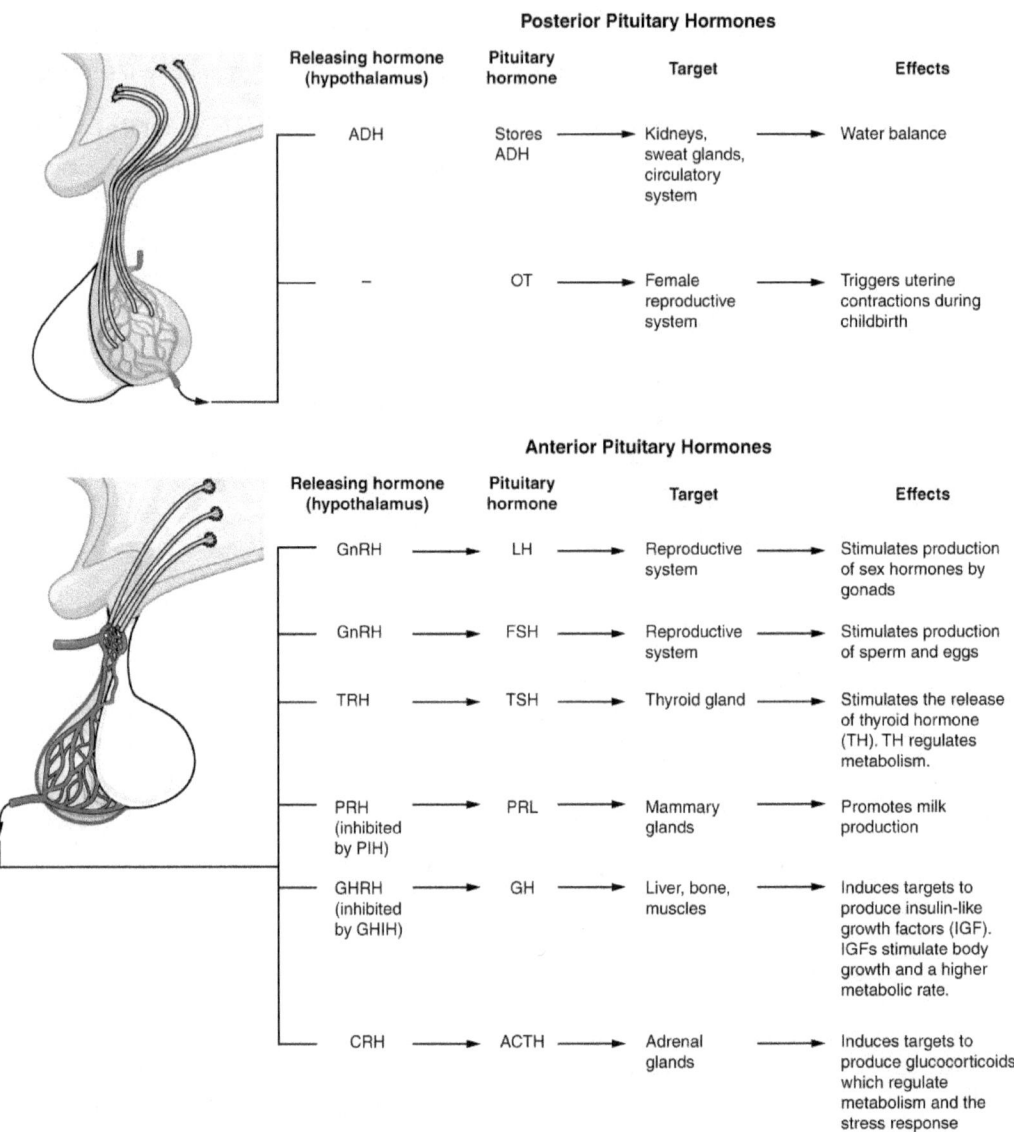

Releasing hormones from the hypothalamus and the effects on posterior and anterior pituitary

Releasing hormone from the hypothalamus finds its target (posterior or anterior pituitary cell). It binds to the receptor, where a chemical messenger instructs the cell to release the desired hormone. The secreted hormone targets a tissue (e.g., the thyroid gland) and instructs the tissue to produce a substance.

Endocrine Glands

Structure and function of major endocrine glands

Humoral glands directly respond to blood levels of ions and nutrients, such as the parathyroid hormone's response to low blood calcium levels.

Neural glands release hormones when a nerve impulse or an action potential is stimulated. These glands are involved primarily with the fight-or-flight response. Hormonal glands release hormones when stimulated by other hormones from another gland.

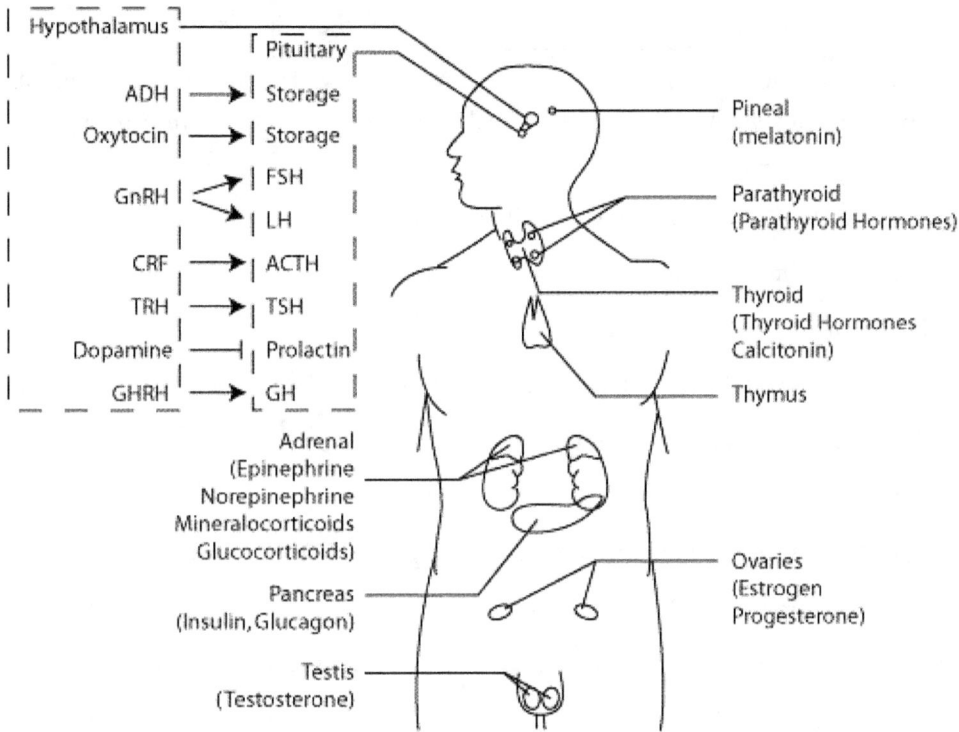

Endocrine glands and associated hormones

Hypothalamus monitors the external and internal conditions of the body. It regulates the internal environment through the autonomic nervous system, affecting heartbeat, temperature, and water balance.

Hypothalamus contains neurosecretory cells linking it to the pituitary gland, which controls glandular secretions. The hypothalamus secretes *ADH* (vasopressin), *oxytocin,* and *GnRH* (gonadotropin-releasing hormone).

Pituitary gland is situated at the back of the brain and synthesizes several hormones for growth. The pituitary gland is connected to the hypothalamus by a stalk-like structure and can store hormones produced by the hypothalamus.

The pituitary gland comprises the *posterior pituitary* and *anterior pituitary*.

Posterior pituitary does not synthesize hormones. Instead, it stores vasopressin and oxytocin produced by the hypothalamus and secretes them into the bloodstream. Posterior pituitary contains neurosecretory cells originating in hypothalamus and responding to neurotransmitters.

Anterior pituitary

Anterior pituitary (adenohypophysis) regulates hormone production from other glands.

Hypothalamus regulates stimulation of the anterior pituitary. The hypothalamus controls the release of anterior pituitary hormones through a *portal system* with two capillary systems connected by a vein.

Anterior pituitary produces seven types of hormones:

    1) thyroid-stimulating hormone (TSH)

    2) adrenocorticotropic hormone (ACTH)

    3) gonadotropic follicle-stimulating hormone (FSH)

    4) gonadotropic luteinizing hormone (LH)

    5) prolactin

    6) melanocyte-stimulating hormone (skin color change in fishes, reptiles, amphibians)

    7) growth hormone (GH), known as somatotropin

Pituitary gland regulation is via a *negative feedback mechanism* and secretion of releasing and inhibiting hormones. The hypothalamus produces hypothalamic-releasing and hypothalamic-inhibiting hormones that pass to the anterior pituitary by the portal system.

Releasing hormones originate in the hypothalamus, targeting cells in the anterior and posterior pituitary glands to stimulate the production and secretion of hormones.

Conversely, *inhibiting hormones* released from the hypothalamus target cells in the anterior pituitary inhibits a particular hormone's production and secretion. In general, each hormone from the anterior pituitary has a releasing and inhibiting hormone from the hypothalamus that controls its release.

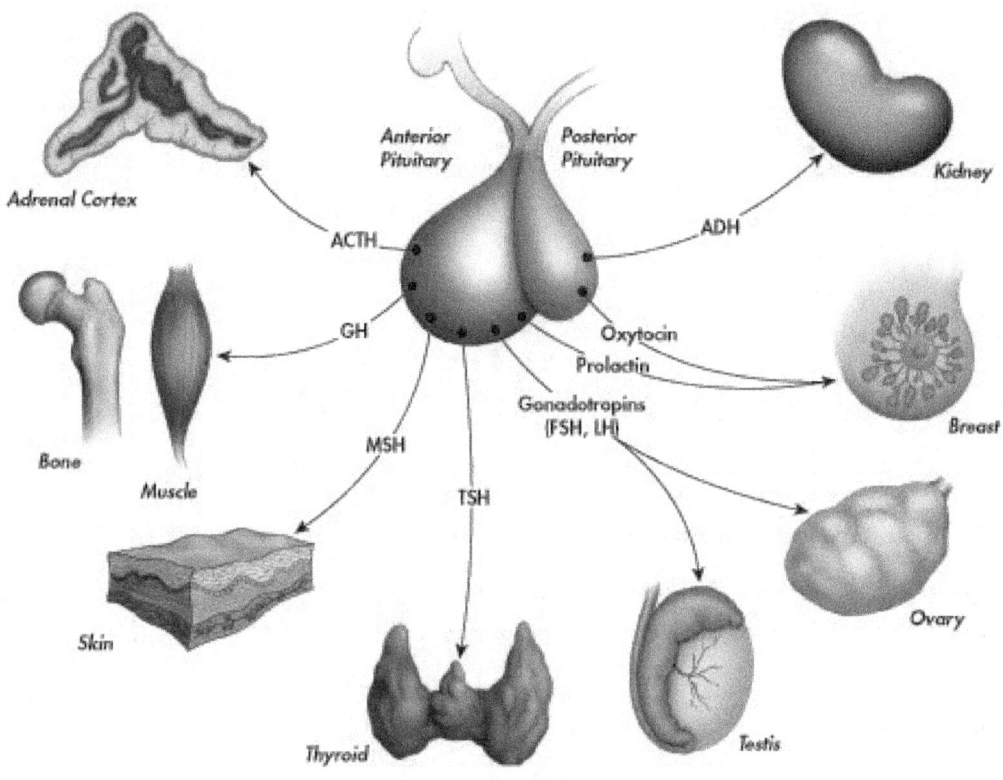

Anterior pituitary hormones

Tropic effects: FSH, LH, TSH, ACTH, ADH

Non-tropic effects: Prolactin, oxytocin, MSH

Non-tropic and tropic effect: GH

Tropic hormones have *other* endocrine *glands* as targets.

Thyroid gland

Thyroid gland is in the neck, attached to the ventral surface of the trachea below the larynx.

Anterior pituitary gland stimulates the thyroid, which secretes *thyroid-stimulating hormone* (TSH). Thyroid hormones increase metabolism and require iodine to function adequately.

Thyroid gland follicles produce two hormones: thyroxine (T4) and triiodothyronine (T3). These hormones possess four and three iodine atoms, respectively. Iodine is necessary for growth and neurological development in children and increases basal metabolic rates in the body.

Iodine, actively transported into thyroids, reaches concentrations 25 times greater than in blood.

Iodine deficiency causes the enlargement of the thyroid (*goiter*).

Goiter is easily prevented by supplementing with fortified salt containing iodine.

Thyroid gland produces *calcitonin*, which decreases the calcium levels in the blood.

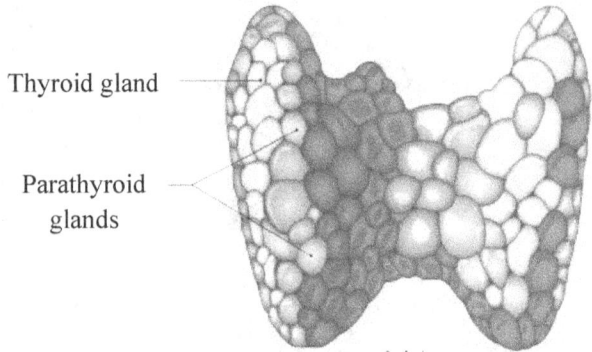

Posterior view of thyroid showing parathyroid glands

Thyroid disorders and metabolic rates

Hyperthyroidism (Graves' disease) is when the thyroid gland is enlarged or overactive. The eyes protrude because of edema in the eye socket tissue as an *exophthalmic* goiter.

Additional symptoms include an increased metabolic rate and sweating. Removal or destruction of some thyroid tissue by surgery or radiation often cures it.

Hypothyroidism is caused by decreased thyroid gland secretion and lowers heart and respiratory rates.

Other thyroid disorders are *achondroplasia* (dwarfism) and *progeria* (premature aging).

Cretinism is a condition of stunted physical and mental growth in people suffering from hypothyroidism since birth. Thyroid treatment must be started in the first two months of life to prevent developmental delays.

Four *parathyroid glands* are embedded in the thyroid glands posterior surface in a conformation resembling four peas.

Parathyroid glands produce *parathyroid hormone* (PTH).

Low calcium (Ca) levels stimulate the release of the parathyroid hormone, which increases calcium levels by stimulating osteoclasts to release calcium from the bone.

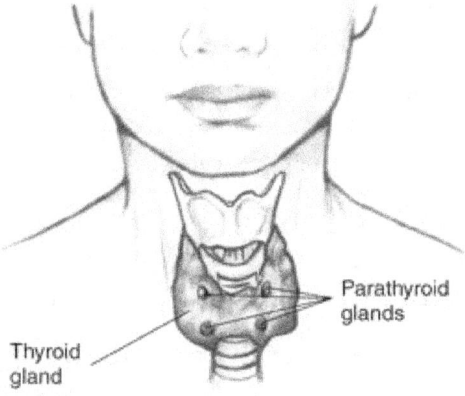

Anterior view of the thyroid gland. Parathyroid glands are on the posterior surface

Adrenal glands for sex hormones and stress responses

Two *adrenal glands* are on top of each kidney. Each gland has two sections: an outer *adrenal cortex* and an inner *adrenal medulla*. The hormones released from the adrenal cortex provide a sustained stress response.

Adrenal cortex secretes *glucocorticoids* and *mineralocorticoids*, which are steroid hormones. It secretes a small amount of male and female sex hormones in each sex. The adrenal medulla releases *epinephrine* and *norepinephrine*, which provide an immediate stress response (as opposed to the sustained response provided by the hormones from the adrenal cortex).

Hypothalamus exerts control over each adrenal gland. Nerve impulses travel via the brain stem through the spinal cord to sympathetic nerve fibers to the medulla.

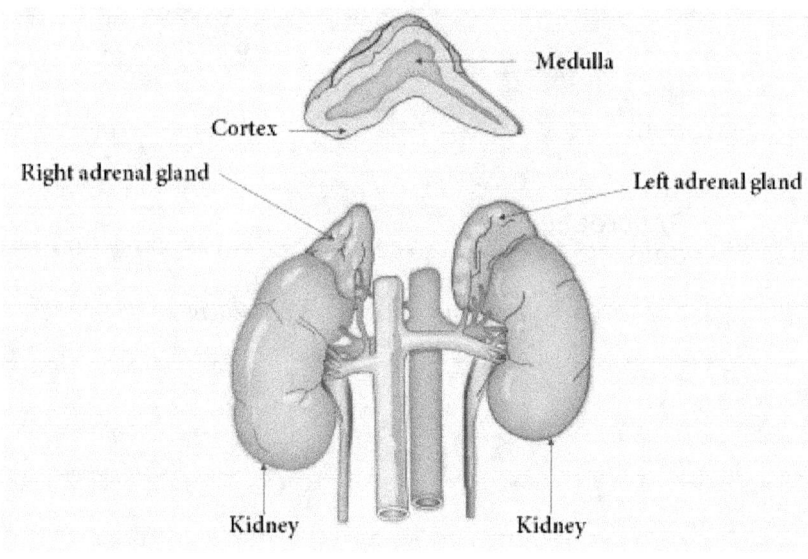

Adrenal glands

Hypothalamus uses ACTH-releasing hormone to control anterior pituitary secretion of ACTH. This hormone stimulates the adrenal glands to release *dehydroepiandrosterone* (DHEA) and *cortisol*. Adrenal hormones increase during times of physical and emotional stress.

Pancreas functions as an exocrine and endocrine gland

Pancreas lies transversely in the abdomen between the kidneys and near the small intestine duodenum. The pancreas is composed of exocrine and endocrine tissue. Exocrine tissue produces and secretes digestive juices into the small intestine via the ducts.

Pancreatic islets of Langerhans are endocrine tissues that produce *insulin* and *glucagon.*

Islets of Langerhans contain two cell types: alpha cells and beta cells.

Alpha cells of the islet secrete glucagon.

The release of glucagon is catabolic and occurs when the energy charge is low, working to raise blood glucose levels. The term energy measures the status of biological cells related to ATP, ADP, and AMP concentrations.

Beta cells secrete insulin, secreted anabolically and released when the energy charge is high, where beta cells work to lower blood glucose levels. Insulin stimulates the liver and other body cells to absorb glucose.

Body cells utilize glucose; therefore, its level is subject to homeostasis and tightly regulated.

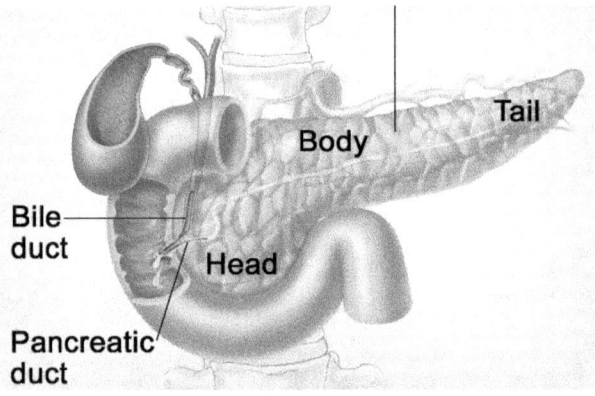

Pancreas anatomy and associated structure

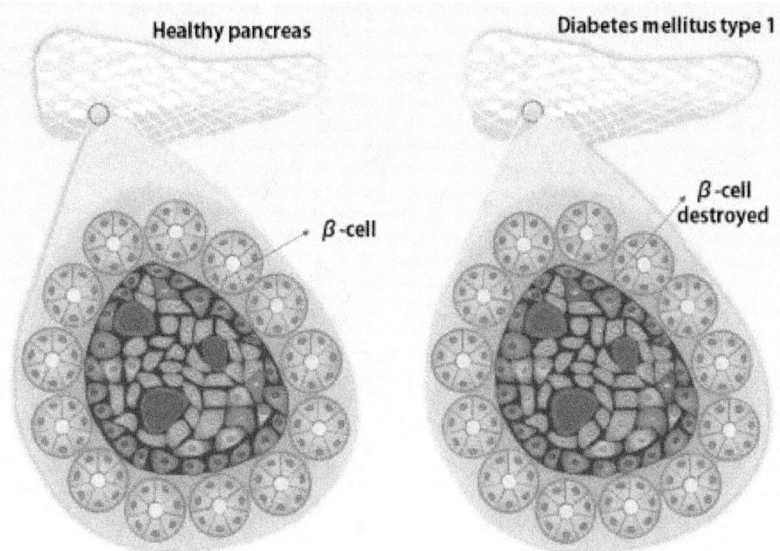

Pancreatic Islets of Langerhans: beta cells secrete insulin in non-diabetic patients

Male *testes* are in the scrotum and function as the human gonads, producing *androgens*, including the male sex hormone *testosterone*.

Testosterone stimulates male secondary sex characteristics, such as large vocal cords, increased muscle mass, and facial hair.

Female sex hormones include estrogens and progesterone, secreted by *ovaries* (female gonads).

Estrogen secreted at puberty stimulates the maturation of ovaries and other sexual organs.

Progesterone is a steroid hormone needed for menstrual cycle, pregnancy, and embryogenesis.

Pineal and thymus glands

Pineal gland, near the center of the brain, produces *melatonin*, primarily at night.

Melatonin establishes *circadian rhythms*, the basis for a 24-hour physiological cycle.

Pineal gland may be involved in human sexual development; children with a damaged pineal gland due to a brain tumor tend to experience puberty earlier.

Thymus is a lobular gland that lies beneath the sternum in the upper thoracic cavity.

Thymus hormones (*thymo-*, *thymic*) stimulate development of T cells for an immune response.

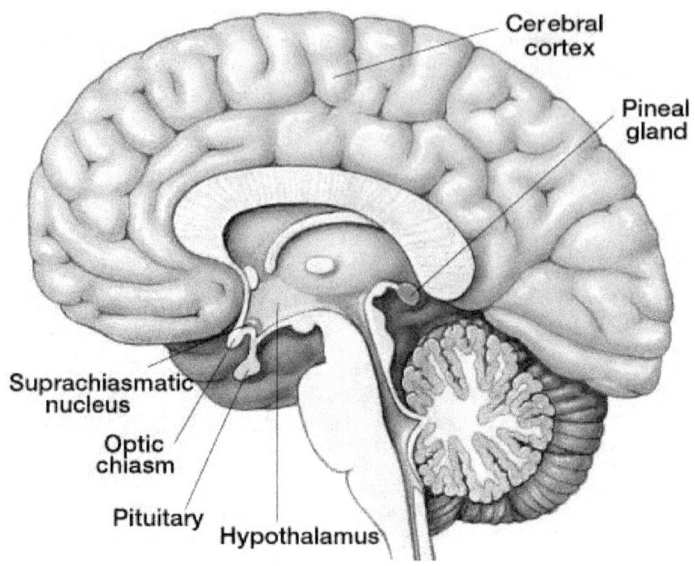

Pituitary gland, hypothalamus, and pineal gland

Thymus is the largest and most active during childhood; it shrinks and becomes fatty with age.

Some lymphocytes originating in bone marrow pass through the thymus and become T lymphocytes.

Thymus produces and secretes thymosins, which aid in differentiating T cells and may stimulate other immune cells.

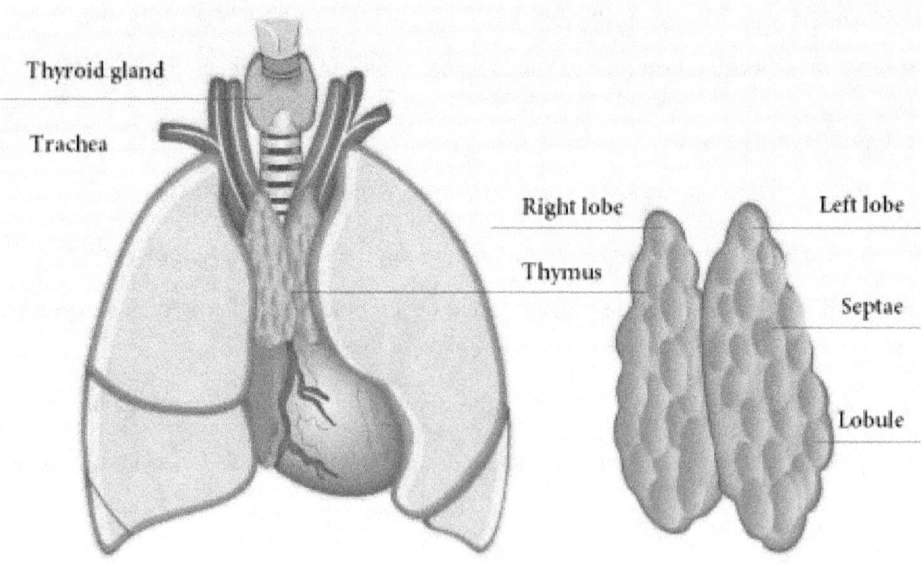

Thymus gland stimulates the development of T cells

Classifying Hormones

Major classifications of hormones and modes of action

Three major classes of hormones: peptide, steroid, and amino acid-derived hormones.

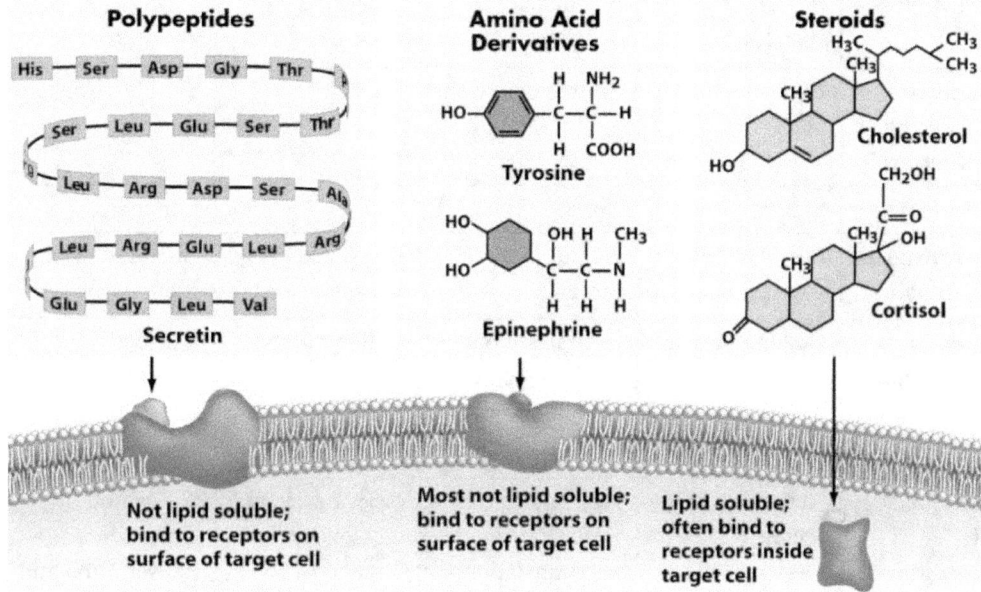

Three classes of hormones and a schematic of their mode of action

Peptide hormones have amino acids like peptides or proteins with receptors on cell surfaces.

Their mechanism of action utilizes the secondary messenger system.

They affect their target organs rapidly; however, their effects are temporary. Calcitonin is an example of a peptide hormone that stimulates osteoblasts to decrease plasma calcium levels as bone density increases.

Steroid hormones contain cholesterol. Their receptors are in the cytosol (or nucleus) of a cell.

Steroids pass through the phospholipid bilayer of the cell membrane. Once the steroid hormone binds to an intracellular receptor, the hormone-receptor complex migrates to the nucleus, and the complex binds to a DNA target to affect gene transcription.

Steroid hormones affect their target organs slowly, but their effects are long-lasting. An example of a steroid hormone is the growth hormone.

Amino acid-derived hormones are the third class derived from the amino acid tyrosine. Amino-derived hormones are generally small molecules. They are catecholamines (e.g., epinephrine, norepinephrine, dopamine).

Peptide, steroid and amino acid-derived hormones

	Peptide hormones	Steroid hormones	Amino acid derivatives	
			Catecholamines	Thyroid hormones
Synthesis and storage	Made in advance; stored in secretory vesicles	Synthesized on-demand from precursors	Made in advance; stored in secretory vesicles	Made in advance; precursor stored in secretory vesicles
Release from the parent cell	Exocytosis	Simple diffusion	Exocytosis	Simple diffusion
Half-life	Short	Long	Short	Long
Transport in blood	Dissolved in plasma	Bound to carrier proteins	Dissolved in plasma	Bound to carrier proteins
Location of receptor	Cell membrane	Cytoplasm or nucleus; some have membrane receptors	Cell membrane	Nucleus
Response to receptor-ligand binding	Activation of second messenger systems; may activate genes	Activates genes for transcription and translation; may have non-genomic actions	Activate second messenger systems	Activation of genes for transcription and translation
General Target Response	Modification of existing proteins and induction of protein synthesis	Introduction of new protein synthesis	Modification of existing proteins	Induction of new protein synthesis
Examples	Insulin, parathyroid hormone	Estrogen, androgens, cortisol	Epinephrine, norepinephrine, dopamine	Thyroxine (T_4)

Hormonal Modes of Action

Insulin regulates blood glucose levels

Most hormones are peptide hormones. They are initially synthesized as larger *preprohormones*, which are cleaved to inactive *prohormones* in the lumen of the rough ER. The prohormone is cleaved to form the active hormone in the Golgi apparatus. In the Golgi, they may be modified with carbohydrates.

Insulin is a peptide hormone secreted by the beta (β) cells of the islets of Langerhans in the pancreas. Its secretion is increased during the absorptive state and decreased during the post-absorptive state. Insulin targets are muscle, adipose, and liver tissues.

The main roles of insulin are to 1) stimulate the movement of glucose from the extracellular fluid into the cells by facilitated diffusion, 2) stimulate glycogen synthesis, and 3) inhibit glycogen catabolism. Insulin is an anabolic building hormone and inhibits protein degradation. It promotes cell division and differentiation because it is required to produce *insulin-like growth factors* (IGF-I), which are vital for regulating normal physiology. An increase in plasma glucose or amino acid concentration controls insulin.

Glucose-dependent insulinotropic peptide (GIP) is a hormone secreted in the GI tract to stimulate insulin secretion. Parasympathetic nerve fibers stimulate insulin secretion.

Peptide hormones' mode of action

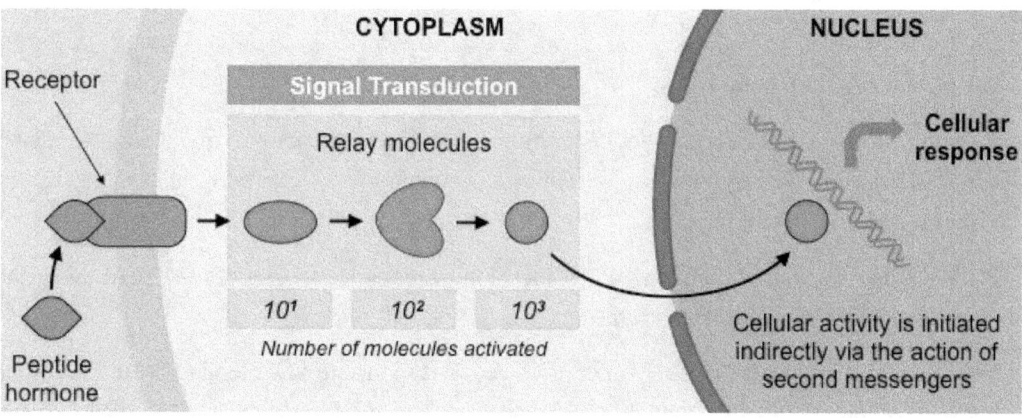

Peptide hormones bind to a plasma membrane receptor as a ligand and initiate a second messenger cascade to amplify the cellular response. The hormone may initiate phosphorylation or dephosphorylation of molecules in the cytoplasm as the mechanism for the cellular response.

Hypoglycemia refers to low plasma glucose levels resulting from an excess of insulin (beta cells) or glucagon deficiency (alpha cells). *Glucagon* is a peptide hormone secreted by alpha (α) pancreas cells. Its target is the liver tissue, and its actions are antagonistic to insulin.

Glucagon increases glycogen breakdown and gluconeogenesis to increase the plasma concentration of glucose during the post-absorptive state or when plasma glucose is low (hypoglycemia). Sympathetic nerves stimulate glucagon secretion.

Atrial natriuretic hormone (ANH) is a peptide hormone secreted by cardiac (heart) cells when the atria of the heart are stretched due to increased blood volume. ANH inhibits the secretion of renin by the kidneys, inhibits the secretion of *aldosterone* from the adrenal cortex, and decreases sodium reabsorption; when sodium is excreted along with water, the blood volume and pressure decrease.

Antidiuretic hormone (ADH) is a peptide hormone produced in the hypothalamus. Antidiuretic hormone (ADH) increases water reabsorption by increasing the permeability of the nephron's collecting ducts, which results in water reabsorption and increased blood volume and pressure. ADH is released when the blood has low water content (high osmolarity). Caffeine blocks ADH, tricking the brain into thinking the body is over-hydrated. This causes increased fluid output, so coffee drinkers may often urinate.

Calcitonin is a peptide hormone produced by the thyroid gland. Calcitonin lowers calcium levels in the blood by inhibiting calcium release from bone. Calcitonin increases deposits in the bone by reducing the activity and number of *osteoclasts* (the type of bone cells that resorbs bone tissue). Calcium is necessary for blood clotting. If blood calcium is lowered, the release of calcitonin is inhibited.

Hormones regulate homeostasis

Parathyroid hormone (PTH), a peptide hormone produced by the parathyroid gland, stimulates the absorption of Ca^{2+} by activating vitamin D, retaining Ca^{2+}, excreting phosphates by the kidneys, and demineralizing bone by promoting the activity of osteoclasts.

PTH is antagonistic to calcitonin. When the blood calcium level reaches the right level, the parathyroid glands inhibit PTH synthesis.

The body goes into tetany if PTH is not produced in response to low blood Ca^{2+}. In *tetany*, the body shakes uncontrollably from involuntary, continuous muscle spasms. Ca^{2+} is vital to proper nerve conduction and muscle contraction.

Gonadotropins are peptide hormones produced in *adenohypophysis*.

Two main gonadotropins, *follicle-stimulating hormone* (FSH) and *luteinizing hormone* (LH), act on the gonads (ovaries and testes) to secrete sex hormones.

FSH stimulates the maturation of ovarian follicles in females, and in males, it acts on the Sertoli cells of the testes to stimulate sperm production (spermatogenesis).

LH triggers ovulation and the formation of the corpus luteum in females. In males, it stimulates the interstitial cells of the testes to produce testosterone.

Gonadotropin-releasing hormone (GnRH) is released by the hypothalamus and stimulates gonadotropin production.

Oxytocin is a peptide hormone produced in the hypothalamus that stimulates uterine muscle contraction in response to uterine wall nerve impulses markedly during childbirth. It stimulates the release of milk from mammary glands for nursing.

Prolactin, a peptide hormone produced in adenohypophysis, is secreted after childbirth; it causes the mammary glands to produce milk and plays a role in carbohydrate and fat metabolism. The neurotransmitter dopamine inhibits prolactin.

Gastrin is a peptide hormone used during digestion in the stomach; stimulating HCl secretions.

Secretin is in the small intestine and is activated when acidic food enters the stomach. It neutralizes chyme's (i.e., partly digested food) acidity by secreting alkaline bicarbonate.

Cholecystokinin (CCK) in the small intestine causes contractions of the gallbladder and bile release, which is involved in the digestion of fats.

Growth hormone (GH), or somatotropic hormone, is a peptide hormone produced in the adenohypophysis that promotes skeletal and muscular growth. GH stimulates the transport of amino acids into cells and increases ribosomes' activity. GH promotes fat metabolism rather than glucose metabolism.

When there are low plasma levels of GH, *growth hormone-releasing hormone* (GHRH) is released from the hypothalamus, and GHRH stimulates GH production.

Gigantism is a condition caused by the over secretion of growth hormone during childhood and results in a person being significantly taller and bigger than a typical human.

Acromegaly occurs when too much growth hormone is produced during adulthood, resulting in disproportioned growth of some body regions (the parts that still respond to growth hormones).

Adrenocorticotropic hormone (ACTH) is a peptide hormone that stimulates the adrenal cortex to release glucocorticoids and cortisol, steroid hormones involved in regulating glucose metabolism.

Steroid hormones' mode of action

Adrenal cortex and the gonads produce steroid hormones synthesized from cholesterol in smooth ER. They are lipids and can freely diffuse across membranes but require protein transport molecules to dissolve in the blood.

Steroid hormones have the same complex of four carbon rings but have different side chains.

Steroid hormones include the glucocorticoids (e.g., cortisol) and mineralocorticoids (e.g., aldosterone) of the adrenal cortex. They include the gonadal hormones estrogen, progesterone, and testosterone. The placenta produces estrogen and progesterone.

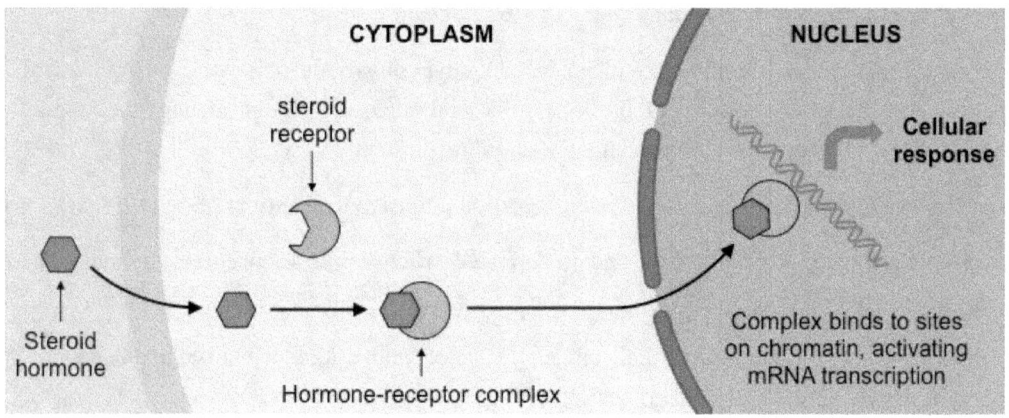

Steroid hormones pass the plasma membrane and bind to an intracellular receptor which migrates as a complex into the nucleus to affect gene transcription

Glucocorticoids are stress hormones that help regulate blood glucose levels. They raise blood glucose levels by stimulating gluconeogenesis in the liver, affecting fat and protein metabolism.

Like glucocorticoids, *cortisol* increases energy by raising blood glucose levels. Cortisol inhibits the immune system and exerts antigrowth effects by stimulating protein catabolism. Cortisol and corticosterone affect the metabolism of glucose and other organic nutrients. Cortisol counteracts the inflammatory response and helps to medicate arthritis and bursitis.

When the body is under stress, corticotropin-releasing hormone (CRH) from the hypothalamus is released, which triggers ACTH from the adenohypophysis to be released.

Aldosterone, a mineralocorticoid produced in the adrenal cortex, participates in mineral balance by regulating the kidney's Na^+, K^+ and H^+ ions. Its primary role is helping the kidneys move sodium and water from urine into the bloodstream, thus regulating the body's sodium and potassium balance.

Additionally, aldosterone reduces the sodium sensitivity of taste buds, and it acts on sweat glands to reduce sodium loss during perspiration. Aldosterone is stimulated by decreased blood volume and by increasing Na^+ reabsorption.

Hyposecretion (i.e., diminished secretion) of glucocorticoids and mineralocorticoids results in *Addison's disease*. When ACTH is in excess, it can lead to melanin buildup. The lack of cortisol results in low glucose levels. This can lead to severe fatigue, perpetuated and worsened by stress. The lack of aldosterone lowers sodium levels; the person has low blood pressure and dehydration. Untreated, Addison's disease can be fatal.

Hypersecretion (i.e., excessive secretion) of corticosteroids results in *Cushing's syndrome*. Excess cortisol changes carbohydrate and protein metabolism and causes a tendency toward diabetes mellitus. As a result, muscular protein decreases, and subcutaneous fat collects, creating an obese torso, while arms and legs usually remain proportioned. A "puffy" appearance typically characterizes sufferers of this syndrome.

Gonadocorticoids are another group of steroid hormones produced in the adrenal cortex. They are responsible for the onset of puberty and the onset of the female libido.

Androgens and estrogens

Adrenal *androgens*, responsible for developing male sex characteristics, are produced in the adrenal cortex, and regulated by ACTH. The most potent androgen, testosterone, is produced primarily in the testes.

Adrenal androgens are weak steroids, and some function as precursors to testosterone (e.g., DHEA, which is androstenolone). In addition to influencing male development, androgens play some role in female puberty and the adult female. The renin-angiotensin-aldosterone system controls mineralocorticoid secretion. Under low blood volume and sodium levels, the kidneys secrete renin, cleaving angiotensin I and promoting a cascade that increases blood pressure.

Testosterone is the primary androgen secreted by the testes. Testosterone is mainly responsible for the male sex drive. Anabolic steroids are synthetic variants of testosterone used to treat some hormone issues in men. Testosterone affects the sweat glands and the expression of the baldness gene, among other characteristics and functions of the body.

Estrogen, a female sex hormone secreted by the ovaries, is necessary for oocyte development. It is responsible for developing female secondary sex characteristics, including forming a layer of fat under the skin and a larger pelvic girdle. Estrogen and progesterone regulate breast development and uterine cycle regulation.

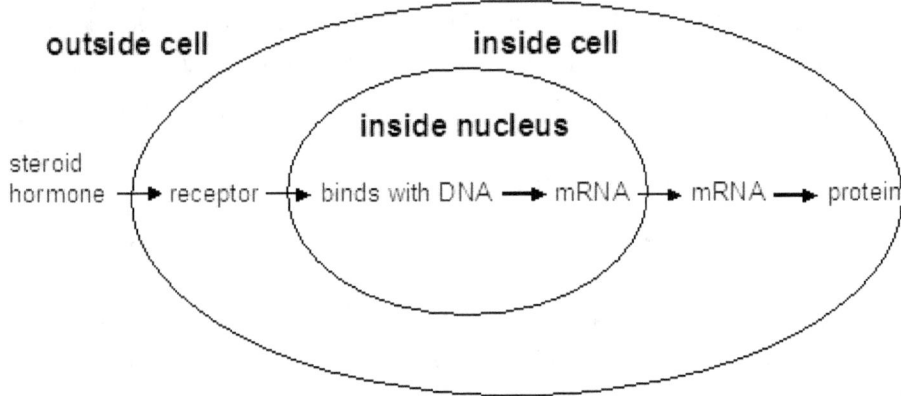

Steroid hormone pathway mechanism

Amino acid-derived hormones mode of action

Amino acid-derived hormones are usually derivatives of the amino acid tyrosine. Enzymes form *tyrosine derivative*s in the cytosol or on the rough ER. The adrenal medulla secretes the amino acid-derived hormones *epinephrine* (adrenaline) and *norepinephrine* (noradrenaline), which stimulate "fight or flight" responses. They are *stress hormones* because both hormones bring about body changes corresponding to an emergency.

Fight-or-flight response initiates glycogen-to-glucose conversion, vasoconstriction of the internal organs and skin, vasodilation to the skeletal muscles, and increased heartbeat. This causes the blood glucose level and the oxygen content to rise and increases metabolic rate. The bronchioles dilate, and the breathing rate increases.

Blood vessels to the digestive tract and skin constrict, while blood vessels to the skeletal muscles dilate and the cardiac muscle contracts forcefully, causing the heart rate to increase.

Adrenal medulla secretes more epinephrine than norepinephrine. Both hormones are catecholamines. *Catecholamines* solubilize in water, dissolve in blood, bind to receptors on the target tissue, and mainly act via the secondary messenger system.

Norepinephrine is formed from amino acid tyrosine and *epinephrine* from norepinephrine. Although the effects of these two catecholamines are similar, there are differences.

Norepinephrine constricts almost all the body's blood vessels, while epinephrine constricts only the minute blood vessels and dilates the larger blood vessels of the liver and skeletal muscle.

Epinephrine increases metabolic rate through its calorigenic effect and stimulates the catabolism of glycogen and triacylglycerols. It increases energy by raising glucose and oxygen content in the blood. It is released when the autonomic nervous system must respond to stress.

Other amino acid-derived hormones include the two iodine-containing hormones, *thyroxine* (T_4) and *triiodothyronine* (T_3), secreted by the follicles of the thyroid glands. T_4 is secreted in larger amounts but is mainly converted to T_3, the active form.

Thyroid hormones (TH) are lipid-soluble, require a protein carrier in the blood, and bind to receptors in the nucleus. TH regulates oxygen consumption, growth, and brain development.

Thyroxine controls the body's metabolic rate, energy consumed, and protein volume. Thyroxine is released when there is a low concentration of it in the blood.

Hyperresponsiveness is hypersecretion of thyroid hormones, leading to hyperresponsiveness to epinephrine and increased heart rate.

Although tyrosine is the primary amino acid from which this class of hormones is derived, other amino acids are hormone precursors. For example, the amino acid tryptophan is the precursor to melatonin.

Melatonin, produced in the pineal gland, aids in maintaining balanced circadian rhythms (daily biological cycles) and sleep patterns.

Glutamic acid is an amino acid precursor to *histamine*, a hormone part of the body's natural allergic response. Histamine plays a vital role in the immune system.

Hormone Distribution, Secretion and Effects

Cellular mechanisms of hormone action

Lipid-soluble hormones cross the plasma membrane and directly activate genes.

Water-soluble hormones are unable to cross the plasma membrane. Instead, they bind to membrane receptors on the outside of cells. Secondary messengers (e.g., tyrosine kinase or G-coupled proteins) relay the signal inside the cell. An example of a secondary messenger is cyclic AMP (cAMP). An amino acid hormone binds to a membrane receptor in a cAMP pathway.

G-protein is activated alongside adenylate cyclase, and cAMP is produced.

In the *phospholipid pathway,* an amino acid hormone binds to a membrane receptor, activating a G-protein. *Phospholipase C* is activated, and the membrane phospholipids split into two secondary messengers: *diacylglycerol* (DAG) and *inositol triphosphate* (IP$_3$). DAG triggers a protein kinase cascade, and IP$_3$ releases Ca^{2+} from the ER.

Hyposecretion is when a gland secretes insufficient hormones because it cannot function normally; the disorder is *primary hyposecretion.* Causes include a genetic lack of an enzyme, dietary precursor deficiency, or infection.

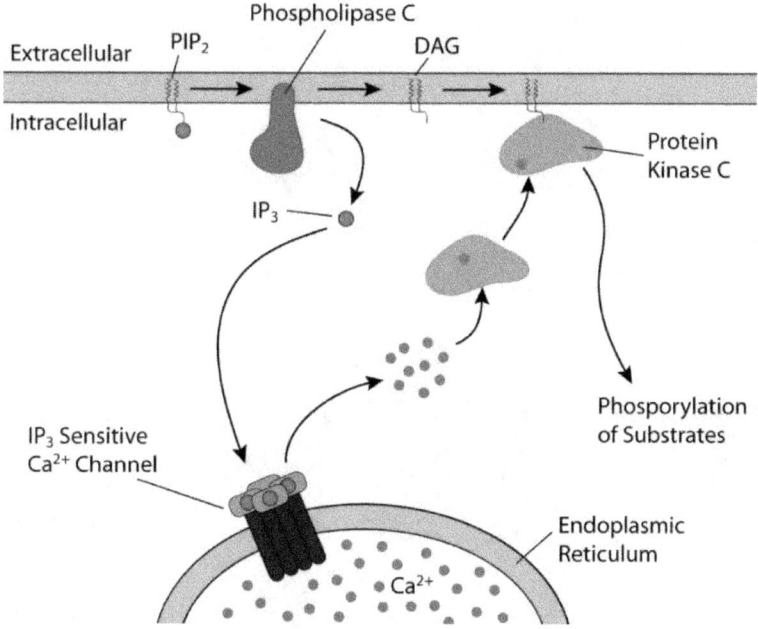

Phospholipid pathway: cleavage to IP$_3$ and DAG to release calcium for the ER

Primary hypersecretion is when a gland secretes too much hormone.

Secondary hypersecretion is the excessive stimulation of a gland by its tropic hormone.

Hyporesponsiveness is when target cells do not respond to a hormone due to a deficiency of receptors, a defect in the signal transduction mechanism, or a deficiency of an enzyme that catalyzes the activation of the hormone. For example, in diabetes mellitus, the target cells of the hormone insulin are hyporesponsive.

Hormone distribution through blood and lymph fluid

Hormones travel long distances via the blood and lymph.

Unbound (peptide) hormones are water-soluble hormones that dissolve in plasma blood.

In contrast, *bound hormones* (*steroids*) circulate in the blood while bound to plasma proteins (e.g., serum carrier or transport proteins). Free hormones diffuse across capillary walls to encounter their target cells.

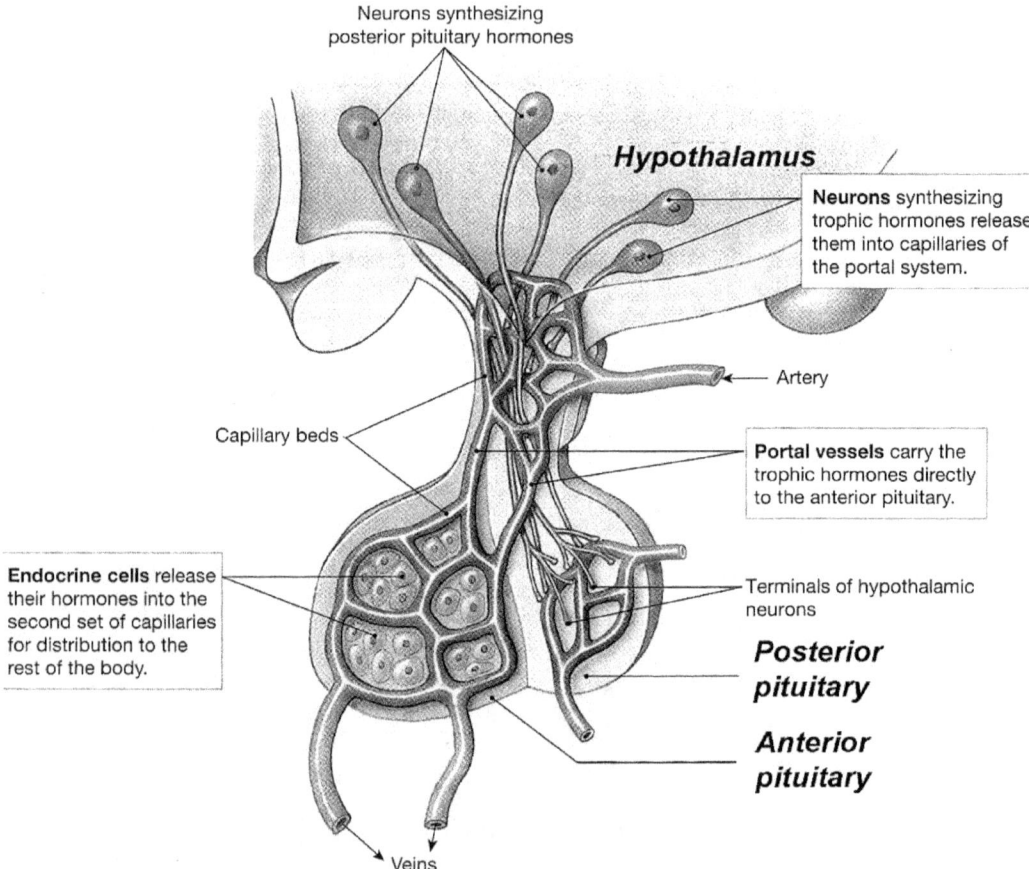

Hypothalamus, posterior and anterior pituitary axis

Hypothalamic-hypophyseal and hepatic portal circulation

Hypothalamic-hypophyseal portal circulation permits the transport of neurohormones by the hypothalamus' neuroendocrine cells directly to the pituitary cells.

Usually, these hormones are excluded from the general circulation. In this system, capillaries from the hypothalamus go through the plexus of veins around the pituitary stalk and into the anterior pituitary gland.

Hepatic portal circulation allows for the transport of hormones from the Islets of Langerhans in the pancreas. The hormones of the pancreas include insulin and glucagon.

Various nutrients are absorbed from the intestine and transported into the liver through this pathway. This pathway occurs before general circulation occurs.

In this system, capillaries originating from the gastrointestinal tract and the spleen merge to form the portal vein. The vein enters the liver and divides to form portal capillaries.

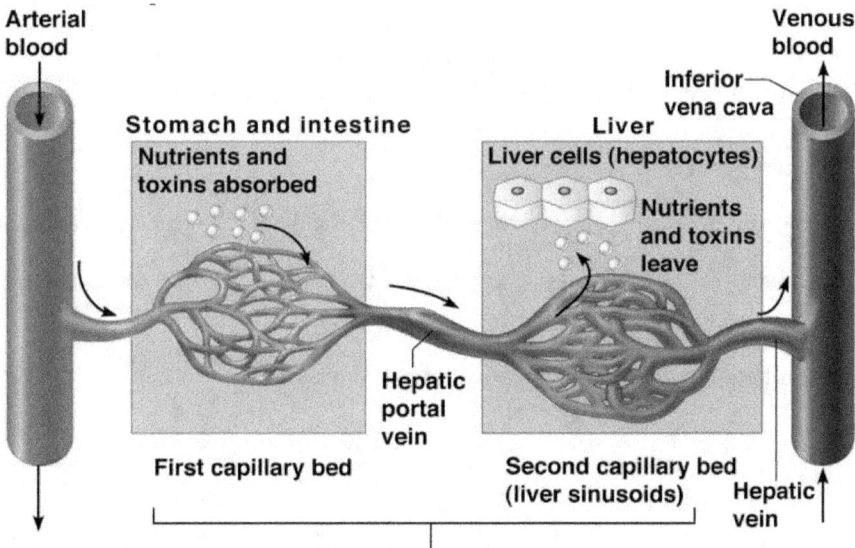

Hepatic portal circulation

Target tissue specificity of hormones

Hormones reach tissues via the blood, but cells with specific receptors are hormone targets.

Specificity depends on the unique receptors on the target cells and the lack of receptors on non-target cells for the hormone. Hormones bind to cells with receptor sites for that hormone.

Peptide hormone receptors are on the cell's surface, while steroid hormones bind receptors in the cytoplasm (or nucleus).

Cells can *upregulate* (i.e., increase production) or *downregulate* (i.e., decrease production) the expressed receptors. Low hormone concentration may be compensated for by increasing receptor numbers. In contrast, a high hormone concentration decreases the number of receptors.

Receptors for peptide hormones and catecholamines are present on the plasma membrane's extracellular surface, while those for steroids are mainly in the cytoplasm.

Hormones that bind to surface receptors can influence ion channels, enzyme activity, G proteins, and secondary messengers. Genes can be activated or inhibited, resulting in a change in the synthesis rate of proteins encoded by these genes.

Some hormones can reduce the number of receptors available for a second hormone, resulting in decreased second hormone effectiveness.

Hormones that block the second hormone are *antagonists,* and this process is *antagonism.*

A hormone can increase the receptors for a second hormone, increasing the latter's effectiveness, a process of *permissiveness.*

Cell-to-cell signaling pathways allow hormones to bind to various target cells. In *endocrine signaling*, hormones are distributed into the blood and bind to long-distance target cells.

Autocrine and paracrine signals

Autocrine signals are local chemicals that cells release and bind to receptors on the same cell.

Paracrine signals act through short distances on other cells. Signals involve messengers with short lifespans since a short distance needs to be covered.

Neurotransmitter secretions are a type of paracrine signaling.

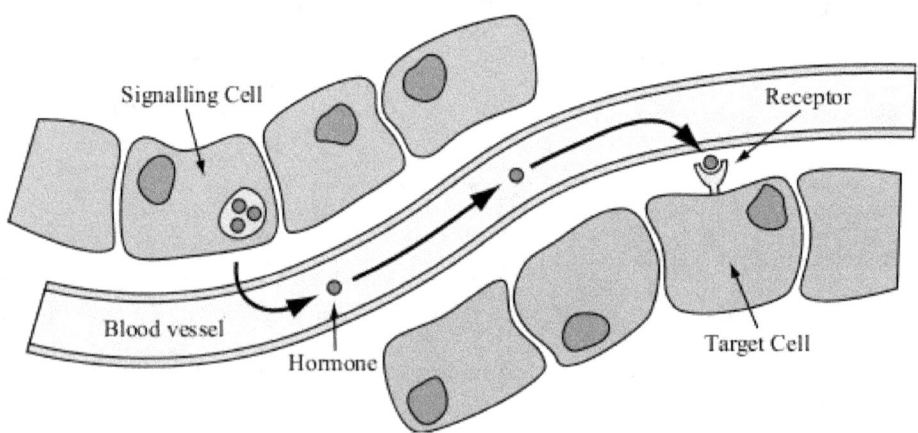

Hormones are released from a gland, travel in the blood and affect a target cell that has the receptor

Some signals locally affect neighboring cells and do not travel through the bloodstream.

Prostaglandins are potent chemical signals produced within cells from arachidonate, a fatty acid. Prostaglandins cause the uterus to contract and are involved in menstrual discomfort. The effect of aspirin on reducing fever and controlling pain is due to its effect on prostaglandins.

Growth factors promote cell division and mitosis.

*Pheromone*s are chemical signals that act at a distance between individual organisms. Ants produce a pheromone trail for other ant colony members to find food. Female silkworm moths release pheromones to lure male moths from miles away. Axillary secretions from the armpits of men and women are thought to affect the opposite sex. Some women may prefer men's axillary odor with a different plasma membrane protein. Women may synchronize their menstrual cycles with other women living nearby.

Notes for active learning

Endocrine and Neural Integration

Neuroendocrinology intersects the nervous and endocrine systems

Secretion of some hormones is under the control of the nervous system.

This was first recognized in the brain's role (specifically the hypothalamus) in stimulating the pituitary gland to release hormones. The nervous system controls hormone release based on the body's current state.

For example, control through the hypothalamus is seen when blood glucose levels are higher from stress. The endocrine system is significantly slower than the nervous system, and hormones can modulate the nervous system. For example, low estrogen levels during menses tend to lead to mood disruptions, characteristic of premenstrual syndrome (PMS).

Neurons secrete *hypophysiotropic hormones* in response to action potentials. These hormones are named after the anterior pituitary hormone that it controls.

Endorphins, technically a neuro-hormone, inhibit the perception of pain.

Endocrine integration with the nervous system by feedback control

Hormonal effects are controlled by negative feedback and antagonistic hormone actions.

Negative feedback is where the product of a process decreases the rate of that process.

Long-loop negative feedback is when the last hormone in a chain of control exerts negative feedback on the hypophysis-pituitary system.

If an anterior pituitary hormone exerts a negative feedback effect on the hypothalamus, it is *short-loop negative feedback*. This mechanism is seen in pituitary hormones that do not influence other endocrine glands. For example, the pancreas produces insulin when blood glucose rises, causing the liver to store glucose. When glucose is stored, blood glucose level decreases, and the pancreas stops insulin production.

Antagonistic actions of hormones are essential factors in regulation. For example, the effect of insulin is offset by the pancreas' glucagon production. The thyroid hormones lower blood calcium levels, while the parathyroid hormones raise blood calcium levels.

The concentration of a hormone in the plasma depends on its secretion and removal rates. The kidneys can excrete hormones or are metabolized by the target cells. Plasma concentrations of ions (or nutrients) may control the secretion of a hormone, and the hormone may control the concentration of its regulators through negative feedback.

When nerve cells in the hypothalamus determine that blood is too concentrated, ADH is released, and the kidneys respond by reabsorbing water. As the blood dilutes, ADH is no longer released, an example of negative feedback.

Oxytocin is made in hypothalamus and stored in the posterior pituitary; it is *positive feedback* as it increases intensity. Positive feedback does not maintain homeostasis.

During the normal control of hormones, *humoral glands* directly respond to chemical levels in the blood (e.g., parathyroid responds to low blood calcium).

Neural glands release hormones when stimulated by nerves (fight-or-flight response).

Hormonal glands release hormones when stimulated by other hormones (tropic hormones).

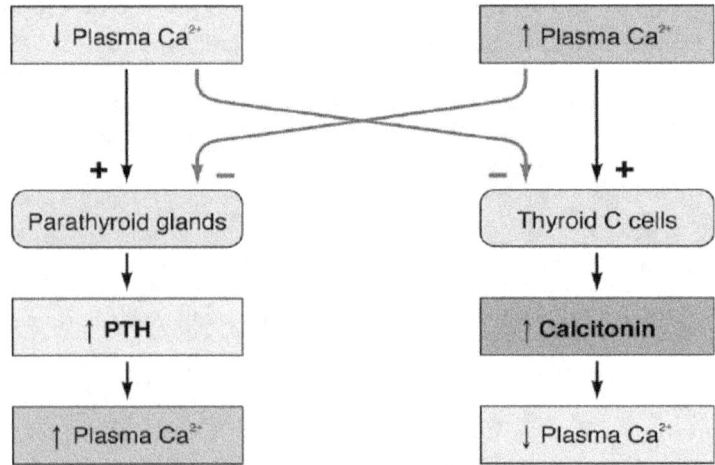

Positive and negative feedback loops to regulate plasma Ca^{2+} levels

Regulation by second messengers

Secondary messenger system utilizes non-steroid hormones. In this system, the hormone binds to a membrane receptor but does not enter the cell. When the hormone binds to a membrane receptor, it initiates some reactions that activate an enzyme.

Hormone receptor binding causes the adenylate cyclase in the membrane to be activated. This activation converts ATP to cAMP, and cAMP activates protein kinases. Protein kinases activate various enzymes, stimulate cellular secretions, and open ion channels.

Peptide hormones cannot enter a cell independently and use vesicles to cross the membrane. Typically, they act on the surface receptors via secondary messengers.

Peptide hormones bind to a receptor protein on the plasma membrane, a receptor-mediated endocytosis process. For example, epinephrine is a peptide hormone that binds to a receptor protein. A relay system leads to the conversion of ATP to cAMP.

Peptide hormones are the first messengers, while cAMP and calcium are the second.

Second messenger may initiate an enzyme cascade. Activated enzymes can be used repeatedly, resulting in a thousand-fold response. These hormones may serve as neurotransmitters.

Nucleotide cAMP is produced from ATP with the assistance of the enzyme adenylate cyclase, and numerous hormones manipulate the amount of cAMP within the cell. In turn, cAMP affects many cell processes.

Common effect of an increase in cAMP concentration is the activation of the cAMP-dependent protein, protein kinase A. Protein kinase A is commonly found in a catalytically inactive state; however, it becomes active when it binds to cAMP.

When protein kinase A is activated, it phosphorylates many different enzymes, either activated or suppressed by phosphorylation.

For example, glucagon binds to its receptors on the plasma membrane. The bound receptor can interact with the adenylate cyclase through various G proteins. Active adenylate cyclase converts ATP to cAMP, increasing the cell's cAMP content.

Increased cAMP level in the cytosol allows for increased binding of protein kinase A to cAMP, thus making protein kinase A catalytically active. The active protein kinases proceed to phosphorylate various enzymes within the cell, which changes the enzymes' conformation and controls their catalytic behavior. Finally, the levels of the cAMP decrease due to destruction by cAMP-phosphodiesterase and the inactivation of adenylate cyclase.

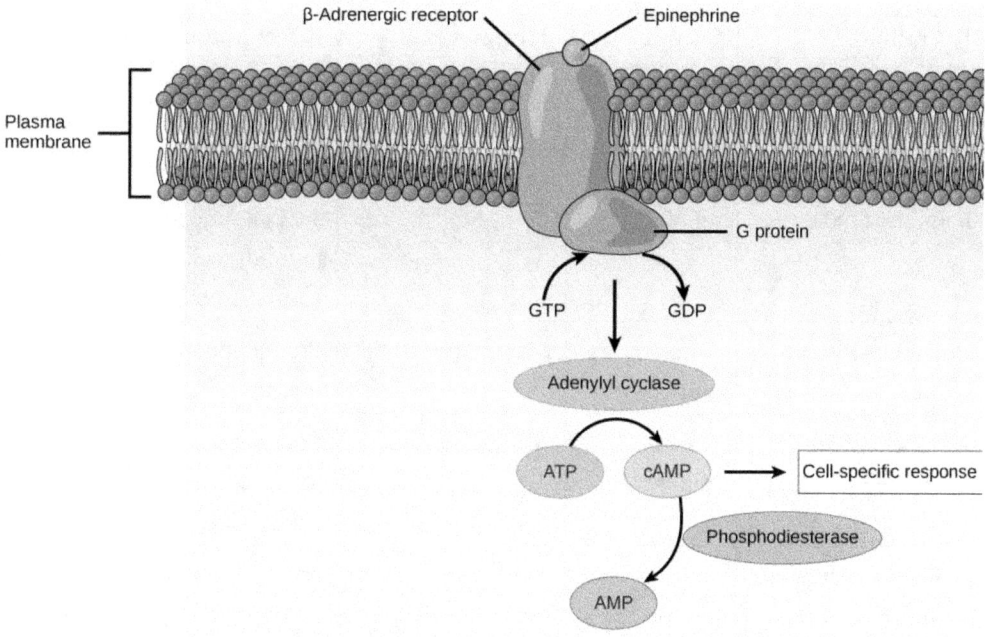

Peptide hormone uses G protein second messenger to phosphorylate cytosolic enzymes

Along with the activity of pre-existing components of the cell, an increase in cAMP can have major effects on the transcription of a gene by phosphorylating transcription factors that regulate gene expression.

Tyrosine kinase is another secondary messenger molecule. Protein kinases are often the receptors for protein hormones. The kinase activity of receptors results in the phosphorylation of various tyrosine residues on other proteins. For example, insulin is a hormone whose receptors are tyrosine kinases.

Steroid hormones bind to the exposed receptor on cell surface to activate tyrosine kinase. This results in a conformational change, which activates kinase domains in the cytoplasmic regions of the receptor. Usually, the receptor phosphorylates during the kinase activation process.

As with cAMP, the activation of the tyrosine kinase cascade causes rapid changes by phosphorylating a variety of intracellular targets, usually enzymes, which become active or inactive after phosphorylation.

In other cases, the binding of a hormone to a surface receptor initiates a tyrosine kinase cascade, even though the receptor might not be a tyrosine kinase. The growth hormone receptor is an example. The interaction of the growth hormone and its receptor leads to the activation of cytoplasmic tyrosine kinases. The results are like *receptor kinases*.

Summary table of hormone secretions, targets and effects

Hormone	Secreted by:	Target	Effect at the target site
Growth hormone (GH)	Anterior pituitary	Bone, muscle, fat	Growth of tissues
Thyroid-stimulating hormone (TSH)	Anterior pituitary	Thyroid	Stimulates the release of T_3/T_4 hormones from the thyroid, which increases the basal metabolic rate
Prolactin (PRL)	Anterior pituitary	Mammary glands	Production of milk in the breasts
Adrenocorticotropic hormone (ACTH)	Anterior pituitary	Adrenal cortex	Stimulates the adrenal cortex to secrete stress hormones called glucocorticoids
Follicle-stimulating hormone (FSH)	Anterior pituitary	Males: seminiferous tubules of testes; Females: ovarian follicle	Males: sperm production Females: follicle growth during menstruation; ovum maturation

Summary table of hormone secretions, targets and effects (*continued*)

Hormone	Secreted by:	Target	Effect at the target site
Luteinizing hormone (LH)	Anterior pituitary	In males: interstitial cells in testes; In females: mature ovarian follicle	Males: testosterone secretion Females: ovulation; estrogen secretion
Triiodothyronine (T_3) & thyroxine (T_4)	Thyroid	All cells	Regulates metabolism
Testosterone	Seminiferous tubules	Gonads (Testes)	Stimulates formation of secondary sex characteristics and closing of epiphyseal plates
Progesterone	Corpus luteum	Uterine endometrium	Preparation for implantation (thickens lining), growth and maintenance of the uterus
Estrogen	Ovarian follicle	Gonads (Ovaries)	Stimulates female sex organs; causes LH to surge during menstruation
Cortisol	Adrenal cortex	All cells	Stress hormone that increases gluconeogenesis in the liver, thus increasing blood glucose levels; stimulates fat breakdown
Aldosterone	Adrenal cortex	Kidney tubules	Increases Na^+ reabsorption and K^+ secretion at distal convoluted tubule and collecting duct; net increase in plasma salt, increasing osmotic potential and blood pressure
Anti-diuretic hormone (ADH)	Posterior pituitary	Distal convoluted tubule (DCT)	Collecting ducts of kidney become highly permeable to water, concentrating the urine

Summary table of hormone secretions, targets and effects (*continued*)

Hormone	Secreted by:	Target	Effect at the target site
Oxytocin (OT)	Posterior pituitary	Uterine smooth muscle	Contraction during childbirth; milk secretion during nursing
Parathyroid hormone (PTH)	Parathyroid	Kidney tubules and osteoclasts	Reabsorption of Ca^{2+} into blood, bone resorption (increases blood Ca^{2+})
Calcitonin	Thyroid	Kidney tubules and osteoblasts	Secretion of Ca^{2+} into urine, bone formation (decreases blood Ca^{2+})
Insulin	β Islets	All cells, liver, and skeletal muscle	Pushes glucose into cells from blood, glycogen formation (decreases blood glucose)
Glucagon	α Islets	Liver and skeletal muscle	Stimulates gluconeogenesis, the breakdown of glycogen (increase in blood glucose)
Epinephrine	Adrenal medulla	Cardiac muscle, arteriole, and bronchiole smooth muscle	Raises heart rate, constricts blood vessels, dilates pupils, and suppresses the immune system
Norepinephrine	Adrenal medulla	Cardiac muscle, arteriole, and bronchiole smooth muscle	Raises heart rate causing glucose to be released as energy and blood to flow to the muscles
Melatonin	Pineal gland	Limbic system	Emotions/behavior; circadian rhythm

Notes for active learning

Notes for active learning

CHAPTER 4

Nervous System

Vertebrate Nervous System Organization

Nervous System Functions

Sympathetic and Parasympathetic Nervous Systems

Reflexes and Feedback Mechanisms

Spinal Cord Anatomy

Endocrine System Integration

Neurons

Nerve Structures

Synapses and Neurotransmitters

Impulse Propagation

Excitatory and inhibitory nerve fibers and summation

Interneurons, Sensory and Efferent Neurons

Vertebrate Nervous System Organization

High-level control and integration of body systems

Three functions of the nervous system are:

- receiving sensory input
- transferring and interpreting impulses
- generating motor output to muscles and glands

Nervous system is a highly organized neural pathway extending to nearly every body part.

Neurons are nerve cells specialized to quickly transmit electrical impulses by forming pathways toward or away from the brain.

Nervous system is organized, so the brain uses neural pathways to interpret environmental stimuli and subsequently direct the appropriate response to the body.

Responses involve other bodily systems (e.g., endocrine, muscular, and cardiovascular).

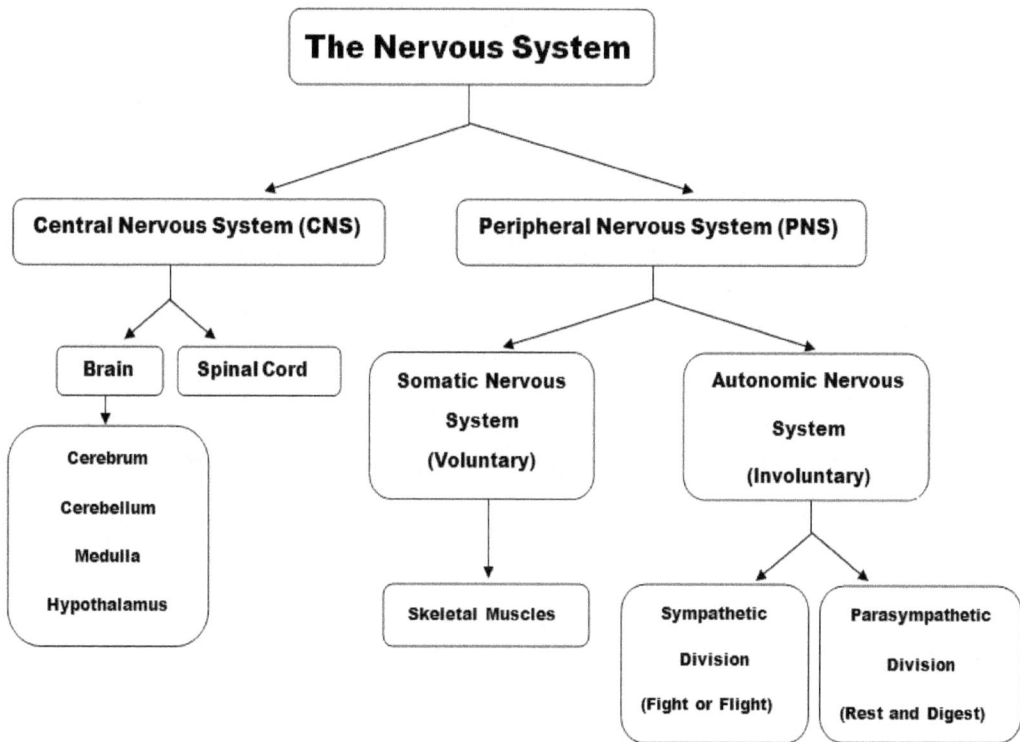

The nervous system divides into the central and peripheral nervous system

Central nervous system vs. peripheral nervous system

Central nervous system (CNS) consists of the brain and the spinal cord, while the peripheral nervous system (PNS) consists of other nerves and ganglia (collections of cell bodies).

PNS contains the *somatic nervous system*, including the pathways of voluntary control over our skeletal muscles, and the involuntary *autonomic nervous system*, including the *sympathetic* (fight or flight) and *parasympathetic* (rest and digest) branches.

PNS sends signals from sensory neurons toward the CNS.

CNS sends signals to muscles and organs via effector neurons to cause specific actions.

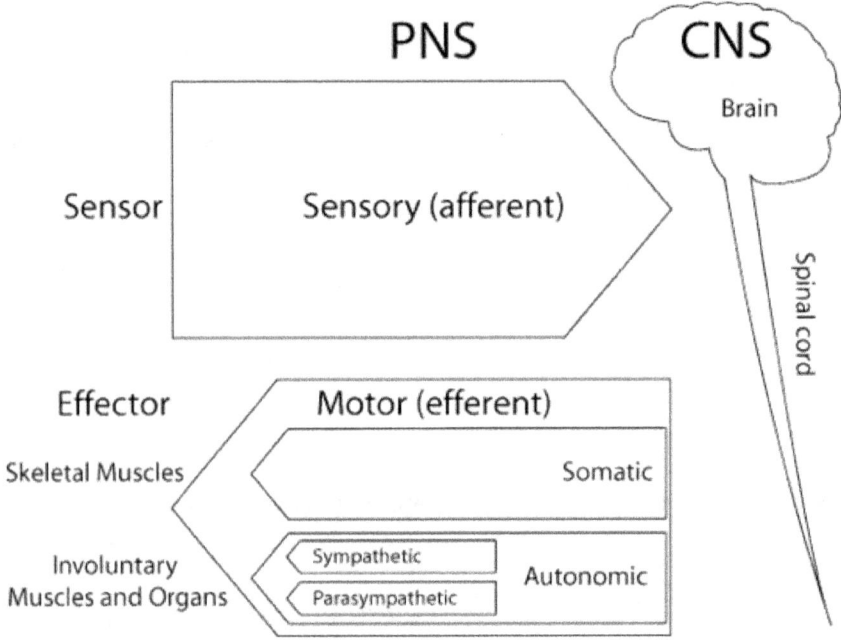

Nervous system is divided into the central nervous system (CNS) and peripheral nervous system (PNS), with afferent and efferent responses to stimuli.

Nervous System Functions

Adaptive capability to external stimuli

The nervous system's highly adaptive capability helps the brain interpret external influences efficiently.

The brain's interpretation of the environment begins at the sensory receptor. The brain communicates the corresponding response using other bodily systems.

Stimulus is energy that activates a receptor. Stimulus energy is first transformed into graded or receptor potentials.

S*timulus transduction* is when a stimulus is transformed into an electrical response.

Each receptor is specific to a stimulus type, an *adequate stimulus*.

Receptors respond to a specified intensity range of stimuli.

However, the nervous system has adapted so that receptors can still be activated when stimuli are not specified for a receptor. This adaptation allows the nervous system to communicate with the rest of the body if a receptor does not appropriately respond to the environment. This example of nonspecific stimulus occurs when the *nonspecific stimulus* is of *high intensity*.

Threshold and all-or-none response

Threshold potential is when a membrane is depolarized to generate an action potential.

A stimulus strong enough to depolarize the membrane is the threshold stimulus.

A stimulus greater than threshold magnitude elicits an action potential of the same amplitude.

This reaction occurs because once the threshold is reached, membrane events are no longer dependent upon the strength of the stimulus.

Action potentials occur maximally or do not occur, generating an *all-or-none* response.

A single action potential cannot convey information about the stimulus magnitude initiating it.

Efferent control

Efferent (or motor) neurons stimulate *effectors* or target cells, eliciting specific responses.

Effectors include muscles, sweat glands, and stomach cells secreting gastrin.

Motor neurons have many dendrites and a single axon. They conduct impulses from the central nervous system (CNS) to muscle fibers or glands.

Efferent system is divided into somatic and autonomic *systems*.

Somatic and autonomic nervous systems

Somatic nervous system innervates skeletal muscles.

It consists of myelinated axons without any synapses. The activity of neurons leads to excitation (e.g., contraction) of skeletal muscles; therefore, they are motor neurons. Motor neurons are never *inhibitory*.

Somatic fibers are responsible for *voluntary movement*.

Autonomic nervous system innervates smooth and cardiac muscles and consists of two neurons connecting the CNS and effector cells.

Synapse between these two neurons is the *autonomic ganglion*.

Nerve fibers between the CNS and the ganglion are *pre-ganglionic fibers*.

Post-ganglionic fibers are between the *ganglion* and the *effector cells*.

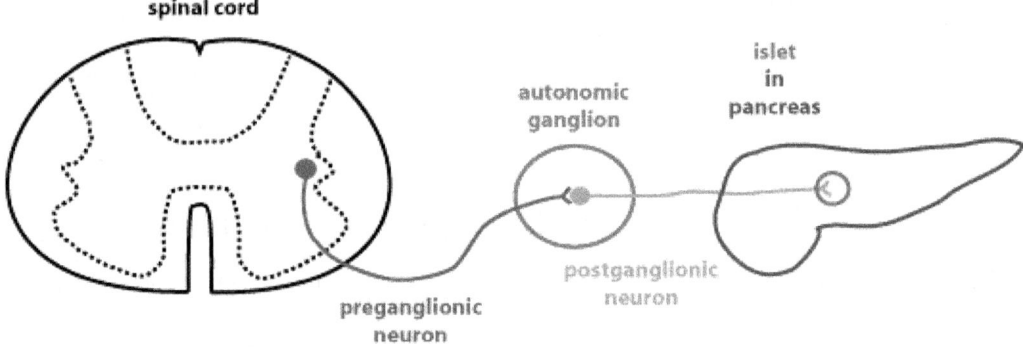

Autonomic nervous system with information traveling from spinal cord to effector cell via pre-ganglionic and post-ganglionic fibers

Negative feedback to achieve homeostasis

Within the autonomic nervous system, impulses are involuntary. Examples of involuntary impulses include respiratory system control and heart rate.

Autonomic nervous system is divided into sympathetic (fight or flight) and *parasympathetic* (rest and digest) systems.

Both systems use negative feedback mechanisms, whereby elevated levels of a compound inhibit its production. For example, the alternating release of the antagonistic hormones insulin and glucagon is essential for homeostatic blood sugar regulation.

Ganglia (i.e., collection of cell bodies) of sympathetic neurons are close to the spinal cord and are arranged to function as a single unit.

Parasympathetic ganglia neurons are close to organs and arranged so parts act independently.

Sympathetic system participates in responses to stress.

Many organs and glands receive dual innervation from sympathetic and parasympathetic fibers.

The two systems have opposite effects (i.e., negative feedback) and work to regulate a response.

Sensory input by the peripheral nervous system

Afferent neurons have sensory dendritic receptors conveying signals from tissues/organs into the CNS.

Somatic system has two pathways in opposite directions. One pathway uses *nerves* (i.e., bundles of axons) to carry sensory information from the peripheral skeletal muscles back to the CNS.

The other pathway works in the opposite direction, allowing humans to consciously use their muscles by sending impulses from the CNS to skeletal muscles.

The receptor is the site of stimulation. Once the receptor receives the stimuli, the sensory neuron carries the impulse to the *integration center*. The integration center connects sensory and motor neurons via synapses inside the CNS. Integration is monosynaptic or polysynaptic.

Monosynaptic integration is when no interneurons (i.e., neurons linking sensory and motor neurons) are involved. It uses a direct synapse from sensory to motor neuron.

Polysynaptic integration requires at least one interneuron. Once the signal reaches the motor neuron, it is carried toward the effector, the site of response to the stimulus.

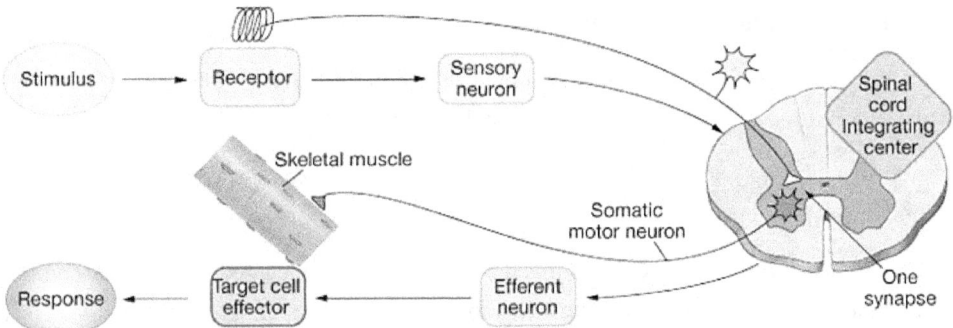

Monosynaptic reflex has a single synapse between the afferent and efferent neurons.

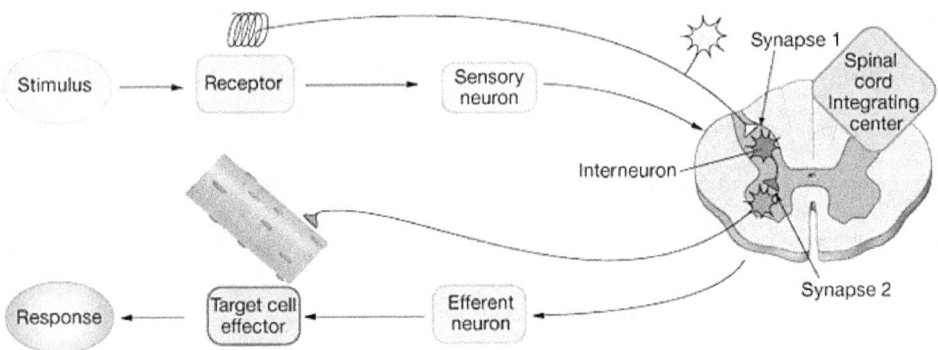

Polysynaptic reflex has two (or more) synapses (i.e., interneurons) between afferent and efferent neurons

Limbic system's structures and purpose

Limbic system is a complex network of tracts in the brain. It incorporates multiple brain areas, such as the medial portions of cerebral lobes, subcortical nuclei, and the diencephalon.

Two major limbic system structures are the *hippocampus* and the *amygdala.*

Limbic system's coordination of multiple brain areas allows for interpreting environmental stimuli and responses.

Hippocampus delivers sensory input to the prefrontal area of the brain. People know past experiences because the hippocampus stores this information in designated association areas.

Amygdala is the brain area that associates emotions with thoughts or experiences. After the amygdala and the hippocampus process sensory information, the advanced prefrontal cortex allows reasoning, preventing humans from acting purely upon basic emotion.

A general interpretation area receives information from the sensory association areas, allowing the quick integration of signals and sending them to the prefrontal area for immediate response. Prefrontal area in the frontal lobe receives input from association areas, reasons, and plans.

Memory and learning

Memory is the brain's ability to retain and recall information.

Learning is when a person retains and utilizes memories.

Prefrontal area in the frontal lobe is active in *short-term memory* (e.g., telephone numbers).

Long-term memory combines semantic (e.g., words) and episodic memory (e.g., events).

Skill memory is the ability to perform motor activities, commonly called "muscle memory."

Hippocampus serves as an intermediary between processed memories and the prefrontal cortex.

Amygdala is responsible for fear conditioning and links danger with certain sensory stimuli.

Long-term potentiation (LTP), strengthening neural pathways in the hippocampus following associated learning, is essential for memory storage.

Some excited postsynaptic cells may die due to excessive glutamate neurotransmitters.

The death of neurons in the hippocampus may be the underlying cause of Alzheimer's disease, gradually causing a person's memory to deteriorate.

Notes for active learning

Sympathetic and Parasympathetic Nervous Systems

Sensory and motor branches of the nervous system

PNS consists of sensory and motor branches. It lies outside the CNS and contains the cranial and spinal nerves. PNS transmits signals to and from the CNS using sensory and motor neurons. 12 pairs of cranial nerves connect to the brain, and 31 pairs of spinal nerves connect to the spinal cord.

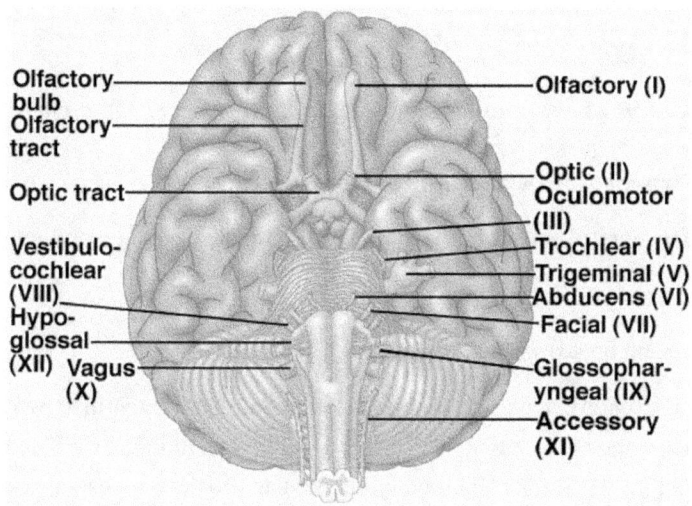

Twelve pairs of cranial nerves labeled with the number and common name

Cranial nerves mostly connect to the head, neck, and facial regions, and *spinal nerves* lie on either side of the spinal cord. Nerves are made from many parallel nerve fibers containing axons and myelin sheaths.

S*pinal roots* are the paired spinal nerves that leave the spinal cord by two short branches.

Dorsal root (or *sensory root*) contains fibers of sensory neurons conducting nerve impulses to the spinal cord.

Ventral root has axons of motor neurons to conduct nerve impulses away from the spinal cord.

Spinal nerves are mixed nerves that conduct impulses to and from the spinal cord. Spinal nerves contain sensory and motor fibers, each fiber type serving its region.

Sensory nerves contain sensory nerve fibers.

Motor nerves contain motor nerve fibers. The cell bodies of neurons are in CNS or ganglia.

PNS is divided into somatic and autonomic systems.

Somatic system is responsible for the voluntary movement of skeletal muscles.

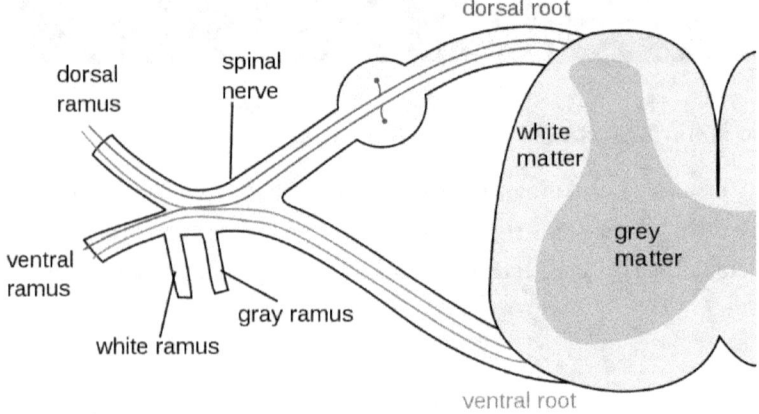

Dorsal root carries impulses to the spinal cord, ventral root carries impulses away

Sympathetic division of the autonomic nervous system

Autonomic system controls involuntary cardiac, smooth muscle, and gland movements.

There are two divisions:

sympathetic and *parasympathetic systems*.

Both systems function involuntarily, innervate internal organs, and utilize two neurons and one ganglion for each impulse. The first neuron has a cell body within the CNS and a preganglionic fiber. The second neuron has a cell body within the ganglion and a postganglionic fiber.

Reflex actions regulate breathing rate and blood pressure to maintain homeostasis.

Sympathetic system controls the fight or flight responses, raising blood pressure and heart rate. Most preganglionic fibers of the sympathetic system arise from the *thoracic-lumbar* (middle) portion of the spinal cord and almost immediately terminate in the ganglia near the spinal cord.

Preganglionic fiber is short, while the postganglionic fiber that contacts an organ is long.

Sympathetic system is vital during emergencies (i.e., "fight or flight" response). The body activates the sympathetic system to accelerate heart rate and dilate the bronchi for defense or fleeing. These responses require a supply of glucose and oxygen.

Sympathetic system inhibits digestion by diverting energy from less necessary digestive functions. It increases blood pressure, dilates the pupils to allow more light into the eye, and breaks down glycogen to release glucose into the blood.

Neurotransmitters released by the postganglionic axon are mainly norepinephrine, similar to epinephrine (adrenaline).

Parasympathetic division of the autonomic nervous system

Parasympathetic system is responsible for rest and digestion responses, lowering heart rate, and promoting non-emergency functions (e.g., digestion, relaxation, sexual arousal).

Parasympathetic system consists of a few cranial nerves and nerves exiting the spinal cord, including the vagus nerve (which innervates the heart and branches to the pharynx, larynx, and some internal organs) and fibers that arise from the sacral region of the spinal cord.

Since the parasympathetic system contains efferent nerves from the cranial and the sacral regions, efferent nerves are *craniosacral* (as opposed to *thoracic-lumbar sympathetic nerves*).

Parasympathetic system is a *"housekeeper system,"* which promotes internal responses, resulting in a relaxed state (e.g., It causes the eye pupil to constrict, promotes digestion, and slows the heartbeat.

Acetylcholine is the neurotransmitter released by the parasympathetic system.

Notes for active learning

Reflexes and Feedback Mechanisms

Reflex arcs as a survival mechanism

Reflexes involve the spinal cord and do not require the brain's participation.

There are two advantages to this. First, the brain is continuously working, and any additional tasks for the brain result in precious resources being diverted. Second, reflexes are designed to be fast responses.

For example, if someone puts their hand on a hot stove, they will not analyze the pain before removing their hand from the heat. As a result of bypassing the brain, the reaction time to these stimuli is faster.

Feedback loops affect flexor and extensor muscles

Feedback loops occur when a system's outputs are fed back into the system as inputs, leading to a change. The two types are positive and negative feedback loops.

Positive feedback is a mechanism that encourages the continuation of a cycle. Examples of positive feedback are uterine contractions, when one contraction leads to oxytocin release and, subsequently, more contractions. Another example is blood clotting, which occurs when platelets are activated at the wound site and attract platelet activation and clumping.

Positive feedback is *not* common because it disrupts *homeostasis.*

Negative feedback counteracts a continuation of a cycle. For example, a drop in blood pressure causes ADH release, increasing blood pressure. Conversely, an increase in blood pressure causes a drop in ADH.

Another example is in the Golgi tendon reflex, a sudden contraction of the quads (extensor muscles) causes negative feedback that relaxes the quads and contracts the hamstrings (flexor muscles).

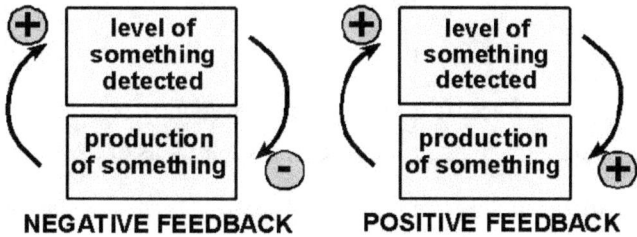

Negative feedback maintains homeostasis, while positive causes perturbation

Reflex arc

Reflex arcs use negative feedback. They are rapid, involuntary responses to stimuli involving two or three neurons, but the brain does not integrate sensory and motor activities.

Instead, the reflex arcs synapse in the spinal cord. Even though the reflex arc bypasses the brain, the brain knows that the response occurred. One example of a reflex arc is immediate withdrawal from a painful stimulus.

Another example of reflexes is the knee-jerk reaction. Tapping the knee tendon causes a sudden stretching of the muscle, and the reflex leads to contraction of that muscle, creating the knee-jerk (negative feedback).

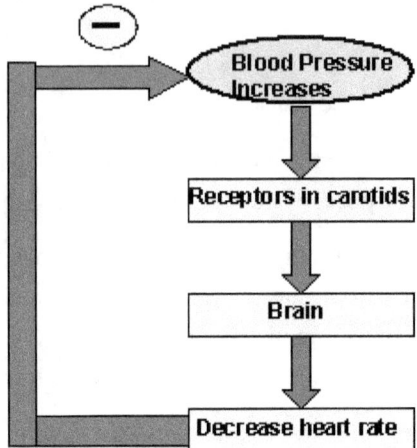

Reflex arcs occur in the following sequence:

1. Sensory receptors generate an impulse in a sensory neuron that moves toward the spinal cord along sensory axons.

2. Sensory axons enter the cord dorsally and pass signals to interneurons.

3. Interneurons pass the signals to motor neurons.

4. Impulses travel along motor axons to an effector.

5. Effectors cause an effect (e.g., muscle contracting) to withdraw from pain stimulus.

Reflex response occurs because the sensory neuron stimulates the interneurons. Some impulses extend to the cerebrum so that a person becomes conscious of the stimulus and reaction.

Reflexes often affect the flexor and extensor muscles. During the knee-jerk reflex, the extensors of the quads are contracted while the flexors of the hamstrings are relaxed.

Spinal Cord Anatomy

Spinal cord function and meninges

In the body's midline, the CNS consists of the brain and the spinal cord. It integrates sensory information and controls the body. CNS is vital because it controls biological processes and conscious thought. Because of the critical importance of the spinal cord and brain, these organs are safely encased within bones.

Cranium protects the brain, and the *spine* protects the spinal cord. Both are wrapped in three connective tissue coverings as *meninges*.

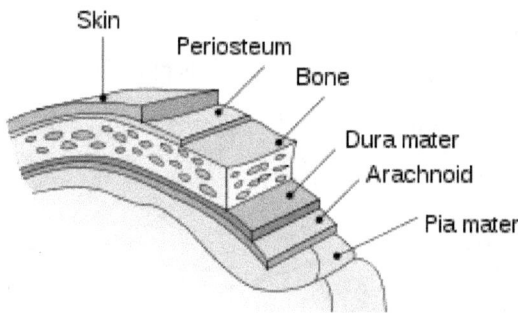

Spaces between meninges have *cerebrospinal fluid* to nourish and protect the CNS. The cerebrospinal fluid is within the central canal of the spinal cord, produced by the *ventricles* of the brain.

Meninges in the CNS have three layers:

    outermost *dura mater*,

    middle *arachnoid* and

    inner *pia mater*.

Subarachnoid space between the pia and the arachnoid space is filled with *cerebrospinal fluid* (CSF), acting as a shock absorber for neural tissue.

Because the brain cannot store glycogen, it depends on a continuous supply of glucose and oxygen from the bloodstream.

The exchange of substances between the blood and extracellular fluid in the CNS is highly restricted via a complex group of blood-brain barrier mechanisms. CSF and the brain's extracellular fluid are in diffusion equilibrium but are separated from the blood.

A group of nerve fibers traveling in the CNS is a *pathway* (or tract). A band of nerve fibers that connect the left and right halves is a *commissure*.

Dorsal and ventral horns for information propagation

Information in the CNS passes along two types of pathways:

1) *Long neural pathways* are neurons with long axons that carry information directly between the brain and spinal cord or between brain regions.

    There is no diminution in the transmitted information.

2) *Multineuronal* (or *multisynaptic*) *pathways* have many neurons or synapses.

New information is integrated into the transmitted information.

Neuron cell bodies have similar function clusters as ganglia in the PNS and nuclei in the CNS.

The spinal cord has two main functions. It provides communication between the brain, the spinal nerves, and the synapses (or synapses if it is polysynaptic) for the reflex arc.

Sensory information *enters* through the *dorsal horn* in the spinal cord.

Sensory information *exits* through *ventral horn* as motor information moves toward periphery.

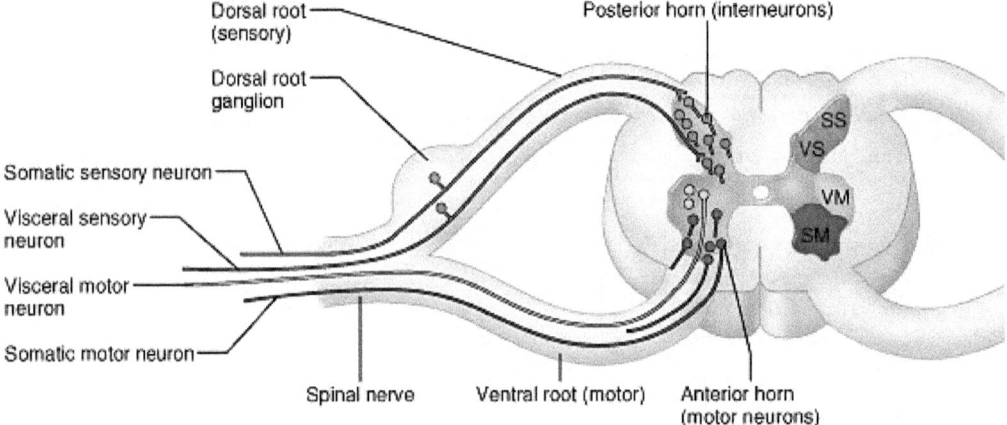

Sensory neuron (dorsal root) and motor neuron (ventral root)

Gray and white matter of the brain and spinal cord

Spinal cord and brain are composed of *gray* and *white matter*.

These areas of matter have unmyelinated or myelinated neurons, whether the neuron's axons have been covered with myelin. This phospholipid substance allows for a faster propagation of axon potentials in neurons.

Gray matter comprises interneurons, cell bodies, dendrites, and glial cells. Unmyelinated cell bodies and short fibers give gray matter its color. In a cross-section, the gray area looks like a butterfly (or the letter H). It contains portions of sensory neurons, motor neurons, and the short interneurons that connect them.

Multiple nuclei make up the *basal ganglia* gray matter in the brain.

Common malfunctions lead to conditions such as Huntington's and Parkinson's disease.

White matter has the long myelinated fibers of interneurons that run in tracts, giving the white matter its color.

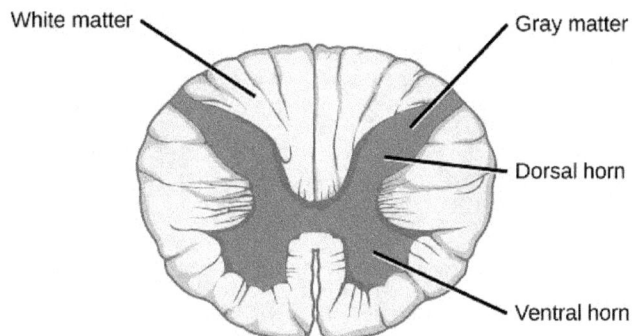

Gray (unmyelinated) matter and white (myelinated) matter comparison

Descending and ascending tracts connect the brain and spinal cord

Tracts conduct impulses between the brain and the spinal nerves;

    ascending tracts are *dorsal* and

    descending tracts from the brain are *ventral*.

Ascending tracts of the lower brain centers relay sensory information to the primary somatosensory area.

Descending tracts from the primary motor area communicate with the lower brain centers.

Near the brain, tracts cross over from one side of the body to the other; therefore, the left side of the brain controls the right side of the body.

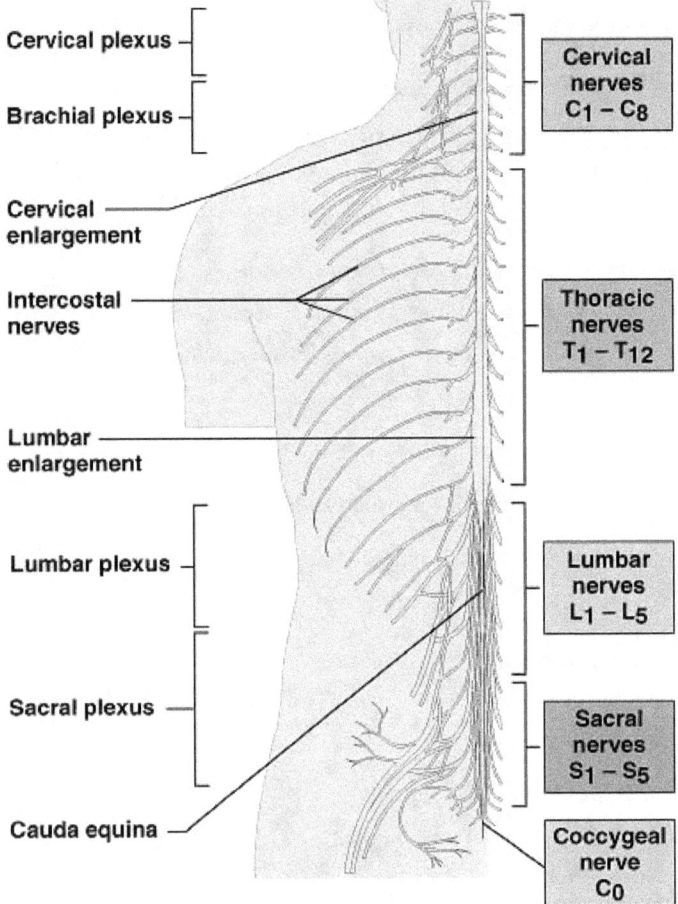

Thirty-one pairs of spinal nerves

Afferent fibers enter from the peripheral system on the *dorsal side* of the spinal cord *via* dorsal roots (containing the dorsal root ganglia).

Efferent fibers leave the spinal cord on the *ventral side* via the ventral roots.

The two roots combine to form a spinal nerve on each side of the spinal cord.

31 pairs of spinal nerves contain:

    cervical – 8 nerve pairs (C1-C8)

    thoracic – 12 nerve pairs (T1-T12)

    lumbar – 5 nerve pairs (L1-L5)

    sacral – 5 nerve pairs (S1-S5)

        coccygeal – a single coccygeal nerve pair

Endocrine System Integration

Integration with endocrine system

Nervous and endocrine systems interact to influence various aspects of human behavior.

Hypothalamus is the brain structure that regulates basic needs and emotional and stress responses. It links the nervous and endocrine systems because it controls the release of hormones by regulating the *pituitary gland*.

An example of an interaction between the nervous and endocrine systems is the release of the hormones *epinephrine* (adrenaline) and *norepinephrine* from the adrenal medulla, triggered by the sympathetic "fight or flight" system.

Epinephrine (adrenaline) and *norepinephrine* are also produced synaptic nerve fiber ends.

The two hormones are highly similar in structure and function and essential in stress response.

> *Epinephrine* is primarily released from the *adrenal medulla* and acts on receptors in the bloodstream.

> *Norepinephrine* is primarily released from synaptic nerve fibers and binds with receptors near the synaptic cleft.

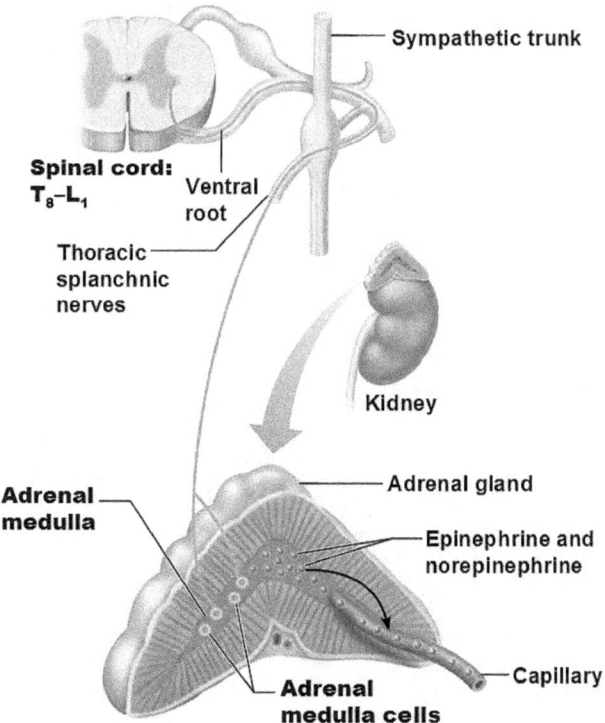

Adrenal medulla of the adrenal gland

Notes for active learning

Neurons

Neuron structure and function

Neurons (nerve cells) generate electric signals that pass from one end of the cell to another. Neurons release chemical messengers, *neurotransmitters*, to communicate with other cells. A neuron conducting signals toward a synapse (the junction where a neuron communicates with a target cell) is a *presynaptic neuron*.

Neurons conducting signals away from a synapse are *postsynaptic neurons*.

Neurotrophic factors are proteins that guide the development of neurons.

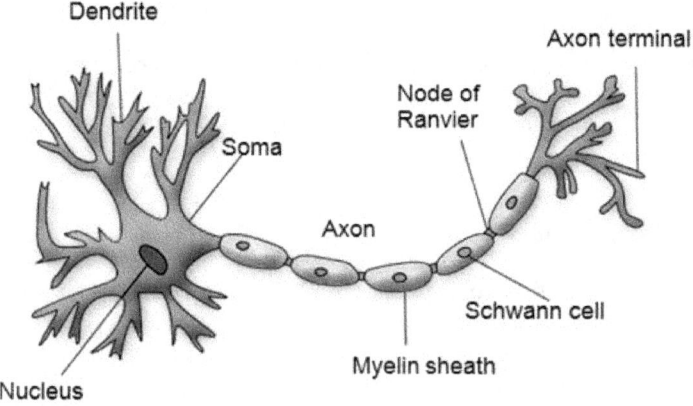

Neurons have dendrites to receive signals that propagate along the axon toward the axon terminal

Neurons outside the central nervous system (CNS) can repair themselves, but neurons within the CNS cannot. In the autonomic nervous system, the transmission of an impulse involves the interaction between at least two neurons.

The first neuron is the *preganglionic neuron*, and the second is the *postganglionic neuron*. Neurons vary in size and shape but have three parts: 1) cell body, 2) dendrites, and 3) axon.

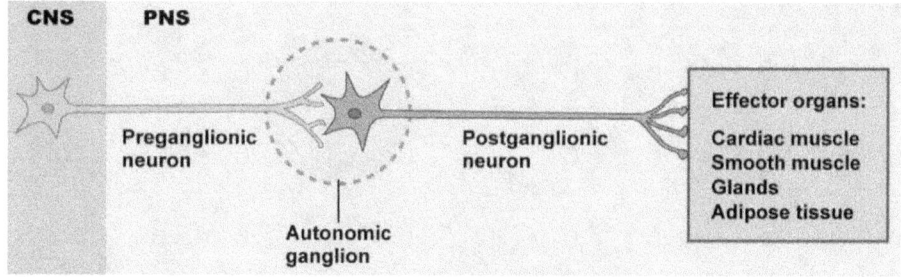

Motor neuron relays signals from the brain or spinal cord to a muscle or gland

Cell body as the site of nucleus and organelles

Because nerve cells are specialized for signal transmission and pathway formation, the form of neurons reflects their function.

Cell body contributes to a neuron's density by containing the neuron's organelles (e.g., nucleus and mitochondria). The cell body has a well-developed, rough endoplasmic reticulum and a Golgi apparatus to synthesize and modify essential proteins for neuronal function.

The cell body of a neuron is similar in form to most somatic cells, except for the *dendrites*.

Dendrite and axon structure and function

Dendrites are the branched receptive areas of a neuron that extend from the cell body.

Dendrites receive information and conduct impulses toward the cell body.

Branching of dendrites increases surface area for receiving signals (e.g., neurotransmitters).

The number of dendrites depends on the function of the neuron. For example, *unipolar neurons* have one dendrite.

Axon: structure and function

Axon differentiates neurons from other cells. The axon is crucial in the neuron's impulse generation and carries outgoing messages from the cell.

A long axon is a *nerve fiber*. A nerve fiber is a single axon, while a nerve is a bundle of axons bound by connective tissue. This axon can originate from CNS and extend to the body's extremities. This effectively provides a pathway for messages from the CNS to the periphery.

Axons send impulses away from cell bodies to stimulate (or inhibit neurons), muscles, or glands.

Axon terminals, secretory regions of the nerve, are at the end of the axon, away from the neuron's cell body. Other names for the axon terminal are the synaptic knob or synaptic bouton.

Neuron's axon terminal is the signal transmission site toward the receptor of another cell.

Nerve Structures

Neuroglia, glial cells and astrocytes

Nervous tissue is made of neurons and neuroglia.

Neuroglia supports and nourishes the neurons.

Glial cells are nervous tissue support cells capable of cellular division. *Oligodendroglia* and *Schwann cells* are glial cells supporting neurons physically and metabolically.

Astroglia regulates the composition of the extracellular fluid in the CNS.

Microglia performs immune functions.

Glial cells include ependymal cells (use cilia to circulate cerebrospinal fluid), satellite cells (support ganglia), and astrocytes (provide physical support to neurons of CNS; maintain the mineral and nutrients balance).

Myelin sheath, Schwann cells, oligodendrocytes

Myelin sheath is a phospholipid layer surrounding a neuron's axon. It insulates the axon, increasing the conductivity of the electrical messages sent through a nerve cell.

Myelin is an excellent insulator because it is fatty and does not contain channels.

By preventing charge leakage, myelin increases the *propagation speed*, making axons *thinner*. It is formed by the membranes of highly specialized, tightly spiraled *neuroglia cells*. These neuroglia cells are Schwann cells or oligodendrocytes.

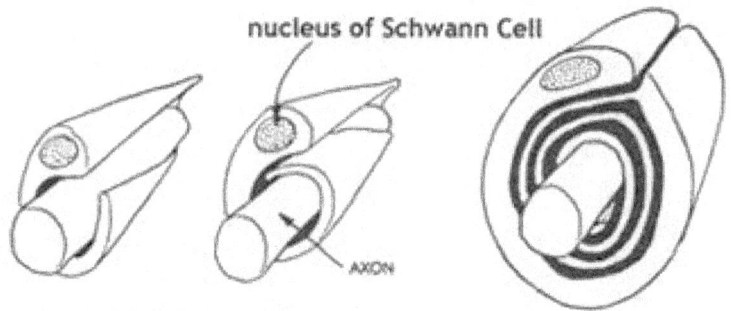

Schwann cell sheath is a phospholipid coat growing around a nerve axon

Schwann cells produce myelin for nerve cells in the *peripheral nervous system* (PNS). Many specialized cells wrap myelin around the neuron's axon, providing an insulating sheath that prevents signal transmission loss.

Oligodendrocytes are the central nervous system analog of Schwann cells. They make myelin sheaths (insulation) around CNS axons. Insulation occurs at intervals, punctuated by openings known as *nodes of Ranvier*, exposing the axon's plasma membrane, and causing an action potential to jump along the nodes of Ranvier.

Only vertebrates have myelinated axons.

Myelinated axons appear as *white matter*, while neuronal cell bodies are *gray matter*.

Many neurodegenerative autoimmune diseases result from a lack of myelin sheath. For instance, in multiple sclerosis, the lack of insulation from a myelin sheath slows or leaks the conductivity of signals across neural pathways, severely decreasing the efficiency of the patient's nervous system.

Nodes of Ranvier

The spaces between adjacent sections of myelin where the axon's plasma membrane is exposed to extracellular fluid are *nodes of Ranvier* (neurofibril nodes). Myelin sheath prevents the flow of ions between intracellular and extracellular compartments.

Therefore, action potentials occur at the non-insulated nodes of Ranvier; *saltatory conduction* is this jump of action potentials from one node to another.

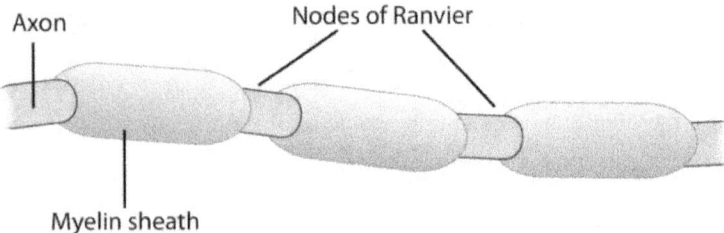

Nodes of Ranvier for saltatory conduction occurring at exposed sections of plasma membrane

Synapses and Neurotransmitters

Impulse propagation between cells

Synapse is the space between the axon bulb and the next neuron's dendritic receptor. A synapse is a junction between two neurons that permits a neuron to pass an electrical (or chemical) signal to another cell.

Synapse consists of a *presynaptic membrane*, a *synaptic cleft*, and a *postsynaptic membrane*.

In a synapse, the presynaptic neuron's electrical activity influences the electrical activity in the postsynaptic neuron. The influence may be excitatory (positive response) or inhibitory (negative response).

Synaptic cleft is a narrow fluid-filled space between presynaptic and postsynaptic membranes.

Neurotransmitters are released within synaptic vesicles from the presynaptic neuron's axon terminal and into the synaptic cleft. The vesicles migrate the synaptic cleft and travel toward the postsynaptic neuron, binding to postsynaptic receptors.

Convergence is when a presynaptic neuron affects a single postsynaptic neuron. This allows information from many sources to *influence the activity of one cell*.

Divergence is when a single presynaptic nerve cell affects several postsynaptic nerve cells, allowing one information source to *affect multiple pathways*.

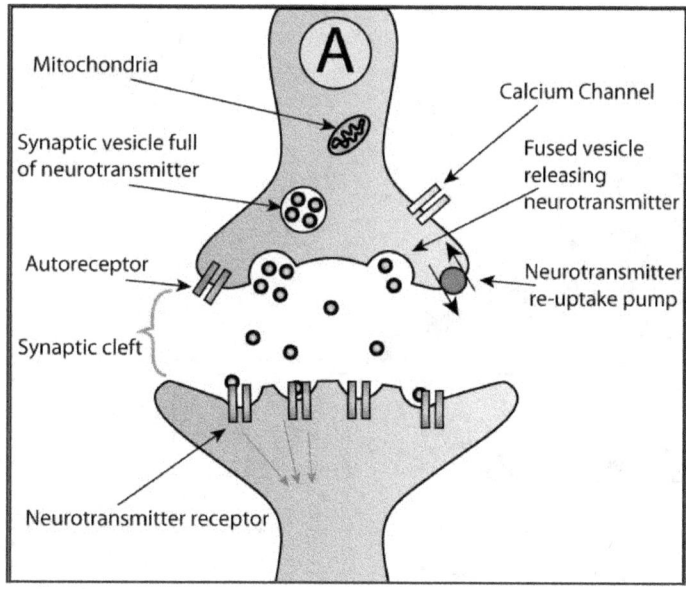

Synaptic cleft between two neurons

Nervous system uses several synapses to create complex pathways for relaying information.

Axodendritic synapses exist between the axon terminal of one presynaptic neuron and one dendrite of the postsynaptic neuron.

Axosomatic synapse resides between the axon terminal of the presynaptic neuron and the cell body of the postsynaptic neuron.

Axoaxonic synapses (rare) can exist between the presynaptic and postsynaptic axon terminal.

Classifying electrical and chemical synapses

Electric synapses have presynaptic and postsynaptic cells joined by *gap junctions*, which allow an action potential to flow directly across the junction.

Due to the short distance and the direct physical link between two neurons, these junctions provide high-speed transmission signals.

Since chemical synapses are usually fast enough for signal transmission, electrical synapses are relatively rare.

Chemical synapse is when the presynaptic neuron axon ends swell as the axon terminal. Extracellular space of the synaptic cleft separates the presynaptic and postsynaptic neurons, preventing a direct propagation of current.

Chemical synapses are unidirectional; a signal can only be transmitted from the presynaptic to the postsynaptic neuron.

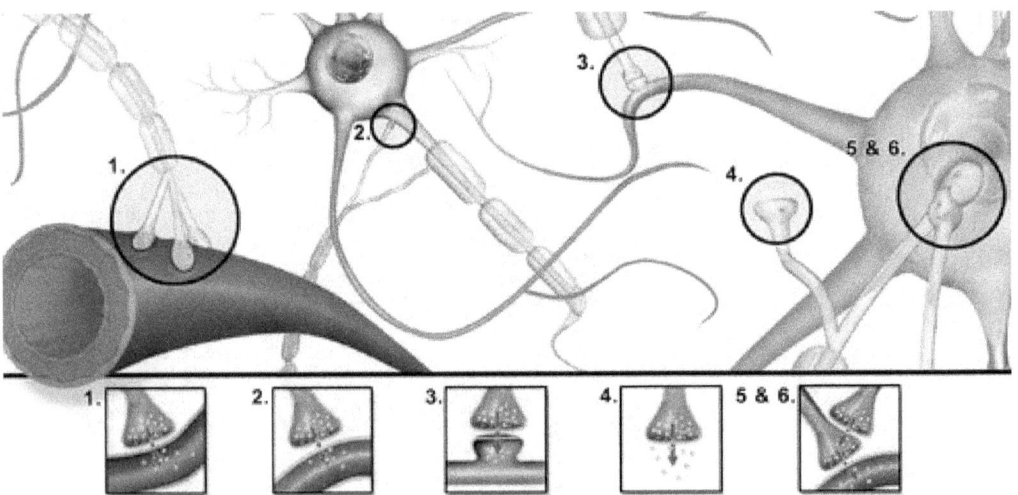

Synapse types: 1) axosecretory – axon terminal secretes directly in the bloodstream, 2) axoaxonic – axon terminal secretes into another axon, 3) axodendritic – axon terminal ends in a dendritic spine, 4) axoextracellular – axon with no connection secretes into the extracellular fluid, 5) axosomatic – axon terminal ends on soma and 6) axosynaptic – axon terminal ends on another axon terminal

Synaptic propagation between cells without signal loss

An action potential travels along the axon and reaches the end of the presynaptic neuron.

Depolarization of the presynaptic membrane opens the voltage-gated calcium channels.

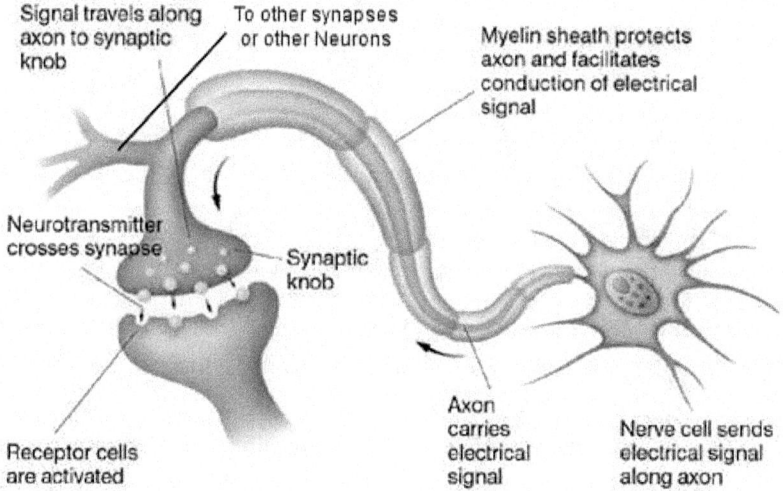

Dendrites receive stimuli, propagate impulses without diminution along the axon, and release neurotransmitters into the synaptic cleft toward the postsynaptic neuron

Calcium ions flow *into* the presynaptic neuron, causing vesicles with neurotransmitters inside the neuron to fuse with the plasma membrane.

Ca^{2+} ions induce reactions, neurotransmitter vesicles fuse with plasma membranes.

Membrane fusion releases the neurotransmitter into the synaptic cleft by *exocytosis*. Synaptic vesicles store neurotransmitters that diffuse across synapse towards postsynaptic membrane.

When an action potential arrives at the presynaptic axon bulb, synaptic vesicles merge with the presynaptic membrane. When vesicles merge with the neuron's plasma membrane, neurotransmitters are discharged into the synaptic cleft.

Neurotransmitter molecules diffuse across the synaptic cleft to the postsynaptic membrane, binding with specific receptors.

Neurotransmitters, presynaptic and postsynaptic membranes

Neurotransmitters are released into the synaptic cleft via *exocytosis*.

Neurotransmitters diffuse via *Brownian* motion (i.e., random, and irregular motion) and bind within the synaptic cleft to specific receptors on the postsynaptic plasma membrane.

Receptors are ligand-gated ion channels that open and let sodium and other positively charged ions into the postsynaptic neuron.

As these positively charged ions enter the postsynaptic neuron, they cause the neuron's membrane to depolarize, resulting in an action potential moving along the postsynaptic neuron.

Calcium ions are pumped into the synaptic cleft from inside the presynaptic neuron. The neurotransmitters are degraded and recycled by enzymes in the synaptic cleft.

Neurotransmitters are chemicals that cross the synapse between neurons or neurons and a muscle or gland. After an action potential has traveled down the axon, it releases neurotransmitters from the presynaptic neuron's axon terminal into the synapse. The axon terminal, or synaptic knob, contains vesicles of neurotransmitters waiting to be exocytosed.

An action potential reaching the synaptic knob causes an influx of calcium, which signals the vesicles to fuse with cell membranes (exocytosis) to release the neurotransmitters into the synaptic cleft.

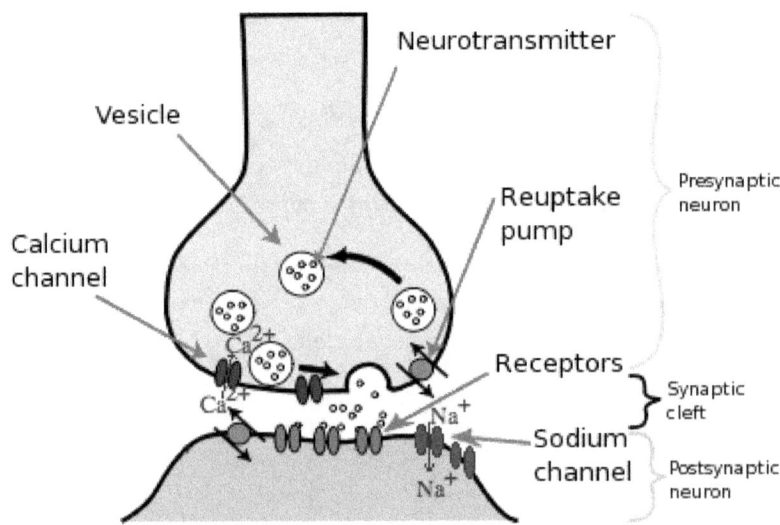

Synaptic transmission with Ca^+ causes the release of neurotransmitters from the presynaptic membrane into the cleft

Postsynaptic neurons and graded potentials

Once the postsynaptic membrane receives the neurotransmitter, the chemicals bind to a receptor (usually on the dendrite) and open ion channels, changing the *membrane potential* of the postsynaptic neuron.

If this *graded potential* stimulus is large enough, it triggers an *all-or-none response*, inducing the propagation of the signal down the axon of the postsynaptic neuron. Enzymes quickly degrade these neurotransmitters, or they are taken up by the presynaptic terminal so that they do not persistently stimulate the postsynaptic neuron.

Classifying neurotransmitters

More than 200 neurotransmitters have been identified.

Acetylcholine (ACh) and *norepinephrine* (NE) are two common neurotransmitters.

Cholinergic fibers release ACh. In some synapses, the postsynaptic membrane contains enzymes that rapidly inactivate neurotransmitters. For example, acetylcholinesterase degrades acetylcholine. Once a neurotransmitter is released into a synaptic cleft, it initiates a response and is removed.

Biogenic amines are neurotransmitters containing an amino group such as *catecholamines* (e.g., dopamine, norepinephrine, epinephrine, serotonin). Nerve fibers that release epinephrine and norepinephrine are *adrenergic* and *noradrenergic*.

Amino acid neurotransmitters are prevalent neurotransmitters in CNS. These include glutamate, aspartate, GABA (gamma-aminobutyric acid), and glycine.

Neuropeptides are composed of amino acids. Neurons that release neuropeptides are *peptidergic* (e.g., beta-endorphin, dynorphin, and enkephalin groups). Nitric oxide, ATP, and adenine function as neurotransmitters.

Many PNS neurons end at neuroeffector junctions on muscle and gland cells. Neurotransmitters released by these efferent neurons activate the target cell.

In other synapses, the presynaptic membrane reabsorbs neurotransmitters for repackaging in synaptic vesicles or molecular breakdown. The brief existence of neurotransmitters in a synapse prevents continuous stimulation (or inhibition) of postsynaptic membranes.

Several drugs affect the nervous system by interfering with (or potentiating) the action potentials by neurotransmitters.

Notes for active learning

Impulse Propagation

Electrochemical gradients

Luigi Galvani discovered in 1786 that an electric current stimulates a nerve. An impulse is too slow to be caused merely by an electric current in an axon.

Julius Bernstein proposed that the impulse is the movement of unequally distributed ions on either side of an axon membrane, the axon's plasma membrane. The 1963 Nobel Prize went to British researchers A. L. Hodgkin and A. F. Huxley, who confirmed this theory.

Hodgkin, Huxley, and other researchers inserted a tiny electrode into the giant axon of a squid. The electrode was attached to a voltmeter and an oscilloscope to trace the change in voltage. The voltmeter measured the difference in the electrical potential between the inside and the outside of the membrane. The oscilloscope indicated any changes in polarity.

Since the plasma membrane is more permeable to potassium ions than sodium ions, there are more positive ions outside the cell; this accounts for some polarity. The large, negatively charged proteins in the cytoplasm (e.g., Cl^-) contribute to the resting potential of -70 mV.

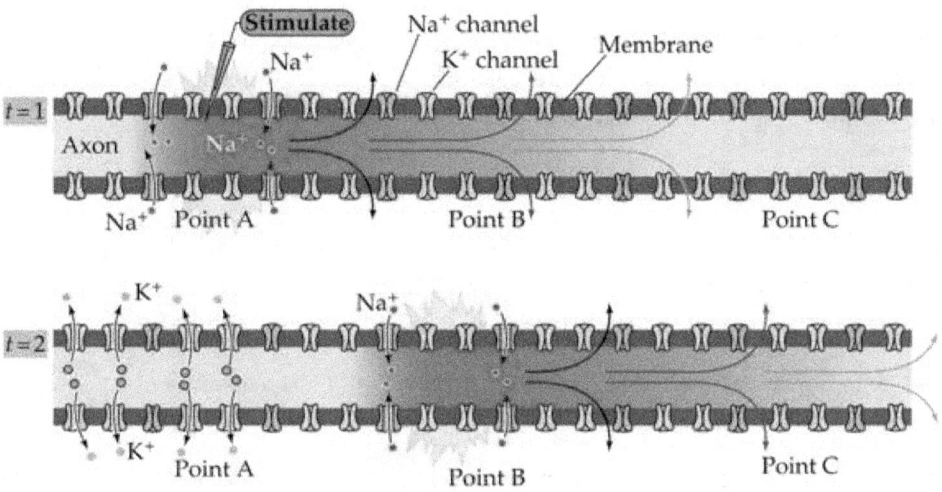

Movement of ions along a synapse changes the voltage across the membrane

When an axon is not conducting an impulse, an oscilloscope records a membrane potential of -70 mV; the inside of the neuron is negative compared to the outside.

Resting potential

Resting potential is the electrical potential across the plasma membrane of a cell's axon that is not conducting an impulse. This polarization is due to the difference in electrical charge on either side of the axon membrane.

Voltage potential magnitude is determined by differences in specific ion concentrations between the intracellular and extracellular fluids and the differences in membrane permeability of different ions as a function of the number of open ion channels for these ions.

Na^+ and K^+ are the most important ions in generating the resting membrane potential. At rest in a living cell, Na^+ is greater outside the cell, while K^+ is greater inside the cell. The ions flow with regard to the *electrochemical gradient*, the combined electrical and chemical concentration differences on each side of a membrane. This difference is attributed to the net flow of charge across the nerve cell's membrane.

Sodium-potassium pump moves three Na^+ ions to the outside of the membrane for every 2 K^+ ions. It moves into the cell along with Cl^- ions inside it, creating a net negative charge inside the cell. Additionally, the plasma membrane is more permeable to K^+ ions as K^+ moves out of the cell more easily than Na^+ moves into the cell, accentuating the relatively negative resting potential inside the neuron.

In general, K^+ moves out of the cell, and Na^+ moves into the cell down their concentration gradients. However, the intracellular concentration of these two ions is kept constant by an active transport system that pumps Na^+ out of the cell and K^+ into it.

All-or-none action potentials, depolarization and repolarization

Action potentials are large, rapid alterations in the neuron's plasma membrane potential. It is the reversal and restoration of the electrical potential across the plasma membrane as electrical impulses pass (i.e., depolarization and repolarization) that use the Na^+/K^+ pump.

Membranes capable of producing action potentials are *excitable membranes* (e.g., membranes of nerve and muscle cells).

When membranes depolarize, sodium channels open, and positive sodium ions rush inside.

During *depolarization*, the ion concentration is opposite from the resting potential. Sodium ions dominate the inside, while potassium ions dominate the outside. In response, the membrane potential moves in a positive direction. The membrane potential goes from about −70 mV at resting potential to +30 mV in the depolarization phase.

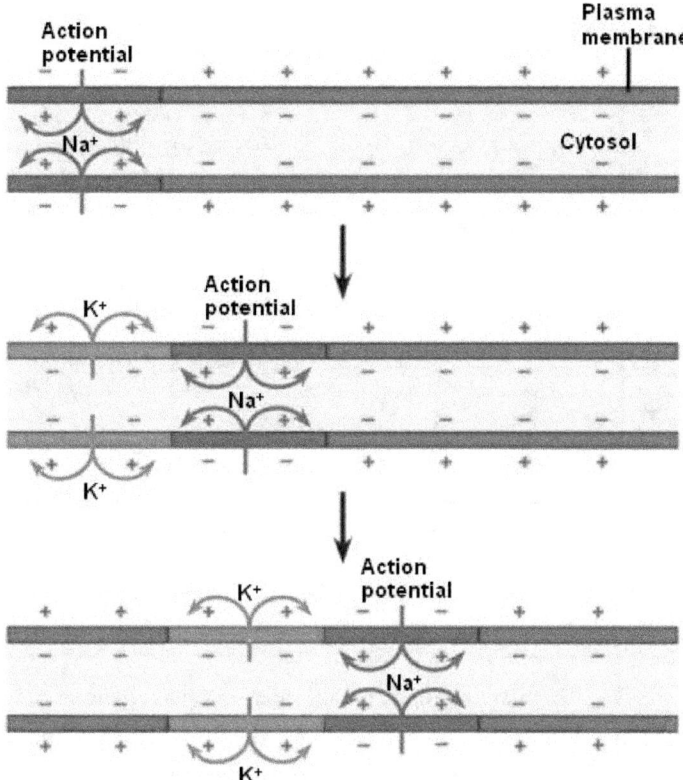

During *repolarization*, potassium channels open, and sodium channels close. The positive potassium ions rush outside, and the membrane potential drops down. Now, sodium ion concentration is higher inside, while potassium ion concentration is higher outside. This is the opposite of the resting state. Thus, the membrane potential returns to its resting value, and the potential returns to –70 mV in the repolarization phase.

Hyperpolarization is an event in the all-or-none axon propagation where potassium channels do not close fast enough. The membrane potential briefly drops below the standard resting potential of around –80 mV.

After an action potential is propagated along the axon of a neuron, there is a period when a second stimulus does not produce a second action potential. This is the *absolute refractory period*, and it occurs because, once the voltage-gated Na^+ channels close, the membrane needs to repolarize before the channels can open again.

Sodium-potassium pump works to re-establish the original resting state (i.e., potassium inside and sodium outside) and maintains unequal distribution of Na^+ and K^+ ions.

Sodium-potassium (Na^+ / K^+) pump is an *active transport* system that moves *Na^+ ions out* and *K^+ ions into* the axon.

Pump continually works because the membrane is permeable to ions, and they spontaneously diffuse toward a lesser concentration.

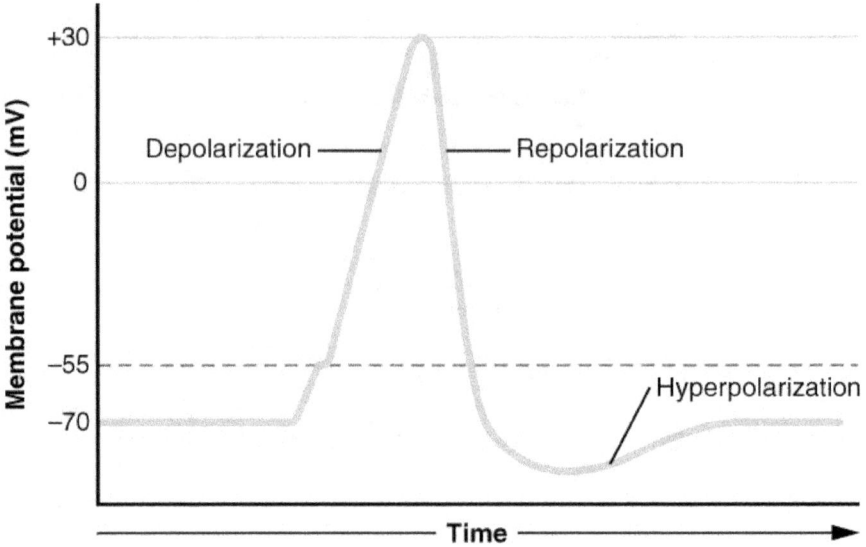

Action potential and voltage changes; depolarization occurs when Na^+ rushes in and K^+ exits the cell; hyperpolarization restores the resting potential with the Na^+/K^+ pump

Resting potential of –70 mV is restored, and the neuron cannot generate another action potential. Following absolute refractory, a second action potential can be produced only if the stimulus strength is greater than usual. This is *relative refractory* and results from hyperpolarization.

Relative refractory period begins after hyperpolarization and lasts until the resting potential is re-established. The refractory period prevents an action potential from reversing direction, even though theoretically, ions are rushing in and diffusing in both directions.

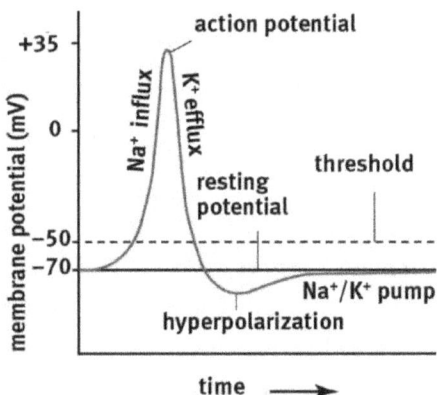

Sufficient depolarization greater than the threshold leads to an action potential

Na^+ ion channels are blocked in local anesthetics, and pain signaling is absent.

Since a neuron is a long cell, it gets depolarized part by part and not all at once. The area of the membrane that gets depolarized has a difference in potential with the adjacent area of the membrane that is still at resting potential, thereby causing a local current. This current then depolarizes the adjacent resting membrane, and an action potential continues. Since the depolarization of an area is followed by a refractory period, the action potential moves unidirectionally.

As water flows through a pipe, the velocity of an action potential across an axon is positively correlated with fiber diameter; a larger fiber offers less resistance, and thus, a greater diameter allows for less resistance to the flow of ions. In addition, myelination of the neuron's axon increases efficiency by preventing ions from escaping, referred to as "charge leakage."

An action potential is all-or-none. If neurotransmitters cause the postsynaptic cell to reach the threshold, action potential is induced in postsynaptic cell by the presynaptic action potential.

Propagation between neurons involves no transmission loss. The postsynaptic action potential is as large as the presynaptic.

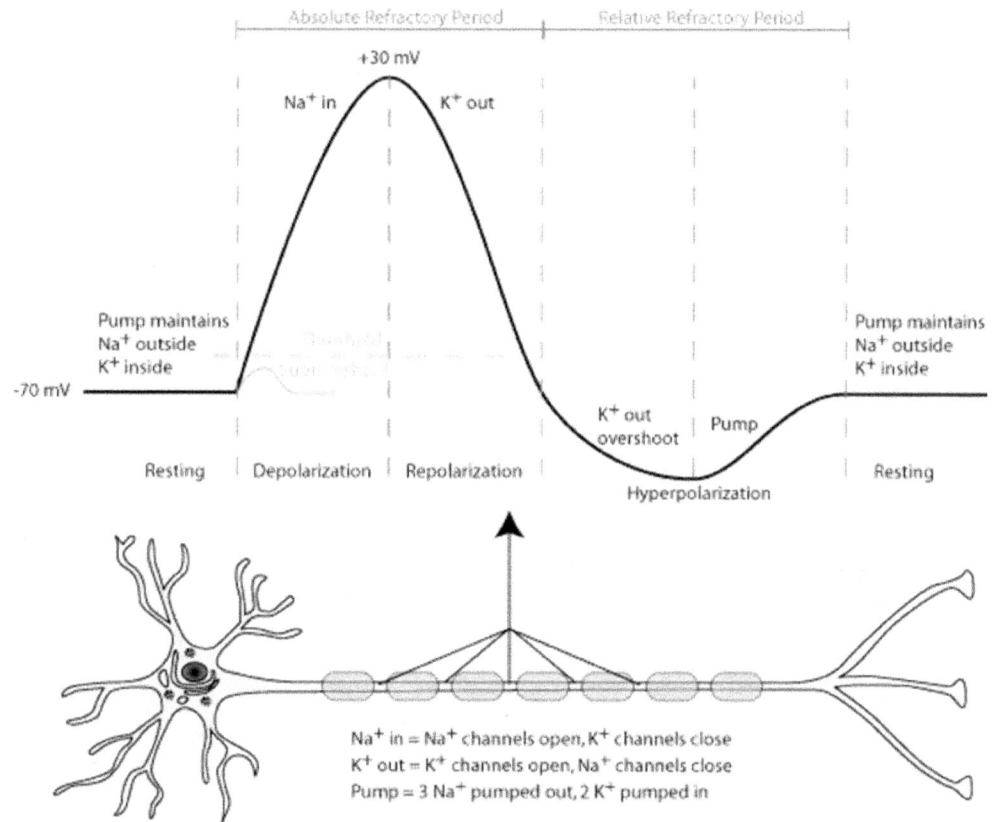

Impulse direction through a neuron is: dendrite → cell body → axon.

Notes for active learning

Excitatory and Inhibitory Nerve Fibers

Membrane potentials

Graded potentials are changes in membrane potential confined to a small plasma membrane region. The magnitude of these potentials is related to the magnitude of the initiating stimulus. When a stimulus (graded potential) depolarizes above a threshold value, an action potential (AP) initiates a signal. If one graded potential just barely makes the threshold value and other overshoots it a lot, both cause the same action potential.

A graded potential is an all-or-none response. From -70 mV up to the threshold of ~ -55 mV (or -70 downward), the graded potential cannot travel, but it can potentially (if it surpasses the threshold) open the voltage-gated channels. If the threshold is exceeded, the action potential travels down the axon by opening other voltage-gated channels. The other gated types cannot spread unless they trigger this AP. Since the AP is an all-or-none response, the strength of a neural signal is based on other factors (frequency of AP firing or how many nerve cells contribute to APs, etc.).

Most synapse interactions are either excitatory or inhibitory. Whether the response is excitatory or inhibitory depends on the type of neurotransmitter or receptor. *Excitatory neurotransmitters* use gated ion channels and are fast-acting.

Inhibitory neurotransmitters affect the metabolism of the postsynaptic cells and are slower.

Neuromodulators modify the postsynaptic cell's response to neurotransmitters by changing the presynaptic cell's synthesis or releasing or metabolizing the neurotransmitter. Neurotransmitters may be taken back into the nerve terminal (active transport), degraded by synaptic cleft enzymes (recycled to presynaptic neuron), or diffuse out of the synapse.

Excitatory and inhibitory chemical synapses

Excitatory chemical synapses occur when activated receptors on the postsynaptic membrane open Na^+ channels. Na^+ ions move into the cell, resulting in depolarization. This potential change in the postsynaptic neuron is an *excitatory postsynaptic potential* (EPSP).

EPSPs are graded potentials.

Inhibitory chemical synapses occur when the activated receptor on the postsynaptic membrane opens Cl^- channels. Cl^- ions move into the cell, resulting in hyperpolarization. The potential change in the postsynaptic neuron is an *inhibitory postsynaptic potential* (IPSP).

Like EPSP, IPSP is a graded potential.

Integration

Integration is the summing up of excitatory and inhibitory signals. If a neuron receives many excitatory signals from one synapse (consecutive neuron firing), the axon probably transmits a nerve impulse. The summing may prohibit the axon from firing if excitatory and inhibitory signals are received.

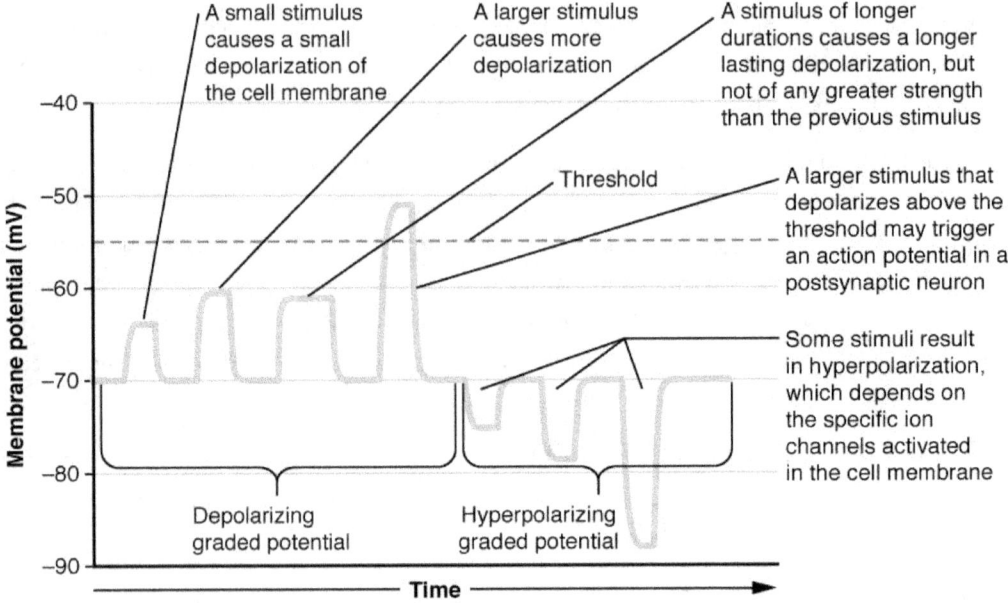

Graded potential includes temporal and spatial summation. Stimuli can be excitatory or inhibitory

One EPSP cannot exceed the postsynaptic neuron's threshold in most neurons. Only the combined effects of many excitatory synapses exceed the threshold and initiate an action potential.

Temporal summation is when several EPSP arrive at separate times creates a depolarization.

Spatial summation is when the number of EPSPs arriving at distinct locations creates depolarization. IPSP shows similar summations, but the effect is hyperpolarization and inhibiting an action potential.

Interneurons, Sensory and Efferent Neurons

Interneurons integrate and transmit signals

Interneurons are typically within the central nervous system structures (i.e., the spinal cord and brain) and account for about 99% of neurons in the body.

Interneurons are multipolar, with many dendrites for receiving information, and a single axon sends the collected information to the synapse.

Interneurons form complex brain pathways throughout the central nervous system, transmit signals to the periphery via *motor neurons*, and function as *integrators* to evaluate impulses for the appropriate response.

The term interneuron refers to small neurons that connect to other nearby neurons (as opposed to *projection neurons* that can connect over long distances).

Interneuron pathways play essential roles in human survival and advancement, accounting for memory and language. They are usually inhibitory, although excitatory interneurons do exist.

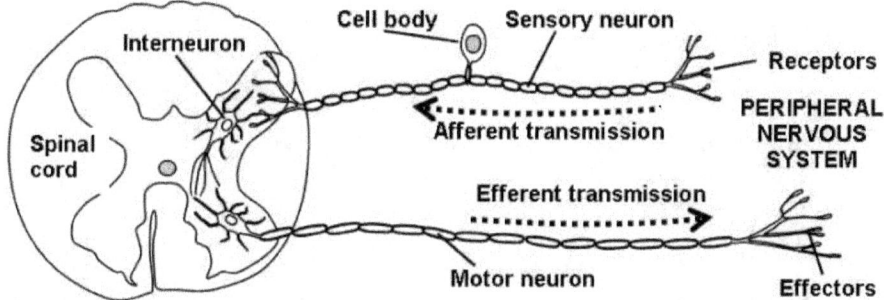

CNS and PNS structures with the direction of propagation shown for afferent sensory neurons (receptors → CNS) and efferent motor neurons (CNS → effectors)

Sensory and effector neurons

Afferent neurons (i.e., sensory neurons) send impulses from the PNS toward CNS. Afferent neurons are unipolar, as a single dendrite collects and transmits information through one axon.

Sensory receptor at a dendrite of an afferent neuron conveys signals from tissues and organs to the brain and spine.

Receptors are specialized endings of afferent neurons or separate cells that affect the ends of afferent neurons and collect information about external and internal environments in various energy forms. Stimulus energy is first transformed into a graded potential (receptor potential).

Stimulus transduction is the process by which a stimulus is transformed into an electrical response. The initial depolarization in afferent neurons is achieved by a *receptor potential* (in receptors) or by a spontaneous change in neuron membrane potential, a *pacemaker potential*.

Efferent neurons (i.e., motor neurons) carry signals away from the CNS to cells of muscles or glands in the peripheral system.

In total, 43 main nerves branch off the CNS to the peripheral nervous system.

Efferent neurons are structurally multipolar and stimulate *effectors*, target cells that elicit a response. For example, neurons may stimulate effector cells in the stomach to secrete gastrin.

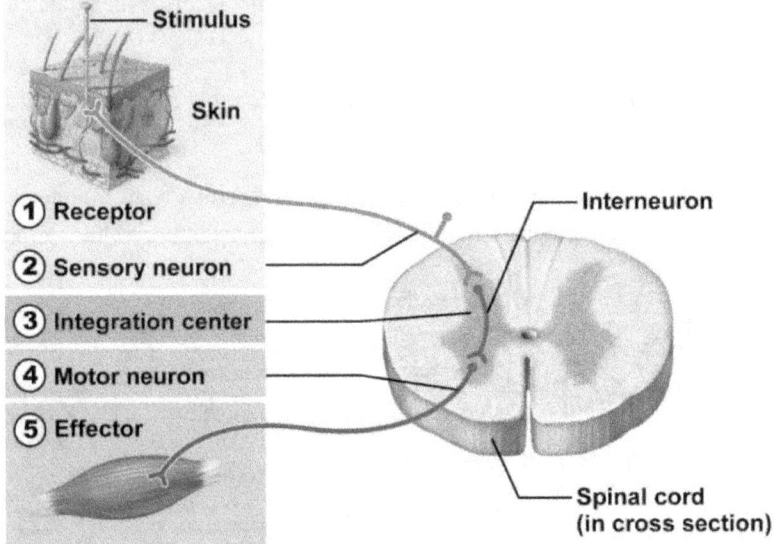

Stimulus is processed through a sensory neuron to the spinal column. An interneuron communicates the information to a motor neuron for a response at the effector.

CHAPTER 5

Sensory Perception and Processing

Perception of Sensations

Sensory Receptors of the Nervous System

Sound Perception and Processing

Vision Perception and Processing

Senses of Touch, Taste, Smell and Balance

Perception Processing

Page intentionally left blank

Perception of Sensations

Psychophysics and experimental psychology

Psychophysics was founded in the mid-1800s by Gustav Theodor Fechner, a German physicist, psychologist, and philosopher. His experiments started the field of psychophysics and the broader field of *experimental psychology*.

Psychophysics is the quantitative study of the relationship between physical and psychological events. Specifically, it refers to studying stimuli and an organism's resulting sensations and perceptions.

The primary areas of study within psychophysics are threshold, Weber's law, signal detection theory, and sensory adaptation.

Threshold and detecting stimuli

The threshold is the intensity that must be exceeded for a reaction or phenomenon.

Sensory threshold refers to the weakest stimulus that can be detected by an organism 50% of the time.

Absolute threshold is the weakest stimulus detected at a certain percentage (often 50%) when there is initially no stimulus.

A typical hearing test, for example, plays beeps at increasing volume levels.

The test-taker is instructed to indicate when first hearing a beep. A hearing test of this variety seeks to measure the absolute threshold for hearing, which is why there is initially no sound.

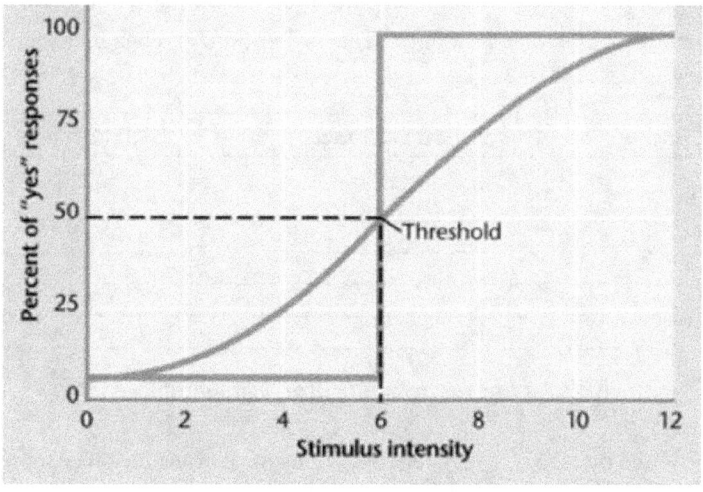

Sensory threshold plotting perception vs. stimulus intensity

Differential threshold is the level at which an organism can perceive a change in an already-detected stimulus and detect it half of the time.

An example is when one notices an increase in a room's temperature.

Differential threshold is the point at which temperature difference is detected and subtracted by the original temperature. It is the intensity magnitude between the original and final stimuli.

Terminal threshold refers to the upper limit at which a stimulus can no longer be detected.

For example, if a person touches a hot stove, the pain would be felt instead of heat because the terminal threshold for temperature has been exceeded.

The highest pitch that a person can hear is the terminal threshold for pitch.

Weber's law of just noticeable differences

Initially proposed for weightlifting, *Weber's law* (named after German physician Ernst Heinrich Weber, founder of experimental psychology) posits that the differential threshold for an individual is dependent on proportion, not the amount.

For example, if a weightlifter notices when one pound is added to the ten-pound weight that he was lifting, then according to Weber's law, he notices that when two pounds are added to a twenty-pound weight. For this reason, Weber's law is the *law of just noticeable differences*.

Weber's law was later applied to sensations. Although it does not hold for sound or high or low-intensity stimuli, Weber's law is generally accurate for sight, touch, taste, and smell.

One experiment in which Weber's law is supported involves having a test subject judge two lines, with one line longer than the other. This is repeated with a *longer set of lines*.

Findings show that the difference in larger lines must be proportional to the smaller lines for participants to notice that one is longer. The proportion of change necessary to notice a difference varies.

	Left is shorter	Right is longer
Obvious	——	——
Less obvious	————	————
Hard to distinguish	——————	——————

Weber's law for detecting proportional differences

The same differential threshold, dependent on proportions, holds for other senses. For example, a dog detects more subtle changes in smell than humans.

Signal detection theory

Signal detection theory aims to uncover the internal and external mechanisms contributing to sensation and perception.

It posits that detecting a given stimulus is partly dependent on the intensity of the stimulus.

For example, a loud noise is more likely to be detected than a soft noise, and a temperature change of 10 °F is more likely to be detected than a change of 2 °F.

Signal detection theory proposes that the psychological state of experiencing the stimuli affects how it is perceived. For example, someone walking alone at night in an unsafe neighborhood likely experiences a soft noise that is subjectively louder than the same noise during the day.

This significant theory notes that past experiences and expectations influence perceptions.

Signal detection theory has applications for researchers seeking to understand sensation by lab experiments. These researchers often begin perception experiments with a *signal detection test*.

In each test trial, a stimulus is presented to or withheld from a participant. The participant is instructed to indicate whether he perceived a stimulus at each trial.

A receiver operating characteristic curve is plotted through repeated trials, providing information to the researchers on detecting various stimuli. This curve provides a unique baseline for each participant and allows researchers to study perception accurately.

Sensory systems are constantly recalibrating based on the environment.

Sensory adaptation

Sensory adaptation is the ability to recalibrate when a constant stimulus persists over time as receptors respond by decreasing their sensitivity to the stimulus. This ability of receptors to adapt is found in all sensory receptors, apart from pain receptors.

For example, a person does not generally notice the sensation of clothes on the skin because skin receptors have adapted to this constant stimulus by reducing their sensitivity.

Similarly, a friend's house may have a specific smell associated with it. However, the people living in the house often cannot detect it because their olfactory receptors have adapted.

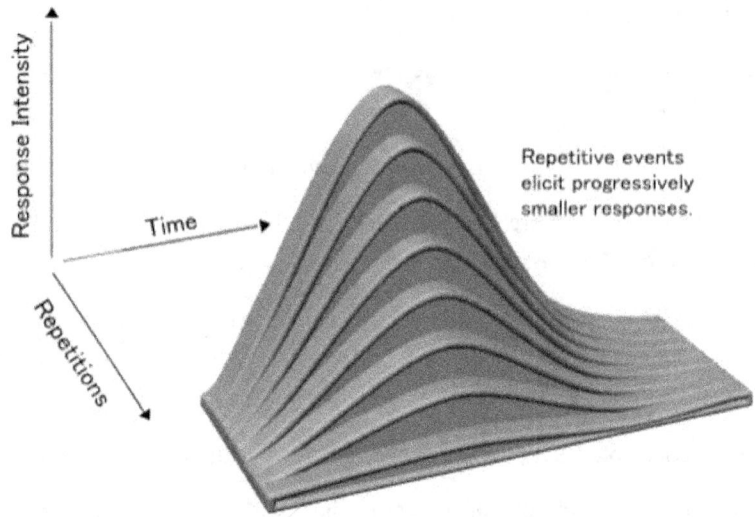

Sensory adaptations illustrate receptors responding by decreasing their sensitivity

Sensory adaptation is observed in the visual system. When in the dark, the concentration of the light-sensing chemical in the rods and cones in the eye increases. This leads to increased sensitivity and the ability to see with acuity.

Dark adaptation occurs in cones within about ten minutes, while rods can take up to thirty minutes to fully adapt.

Sensory Receptors of the Nervous System

Four aspects of stimulus

Sensory systems encode four aspects of a stimulus.

1. *Type* (or modality) is the first aspect of a stimulus. The stimulus is primarily encoded by the receptor type it activates. For example, taste is encoded by taste receptors, while odor receptors encode smell.

2. *Intensity* is the second aspect of stimulus. An increased stimulus produces a larger receptor potential, leading to a higher action potential frequency.

   Stronger stimuli affect a larger area and recruits more receptors.

3. *Location* is the third aspect of a stimulus encoded by the stimulated receptor site.

Acuity is the precision of location, negatively correlated with convergence in ascending neural pathways and the receptive field's size and overlaps with adjacent receptive fields.

The response is highest at the center of the receptive field since receptor density is highest.

Lateral inhibition increases acuity when excited neurons reduce the activity of nearby neurons.

4. *Duration* is the fourth aspect of a stimulus encoded by two types of receptors: rapid adapting receptors and slow adapting receptors.

Rapid adapting receptors respond quickly at the onset of a stimulus but slow down gradually during the remainder of the stimulus.

Slow-adapting receptors maintain responses at or near the initial firing level for the stimulus's duration.

Rapid adapting receptors are critical for signaling rapid change, while slow adapting receptors are essential for signaling slow changes.

Sensory receptors classification

Sensory receptors are nerve endings that respond to an internal or external stimulus.

Three methods classify sensory receptors:

   1) receptor complexity,

   2) location, and

   3) stimulus detected. An example of complex receptors is the encapsulated nerve endings with physical specialization.

Simple receptors are free nerve endings of dendrites as terminal ends without specialization.

Exteroceptors are at or near the skin's surface and respond to stimuli occurring on the body's surface. Exteroceptors encode for tactile sensations and vision, hearing, smell, and taste.

Interoceptors respond to stimuli occurring inside visceral organs and blood vessels. For example, receptors within the GI tract carry signals to the brain relating to feelings of hunger. Interoceptors are associated with the autonomic nervous system.

Proprioceptors respond to internal stimuli occurring in skeletal muscles, tendons, ligaments, and joints and can detect the position of a body part in space.

When classifying receptors by the stimuli they detect, receptors are grouped into five categories.

Mechanoreceptors respond to touch and pressure and rapidly adapt or slow-adapt receptors.

Photoreceptors respond to light.

Thermoreceptors respond to temperature and temperature changes. One thermoreceptor responds to increases in temperature, while another responds to decreases.

Chemoreceptors respond to taste, smell, and changes in blood chemistry. Chemoreceptors are in animals, and chemoreception is the most primitive sense.

Nociceptors respond to pain and tissue damage.

Mechanoreceptors	• Respond to touch and pressure
Photoreceptors	• Respond to light
Thermoreceptors	• Respond to temperature
Chemoreceptors	• Respond to taste, smell, and changes in blood chemistry
Nociceptors	• Respond to pain and tissue damage

Skin contains receptors close to the boundary between the dermis and epidermis. However, mechanoreceptors that respond to pressure are deeper in the dermis.

Proprioceptors, mechanoreceptors, photoreceptors, thermoreceptors, chemoreceptors, and nociceptors are *somatic sensors* in the *somatosensory system*.

Sensory pathways in the brain and spinal column

Sensory units are made of a single neuron and its receptor endings. When stimulated, a sensory unit activates its neuron's receptive field within the brain.

For example, when the retina cells' receptive field is stimulated, associated neurons in the visual cortex of the occipital lobe are activated so that the sensory input is interpreted.

Specific pathways are needed for each of the senses and types of stimuli.

Sensory information passes through the spinal cord to higher brain levels by *ascending pathways*. These pathways transmit information from taste cells to the parietal lobe.

Information from the eyes is transmitted to the occipital lobe.

Information from the ears is transmitted to the temporal lobe.

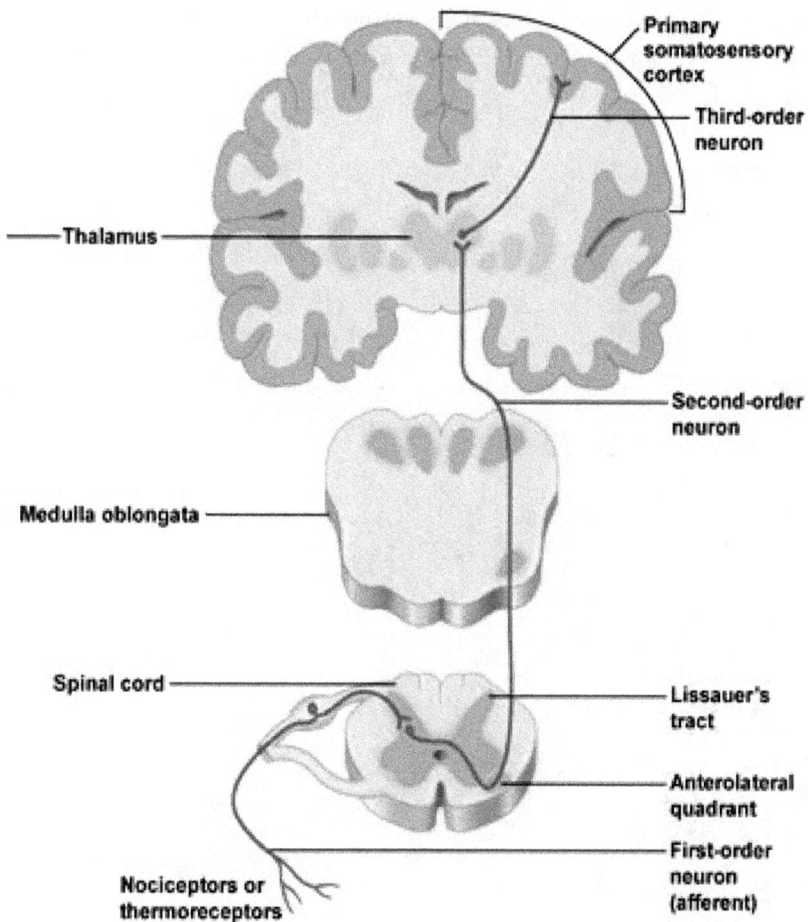

Sensory pathways in the brain and spinal column

Ascending pathways for touch are the posterior column, anterolateral, and spinocerebellar pathways.

- *Posterior column pathway* carries fine touch, vibration, pressure, and proprioceptive (position of body parts) sensations from the skin and joints.

  Information is transmitted to the cerebral cortex's postcentral gyrus via first-, second-, and third-order neurons.

- *Anterolateral pathway* (*spinothalamic tract*) carries pain, temperature, and poorly localized touch sensations.

  Information travels from the skin through the ventral posterolateral nucleus in the thalamus to the somatosensory cortex of the postcentral gyrus.

  The spinothalamic tract consists of two adjacent pathways: an anterior and a lateral pathway. The anterior pathway carries poorly localized touch sensations, while the lateral pathway carries information about pain and temperature.

- *Spinocerebellar pathway* carries sensations of limb and joint position.

  Information from the Golgi tendon organ and muscle spindles is conveyed to the cerebellum.

Posterior column pathway	• Carries fine touch, vibration, pressure, and proprioceptive sensations • Information is sent to the postcentral gyrus of the cerebral cortex
Anterolateral pathway	• Carries sensations of pain, temperature, and poorly localized touch • Information is sent to the somatosensory cortex of the postcentral gyrus
Spinocerebellar pathway	• Carries sensations concerning limb and joint position • Information is sent to the cerebellum

Sound Perception and Processing

Ear structure and function

Human ears have three main parts: *outer ear*, the *middle ear,* and the *inner ear*.

The outer ear is what most people think of when they think of an ear. The outer ear consists of the *pinna* and the *auditory canal*.

Pinna (or *auricle*) is the visible region outside the head that directs and amplifies sound waves.

Auditory canal is the ear opening, lined with fine hairs that filter the air. It contains modified sweat glands that secrete earwax (cerumen) to guard against foreign matter.

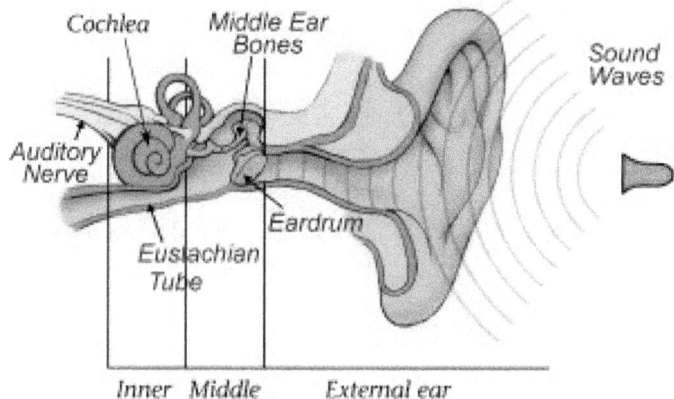

Human ear has external (outer), middle, and inner ear and associated structures

Middle ear cavity is filled with air and contains three tiny bones known collectively as *ossicles*. Bones of the middle ear cavity are the:

    malleus (or hammer), *incus* (or anvil), and *stapes* (or stirrup).

Ossicles convert eardrum vibrations (or *tympanic membrane*) into fluid waves in the inner ear.

Auditory tube (or *eustachian*) extends from the middle ear to pharynx, equalizing the outer ear.

Oval window (or *vestibular window*) is a membrane-covered opening separating the middle and inner ear.

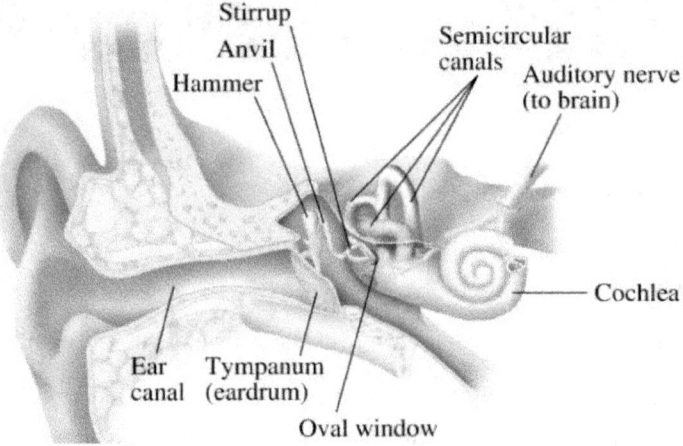

Human ear with ossicles, semicircular canals, cochlea

Inner ear

Inner ear contains the *bony labyrinth*, a hollow cavity in the skull's temporal bone.

Bony labyrinth has two main functional parts: *cochlea* and the *vestibular system*.

Cochlea is spiral-shaped and houses the cochlear duct containing the *organ of Corti*. It has *stereocilia* hair cells.

Afferent neurons from these hair cells form the *cochlear nerve*.

Cochlea's upper compartment is the *scala vestibuli*, a fluid-filled cavity that conducts sound vibrations to the *cochlear duct*.

Cochlear duct transforms vibrational energy into electrical energy and sends signals to the brain.

Vestibular system of the bony labyrinth is composed of *three perpendicular semicircular canals* and critical for the sense of balance.

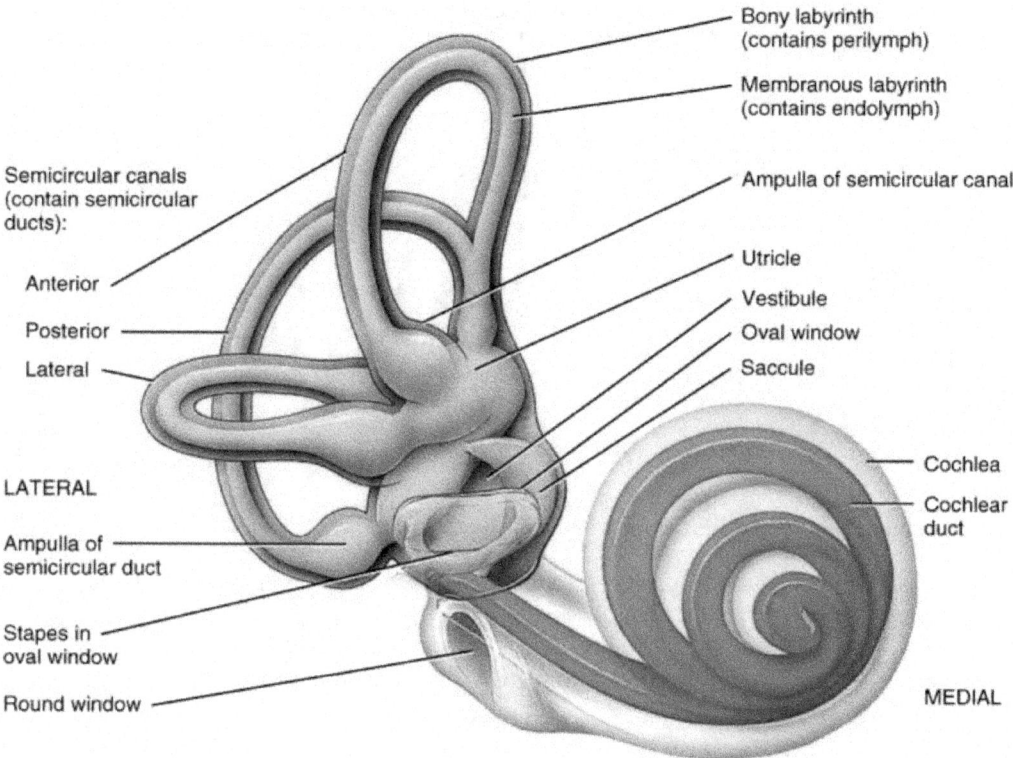

Right inner ear showing cochlea and semicircular canals

Hearing process

The hearing process begins when sound waves enter the auditory canal, hitting the tympanic membrane (eardrum) and causing it to vibrate. These vibrations move to the ossicles.

Sound is amplified about twenty times by the size difference between the tympanic membrane and the oval window. The stapes strikes the oval window's membrane, passing pressure waves to the fluid in the cochlea.

When the stapes strikes the membrane of the oval window, pressure waves move from the vestibular canal to the tympanic canal and across the *basilar membrane*, the base for these hair cells, causing the round window to bulge. This excites the stereocilia, which bend from the vibration of the basilar membrane.

Stereocilia bending generates nerve impulses in the cochlear nerve that travel to the brain stem.

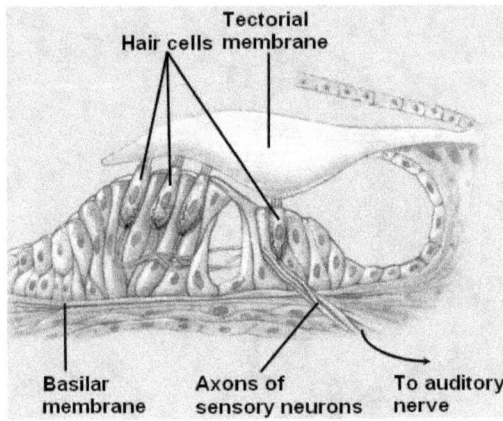

Ear with hair cells and tectorial membrane relationship

Measuring sound and auditory pathways in the brain

When nerve impulses traveling from the cochlear nerve into the brainstem reach the auditory areas of the cerebral cortex, the information is interpreted as sound.

This occurs via the *primary auditory pathway*, which starts in the cochlea and moves through the vestibulocochlear nerve to the superior olivary complex.

A neuron carries the message to the *mesencephalon*, which forms a major component of the midbrain. The primary auditory cortex receives the message.

Source	Sound Level (dB)	Intensity (W/m^2)
Nearby jet airplane	150	1000
Machine gun	130	10
Siren, rock concert (**Threshold of Pain**)	120	1
Subway, power mower	100	1×10^{-2}
Busy traffic	80	1×10^{-4}
Vacuum	70	1×10^{-5}
Normal conversation	50	1×10^{-7}
Mosquito buzzing	40	1×10^{-8}
Whisper	30	1×10^{-9}
Rustling leaves	10	1×10^{-11}
Threshold of hearing	0	1×10^{-12}

Sound perception and associated intensities in decibels

Organ of Corti has a varied structure with areas sensitive to different pitches. The organ's narrow base detects high pitch, while the wide tip detects low pitch. The nerve fibers from these regions lead to slightly different activations in the brain, producing the sensation of pitch.

Sound volume is detected by the magnitude of vibrations. Increased stimulation of receptors is interpreted as louder, while decreased stimulation is interpreted as softer.

The brain detects the tone based on the distribution of the hair cells stimulated, allowing a person to differentiate the sound of a piano from that of a violin, even if the two instruments are playing the same tune at the same volume.

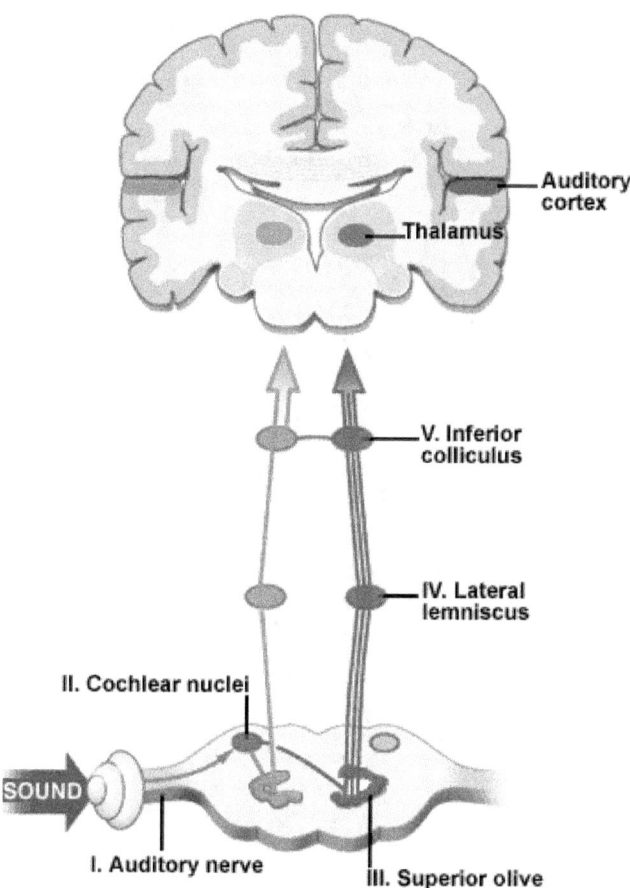

Sound perception pathways with associated anatomy

Notes for active learning

Visual Perception and Processing

Eye structure and function

The human eye is an elongated sphere measuring approximately 2.5 cm in diameter. Although like a camera, the eye is a complex network of interconnected parts.

Orbit contains the eye, a pear-shaped structure formed by several bones.

Sclera is the outer, white, fibrous layer covering most of the eye for protection.

Cornea is the transparent part of the sclera at the front of the eye. It is conceptualized as the "window of the eye." The cornea focuses light on the retina and acts as a protective covering.

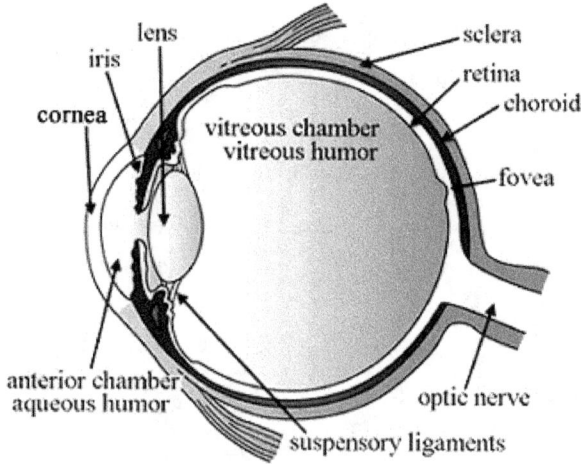

Anatomy of the human eye

Pupil is the black circle in the middle of the eye that dilates and constricts in response to light levels. The size of the pupil determines the amount of light that can enter the eye.

Choroid is the dark brown inner layer of the eye, containing blood vessels and pigments that absorb stray light rays.

The choroid thickens to form a ring-shaped ciliary body, which becomes the *iris*.

Iris is the pigmented area surrounding the pupil. It controls the amount of light entering the eye by dilating and constricting pupils using the *papillary sphincter* and *dilator muscles*.

Sympathetic nerve stimulation *dilates* the pupil to let in more light (e.g., in a dark environment).

Parasympathetic nerve stimulation *constricts* the pupil, allowing less light to enter the eye.

Lens sit behind the iris and aids focusing refracted light onto the retina and divides the eye into two chambers: *aqueous humor* and *vitreous humor*.

Aqueous humor nourishes the cornea and fills the anterior cavity.

Glaucoma results from a blocked outflow of aqueous humor and increases pressure in the eye.

Vitreous humor, which is jelly-like and protects the shape of the eye, fills the posterior cavity.

Lens focuses light onto the retina by *thickening* (*nearby objects*) and *thinning* (*distant objects*).

Retina is a thin layer of tissue behind the lens that interprets visual stimuli. The retina contains blood vessels and cells that sense light.

Fovea centralis is in the retina, which produces color vision in daylight.

Considerable processing occurs in the retina before an impulse is sent to the brain.

Visual acuity and image perception

Myopia (*nearsightedness*) is when people see objects well when they are close but not when they are far away. This is often due to an elongated eyeball that focuses on a distant image in front of the retina.

Radial keratotomy uses surgical cuts and flattening of the cornea to correct low to mild myopia.

Hyperopia (*farsightedness*) is when people see objects well when they are far away but not close. This is often due to a shortened eyeball that focuses images behind the retina.

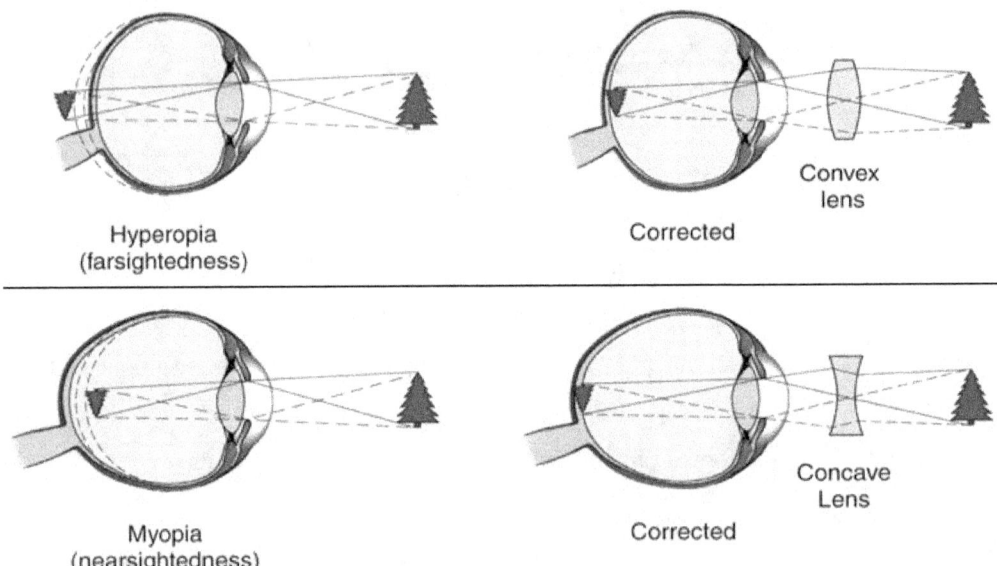

Hyperopia (farsightedness) and myopia (nearsightedness)

Astigmatism occurs when the cornea or lens is uneven, causing blurry images.

Cataracts occur when the lens becomes opaque due to new cells forming within it. Light can no longer enter through the lens. If (due to age) the lens loses its elasticity and can no longer assume a spherical shape, near vision is lost. This type of vision loss is *presbyopia*.

Cones and rods for light and color perception

Vision begins when light becomes focused on photoreceptors in the retina.

Photoreceptor cells sense light by detecting the presence and intensity of light. They are on the back of the retina, which picks up photons of light via the 130,000,000 rods and cones.

Photoreceptors sense light because they contain *photopigments*, which absorb light.

Four types of photopigments:

> rhodopsin,
>
> blue-sensitive pigment,
>
> green-sensitive pigment, and
>
> red-sensitive pigment.

Photopigments are contained within two types of photoreceptors: rods and cones.

Rods and cones have an outer segment joined to an inner segment by a stalk.

Outer segment contains stacks of *lamellae* and membranous disks with rhodopsin molecules.

Rhodopsin molecules contain *opsin* protein and pigment molecules, as retinal and chromatophore molecules, derived from vitamin A.

Cones are responsible for sharp vision and color vision. They are primarily located in the *macula*, an extremely sensitive retina area. They are in the *fovea*, an area within the macula. Three kinds of cones contain blue, green, or red pigment.

Pigments are composed of rhodopsin and opsin, with varying opsin structures allowing for the absorption of different wavelengths of light. Intermediate colors stimulate combinations of cones; the brain interprets the combined nerve impulses as one of 17,000 hues. Humans and other primates are animals that have color vision.

Rods are responsible for *peripheral* and *night vision*. Rods are more *light-sensitive* than cones but do *not* provide detailed images or detect color.

When a rod absorbs light, rhodopsin splits into opsin and retinal, leading to the closure of ion channels in the rod cell plasma membrane, producing signals that result in impulses to the brain.

Rods are grouped outside of the macula in the periphery of the retina.

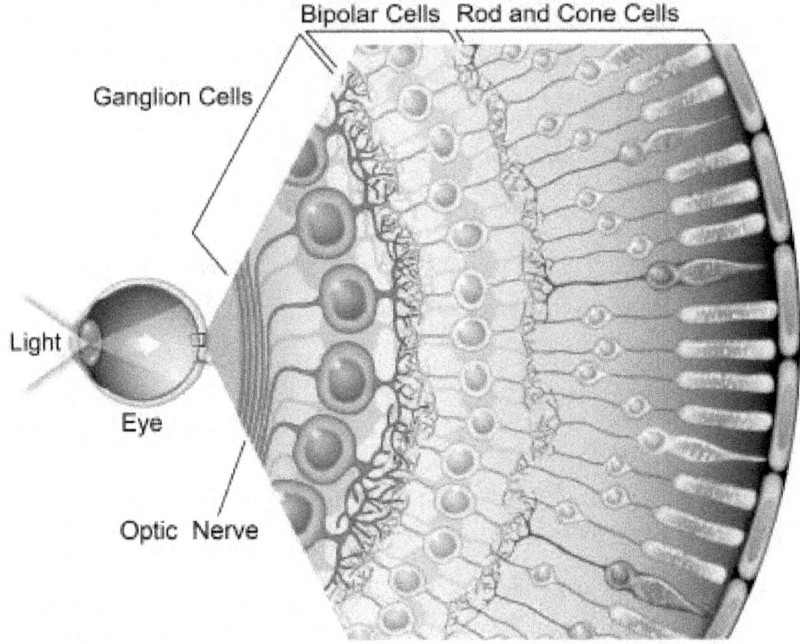

Human eye anatomy of structures with optic nerve and cells noted

Visual image processing

Light rays enter the eye through the cornea, which bends them due to its curved surface, allowing light to pass through the pupil (opening in the center of the iris with the ability to dilate and constrict depending on how much light passes through). Light rays pass through the lens.

Lens shape is controlled by *ciliary muscles*, which relax when viewing distant objects, causing the lens to flatten.

Lens shape becomes rounder when viewing near objects where light rays must bend more. This change is *visual accommodation.*

Once light rays have passed through the lens, they pass through the *vitreous humor.*

Light rays focus on the *retina.*

Due to refraction, the retina image is *inverted 180 degrees*, corrected in the brain.

Once rods and cones have sensed the light within the retina, this sensory information needs to be transmitted to the brain to translate into vision.

Retina has three layers of neurons transmitting this information by rods and cones near the *choroid, bipolar cells,* and *ganglion cells.*

Only rod and cone cells are light-sensitive; light must penetrate the ganglion cells.

When a rod absorbs light, *rhodopsin* splits into *opsin* and *retinal*, leading to a cascade of reactions and ion channel closure in the rod cell plasma membrane. This stops the release of inhibitory molecules from the rod's synaptic vesicles, which starts signals that result in impulses to the brain.

Rods and cones synapse with *bipolar cells*, creating a hyperpolarization that activates the retinal (the pigment molecule) and causes it to change shape.

Retinal activation changes to its resting shape, depolarizing the photoreceptor cell.

Integration of signals by ganglion cells

Bipolar cells pass the information to *ganglion cells*. Through this process, integration occurs.

Many rods can synapse with a *single ganglion cell*, resulting in indistinct vision.

However, each *cone* synapses with one *ganglion cell*, creating clear vision.

There are more rods and cones than nerve fibers leaving ganglionic cells.

If receptive field rod cells are stimulated, ganglion cell is *weakly stimulated* or remain *neutral*.

If the *center* of the receptive field is lit, the ganglion cell is *stimulated*.

If only the edges of the receptive field are lit, the cell is *inhibited*.

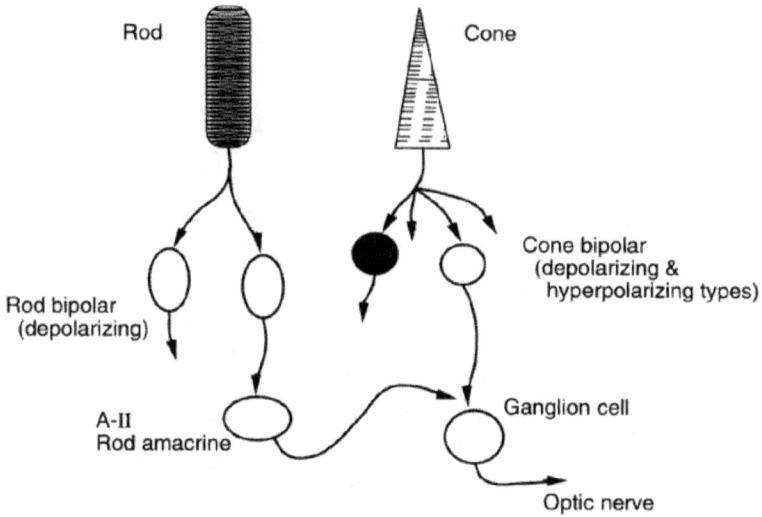

Perception of light (rods) and color (cones) by the human eye

Visual perception was believed to encompass only what the eye saw externally. It was believed that these external stimuli directly produce a perception in the brain.

However, from the discoveries of science, it is now known that this is inaccurate. Information from the eye is a *physiological process*; significant processing of the signals that the eye receives occurs in the brain. To reach the brain, the ganglion cells produce an action potential as the first step in the pathway from the eye to the brain.

Optic nerve

Axons from the ganglion cells form the optic nerve. The *optic nerve* is a pathway that crosses to the opposite side of the brain at the *optic chiasm*.

Information from the right side of the visual field is sent to the left half of the brain, and information stemming from the left side of the visual field is sent to the right half of the brain.

Blind spot is where the optic nerve passes through the retina that lacks rods and cones. The brain combines information from both eyes to compensate for this blind spot.

Information from the optic nerve travels through the optic tract and terminates in the thalamus's lateral geniculate nucleus. Information is sent from the thalamus to the occipital lobe's visual cortex, where a visual association area compares new visual information with old information.

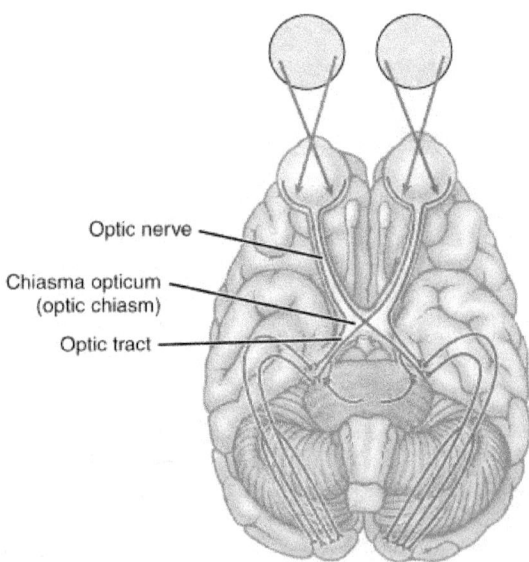

Perception of sight and processing by the brain

Once visual information has been transmitted through this pathway, the brain processes the inverted image from the retina, making it appear upright. The brain combines the two images from each eye to form a 3D image, which judges distance.

Parallel processing

Parallel processing is the brain's ability to process differing quality stimulus simultaneously. This helps a person to perceive the world in a unified way rather than disjointed pieces.

Information is divided into *color, motion, shape*, and *depth* in vision.

Each component is analyzed individually by the brain. This added information is compared with stored memories to identify the stimuli better.

Four components (color, motion, shape, and depth) are integrated to form a complete image without analyzing each component individually.

Some researchers hypothesize that before these separate processes become integrated, they are stored as memories to help the brain recognize the image.

Parallel processing is rooted in cognitive psychology, which studies mental functions and views the brain as a complex computer. The concept of parallel processing can be applied beyond sensation to the other processes within cognitive psychology: attention, memory, perception, language, and metacognition.

Feature detection

Feature detection is how the brain filters visual information for important objects.

Feature detection can be conceptualized as focusing on common elements across instances of an object. For example, if someone sees ten cats, each of a distinct size and color, they know they are cats.

Similarly, regardless of the font, one can identify the letter "a" below.

a a a a a a a

Feature detection examples

It is hypothesized that this process is via *feature detectors*, specialized neurons in the visual cortex that encode certain features such as lines, angles, and movements.

Feature detection occurs for distinctive features simultaneously, making it a type of parallel processing. Feature detectors pass information to higher-level brain cells, which then process this information to form a complete image.

An alternative hypothesis to feature detectors proposes that groups of cells, rather than individual cells, work as a network to detect certain features.

Notes for active learning

Senses of Touch, Taste, Smell and Balance

Sensation of touch

Somatosensation is the comprehensive sensory system of touch, specifically pain, temperature, vibration, and body position.

Somatosensory system receptor types include *nociceptors* (i.e., sense of pain), *proprioceptors* (i.e., position and motion), *thermoreceptors*, and *mechanoreceptors*.

In general, a somatosensory pathway has three long neurons.

First neuron's cell body is in the dorsal root ganglion of the spinal nerve.

Second neuron's cell body is in the spinal cord (or the brainstem). Axons of these neurons cross to the opposite side of the spinal cord (or brainstem) and usually terminate in the thalamus.

Third neuron usually has its cell body in the *ventral posterior nucleus* (VPN) of the thalamus, and it ends in the lateral postcentral gyrus in the parietal lobe of the cerebral cortex, where the processing aspect of somatosensation primarily occurs.

Taste bud anatomy and function

Sense of taste is helpful from an evolutionary perspective. Potentially harmful foods taste bitter, while high-calorie foods taste sweet, increasing an organism's chance of survival. The taste sensation begins with *taste buds*, as they contain the receptors for taste.

Taste buds are primarily on the tongue, specifically along the walls of *papillae*, which are small elevations on the tongue's surface.

Isolated taste buds are on the *hard palate, pharynx,* and *epiglottis* surfaces and with *epithelium*.

Taste buds contain multiple taste cells, which open at a taste pore. Particles of food dissolved in saliva encounter taste receptors.

Taste receptors detect five elements of taste: sweet, sour, salty, bitter, and umami (i.e., savory).

Taste buds for these elements are concentrated tongue regions and organized into independent pathways. The brain takes a weighted average of taste messages to form the perceived taste.

Taste is *chemoreception* because chemical signals are transduced into action potentials.

Elongated taste cells contain hair-like *microvilli* that bear receptor proteins.

Receptor proteins sense certain chemicals. Microvilli release neurotransmitters to send signals to the brain.

Primary sensory axons for taste run through the facial, glossopharyngeal, and vagus nerves. This information is primarily transmitted to the gustatory cortex in the neocortex.

Taste information moves through the thalamus and is received by two frontal lobe regions: the insula and the frontal operculum cortex.

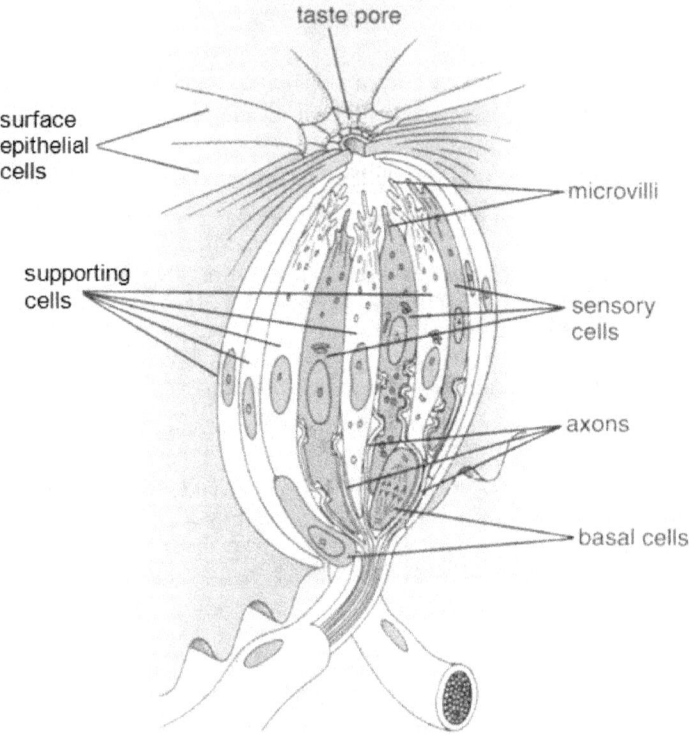

Taste buds and neural processing

Olfactory cells detect smells

Olfactory cells are modified bipolar neurons in the *nasal cavity roof's epithelium (mucous membrane)*. Olfactory cells are a form of *chemoreceptor* because they detect *chemicals*.

Humans have about 40 million olfactory cells that detect over one trillion odors.

Olfactory cells are covered in long, non-motile cilia tufts containing receptor proteins for an odor molecule.

Olfactory cells contain one type of odor receptor; humans have approximately 400 types of olfactory receptors.

When chemicals enter the nostrils, they become trapped in the nasal cavity's mucus, where they dissolve. These molecules bind to the cilia receptors, causing cell depolarization and creating an action potential.

Information is passed to the olfactory cortex within the limbic system through a brain pathway.

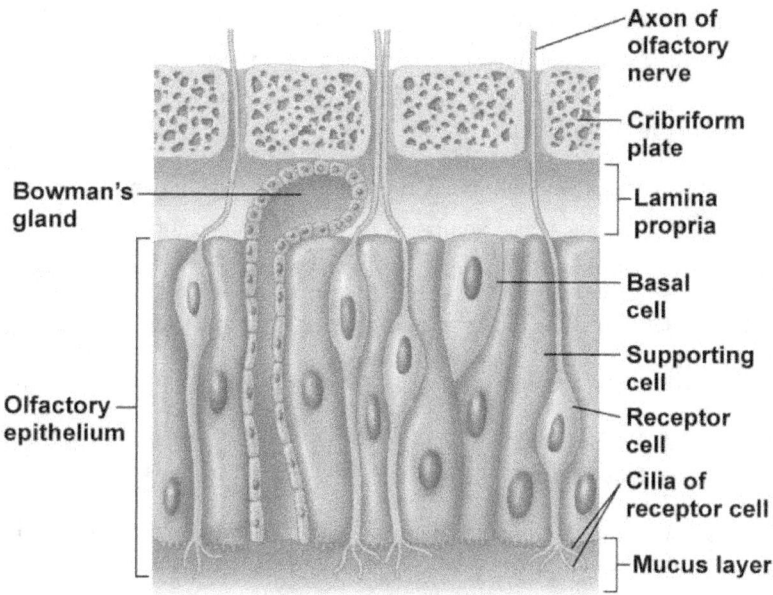

Cells involved in the sense of smell

Sense of smell is supplemented by taste, as the same substances often stimulate the receptors for taste and smell.

A person loses the sense of taste while sick with a cold, often due to olfactory deficiencies.

Pheromones influence behavior

Pheromones are chemicals secreted in sweat and other bodily fluids that influence the body of the organism that is secreting them.

Pheromones are crucial in the *behavior* of many animals, particularly for *sex, fear*, and *food*.

Pheromones play a role in mate attraction; some organisms can release pheromones that attract potential mates from over two miles away.

Pheromones mark territories; dogs and cats spray their pheromone-filled urine on objects.

Research suggests that pheromones influence human behavior. A widely known study conducted by Martha McClintock suggested that women's menstrual cycle could be altered depending on what pheromones the women were exposed to. The methodology of this study has, however, been questioned.

It has been hypothesized that women prefer the smell of men who have genetically encoded immunity (i.e., innate immunity) different from theirs because this results in disease-resistant children.

Olfactory membranes and the *vomeronasal organ* detect pheromones in non-humans.

In adult humans, the vomeronasal organ appears shrunk or absent, suggesting that it is through the normal olfactory process that humans can sense pheromones.

Olfactory pathways in the brain

The olfactory pathway is not yet well understood; however, it is known that once the cilia have detected sensory information, it is transferred to the olfactory bulb through openings in the *cribriform plate*, a part of the skull at the top of the nasal cavity.

*Olfactory bulb*s are at the base of the brain and is in direct contact with the limbic system.

Limbic system is involved in *adrenaline flow*, *emotion*, *behavior*, and long-term memory.

It is hypothesized that the olfactory bulb's connection with the limbic system is why smells are associated with strong emotions and memories.

Input in the olfactory bulb is transferred through the lateral olfactory tract to the primary olfactory cortex. Information travels through the thalamus, where interneurons communicate this information to the orbital frontal cortex, where conscious smell perception occurs.

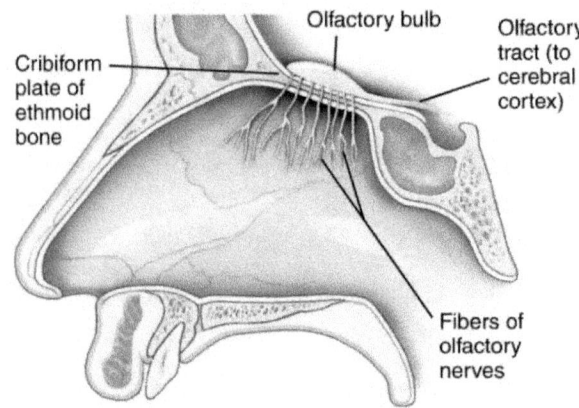

Olfactory pathways

Kinesthetic and vestibular sense

Kinesthetic sense is the body's perception of position, including the movement of joints, muscles, and tendons. Even with eyes closed, the brain can sense where parts of the body are.

Proprioception (kinesthetic sense) provides constant feedback to the brain of the muscles in the body. Much of this information is subconscious.

Proprioceptors provide sensory information about joint angle, muscle length, and muscle tension. Information from the body is transmitted from proprioceptors to the brain's parietal cortex, where information about the position of body parts is interpreted.

The channel through which this transmission of information occurs is still being studied, although it is hypothesized to be a similar pathway to touch.

Vestibular sense is awareness of balance and spatial orientation. Sensory information for this sense primarily originates in the *inner ear*, but visual and proprioceptive information is used.

Dynamic and static equilibrium

Sense of balance is divided into *dynamic equilibrium* and *static equilibrium*.

Dynamic equilibrium is the rotational movement of the head, which utilizes the semicircular canals. The enlarged bases of the canals are *ampullae* (ampulla, singular).

Fluid within the canals causes the stereocilia of the hair cells to bend. The vestibular nerve carries this information to the brain.

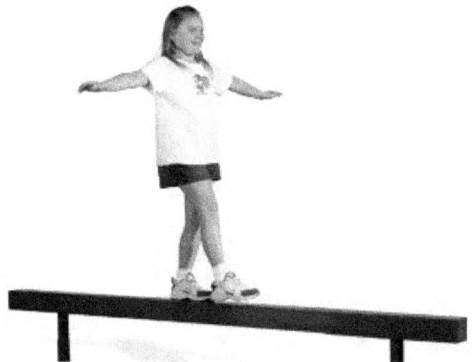

Vestibular sense assists in balance and spatial orientation

Static equilibrium involves vertical and horizontal movement and is detected when the head moves regarding gravity.

Static equilibrium utilizes the utricle and the saccule by the *maculae* (specialized mechanoreceptors) within them.

Utricle and *saccule* are tiny membranous sacs with hair cells.

Utricle is sensitive to *horizontal movements*, while the *saccule* registers *vertical movements*. Small carbon granules that rest on a gelatinous membrane containing hair cells are displaced when movement occurs. This bends the hair cells and indicates the direction of movement.

Information from static and dynamic equilibrium hair cells is transmitted to the parietal lobe. It is integrated with sensory information from other body areas to provide a sense of movement and balance.

Notes for active learning

Perception Processing

Bottom-up and top-down processing

The brain uses both *bottom-up* and *top-down processing* to understand stimuli.

Top-down processing occurs when perceptions are formed by working from a larger concept to more specific information.

Top-down processing is also known as *concept-driven processing* and often occurs *outside of conscious awareness*.

When one sees *an incomplete image* or word (e.g., the image below) but can fill in the missing details, this is a form of top-down processing.

Top-down processing also has applications in the realm of sensation. For example, if a boy walks into a pizza shop and smells something ambiguous, he identifies it as the smell of pizza because of his expectations.

When expectations or prior knowledge influence perception, top-down processing is occurring.

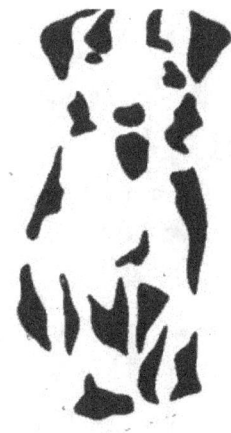

Top-down processing to produce the image of a dog

Bottom-up processing is conceptualized as occurring in the direction opposite to top-down processing. It starts with *sensory information* and then moves to *higher-level processing*.

Bottom-up processing is also known as *data-driven processing*. For example, if someone accidentally places their hand on a hot stove, the reaction is to pull away quickly without consciously deciding to do so. Because processing moved directly from the *stimulus (pain) to action*, bottom-up processing has occurred.

Much debate surrounds how sensory systems rely on top-down versus bottom-up processing.

Researchers have turned to neurobiology to answer these questions. Although much is still unknown, certain brain areas have been found to have more bottom-up connections and others more top-down connections.

Primary visual cortex is believed to contain primarily *bottom-up* connections.

Fusiform gyrus, part of temporal and occipital lobes, is hypothesized for *top-down* processing.

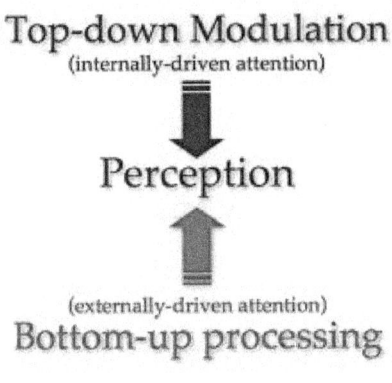

Competing theories of perception

Perceptual organization: depth, form, motion, and constancy

The environment is three-dimensional; thus, a three-dimensional approach is needed to understand it. Therefore, the eyes must measure the three dimensions of height, width, and depth. Organisms can only conceptualize these properties by processing sensory information within the brain.

For example, the brain uses many rules and principles to determine the depth of an object. One rule concern *relative size*, meaning smaller objects tend to be perceived farther away.

Interposition means that objects that block other objects are usually perceived as closer.

Relative clarity is the principle that objects with a clear image are perceived as closer than those with a hazy image. Objects higher in the visual field also tend to be perceived as farther away.

Parallel lines appear to converge with distance, giving the perception of depth. The brain also uses shading to inform depth perception; dimmer objects often seem farther away.

The brain also uses rules and principles to determine the motion of an object. Images of objects traveling toward the eye appear to grow, while those traveling away appear to shrink.

Phi phenomenon is an optical illusion whereby one perceives a continuous motion between objects flashing at a certain speed.

Form perception is identifying a form despite a brand-new image being displayed on the retina.

During visual processing, information is formatted to draw out relevant and detailed information from a stimulus. It is believed to occur in the areas of the brain known as the *ventral* and *dorsal* streams.

Constancy is the ability of the brain to perceive *objects as unchanging*, even when the retinal image changes. For example, people can identify their friends even when seeing them from different angles and do not think they have transformed into different people just because they have turned around.

Gestalt principles

Gestalt is a German term for shape or form. Within psychology, Gestalt usually refers to an organized or unified whole.

The basic principle guiding Gestalt psychology is that the *whole is greater than the sum of its parts,* thus emphasizing *top-down processing*.

Gestalt psychology seeks to understand how organisms *perceive meaning* out of apparently *meaningless stimuli*, particularly visual stimuli. Several Gestalt principles have been proposed to describe how humans perceive "wholes" from parts.

Gestalt principles are generally grouped into similarity, continuation, closure, proximity, and figure categories.

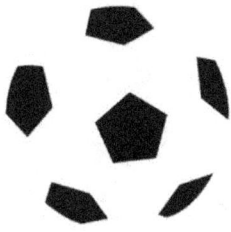

Similarity principle uses similar elements to construct an image

Similarity principle proposes that when an image is made of similar elements, these elements are integrated into groups, and each group is perceived as a single unit.

Principle of continuation asserts that groups aligned with others tend to be perceived as wholes.

Closure principle states that even when an image is incomplete, if enough of the image is present, the mind can fill in the gaps, and the image is perceived as a whole.

Proximity principle proposes that items tend to be perceived as one group when they are close.

Figure principle refers to the tendency to differentiate an object from its surroundings by perceiving the object as a *figure* and the surroundings as a *background*.

Notes for active learning

Chapter 6

Respiratory System

Respiratory System Structure and Function

Lung and Alveoli

Mechanisms of Breathing

Alveolar Gas Exchange

pH and Neural Regulation

Page intentionally left blank

Respiratory System Structure and Function

Gas exchange

Human *respiratory system* includes the structures that conduct air to and from the lungs. It supplies body tissue with oxygen (O_2).

Oxygen pathway in the respiratory system involves *cooperative transport* (i.e., hemoglobin) and *diffusion* within the circulatory system.

Oxygen is taken in from the environment by the lungs. Here, the circulatory system's red blood cells meet the lung's *alveoli*, and oxygen diffuses into the cells.

Red blood cells carry oxygenated *blood towards the body's tissues*.

Carbon dioxide (CO_2) follows a reverse path, traveling in deoxygenated blood from the tissues and back to the lungs. It is expelled into the external environment through the nose (or mouth).

Cellular respiration is the breakdown of organic molecules (e.g., glucose) to produce ATP.

A sufficient supply of oxygen is required for aerobic respiration of the Krebs cycle and electron transport chain to efficiently convert potential energy within food into the energy of ATP.

Carbon dioxide is generated by aerobic cellular respiration and must be removed from the cell. There is an exchange of gases, where carbon dioxide leaves the cell and oxygen enters. Animals have organ systems facilitating respiration and regulating gas transport between the environment and the body's cells.

Breathing involves inspiration (bringing air into the lungs) and expiration (moving air out). In general, gas exchanges involve exchanging gas for another. External respiration involves gas exchange with the external environment at a respiratory surface.

Internal respiration is complex and involves a gas exchange between blood and tissue fluid. The process occurs in the lungs' alveoli (i.e., tiny air sacs).

Oxygen diffuses into the capillaries surrounding the *alveoli*.

Carbon dioxide diffuses out of the capillaries and into the *alveoli*.

Lungs are deep within the thoracic cavity to protect from desiccation. The pathways in the respiratory system connect the lungs to the outside environment.

Human lungs have at least 50 times the skin's total surface area.

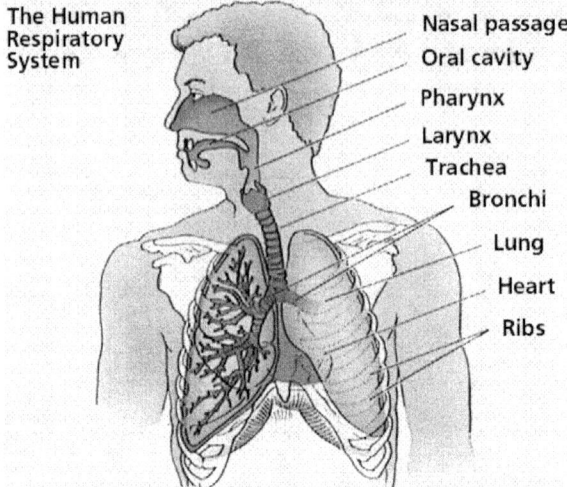

Respiratory system with anatomical structures

Air enters through the nose (or mouth). It is warmed, filtered, and passed through the nasal (or oral) cavity. Air passes through the *pharynx* into the upper part of the trachea, containing the *larynx*, which is held open by cartilage that forms the *laryngeal prominence* (Adam's apple).

Vocal cords are two bands of tissue extending across the larynx's opening. As air passes, these tissues vibrate, creating sounds.

Trachea walls are reinforced with C-shaped rings of cartilage.

Larynx rises as the food is swallowed, and the *glottis* is closed by a flap of elastic, cartilaginous tissue, the *epiglottis*. The soft palate's backward movement covers the nasal passage entrance, directing food downward.

Airways enter the lungs

Airways beyond the larynx are divided into the *conducting zone* and *respiratory zone*.

The trachea divides into two *bronchi*. After passing the larynx, the air moves into the bronchi, which carries air to the lungs.

Bronchi are reinforced to prevent collapse and lined with *ciliated epithelium* and *mucus-producing* cells. *C-shaped rings of cartilage* diminish *as bronchi branch within the lungs*.

Conducting zone has no gas exchange and consists of the tracheal tube, which branches into two bronchi before entering the lungs and branching.

Trachea walls and bronchi contain cartilage for support. *Terminal bronchioles* are the first branches without cartilage.

Each bronchus branches into numerous smaller tubes within the lungs as *bronchioles* that conduct air to *alveoli*, grape-like sac clusters.

Respiratory zone is for gas exchange and has respiratory bronchioles with alveoli attached.

Respiratory bronchioles with capillaries and alveoli for gas exchange are shown.

Oxygen moves from the alveoli to the red blood cells, while carbon dioxide moves from the red blood cells (or dissolved in the plasma) to the alveoli for expiration by the lungs.

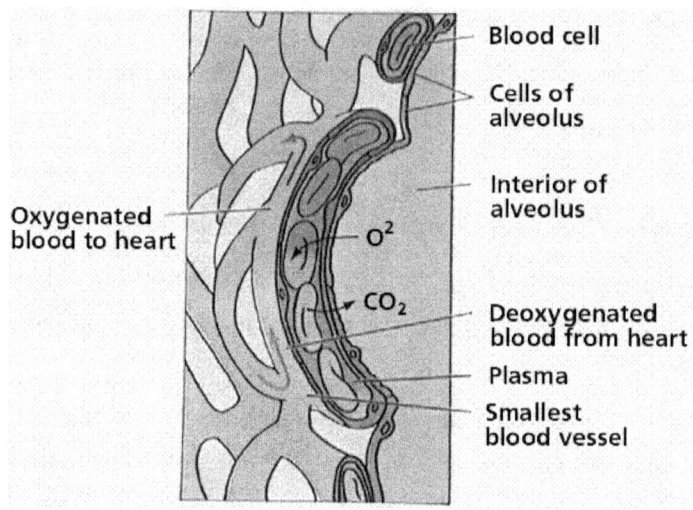

Respiratory bronchioles with capillaries and alveoli for gas exchange.

Protection against disease and particulate matter

Respiratory system has several mechanisms to protect against disease and particulate matter.

Nasal cavity contains visible hairs as *vibrissae*. Nostril hairs filter out coarse particles.

Paranasal sinuses secrete mucus, passing through the mucous glands into the lamina propria and the respiratory mucosa, where the mucous traps foreign particles and pathogens.

Respiratory mucosa's epithelial cells secrete *defensins*, natural antibiotics that aid in defense against invading microbes.

Serous glands supply the *lamina propria* with water fluid containing lysozyme (antibacterial enzyme). Macrophages, which engulf pathogens, are present.

Respiratory mucosa is a part of the nasal cavity's *ciliated epithelial* lining.

Cilia on the mucous lining of the respiratory tract sweep pathogens and particles out of the body by creating a slight current.

Nasal cavity wall contains three projections: *superior*, *medial*, and *inferior turbinate* (or *conchae*), which increase the surface area of the nasal mucosa.

Heavier non-gaseous components are deflected into mucosal surfaces as air passes. The entire respiratory tract has a warm, wet, mucous membrane lining exposed to environmental air.

Airways and pressure difference between the lungs and atmosphere are essential factors in airflow in and out of the lungs. Many diseases can affect the condition of the airways.

Respiratory ailments

Strep throat is a severe infection caused by *Streptococcus pyogenes*, resulting in a high fever, increased difficulty swallowing, and a substantial risk of systemic infection.

Sinusitis is a sinus infection; 1–3% of upper respiratory infections are accompanied by sinusitis.

Asthma narrows the airways by causing allergy-induced spasms of surrounding muscles or clogging the airways with mucus.

Tonsillitis is when tonsils and adenoids of the pharynx become inflamed as an initial defense.

Laryngitis is an infection of the larynx, causing hoarseness and an inability to speak. However, persistent hoarseness without any upper respiratory infection is one of the warning signs of laryngeal cancer.

Lung cancer, formerly more common in men, now surpasses breast cancer as a cause of death in women. It is often due to smoking. Lung cancer develops in the lung tissue in steps. First, the thickening and callusing of the cells lining the bronchi begins. In addition, cilia are lost, so it becomes impossible to prevent dust and dirt from settling in the lungs. Next, cells with atypical nuclei appear in the callused lining.

Bronchitis is an inflammatory response that reduces airflow and is caused by long-term exposure to irritants such as cigarette smoke, air pollutants, or allergens.

Acute bronchitis is an infection of primary and secondary bronchi, usually preceded by a viral upper respiratory infection.

Chronic Obstructive Pulmonary Disease (COPD) is chronic bronchitis or the production of excessive mucus in bronchi that obstructs the airways.

Pneumonia is usually caused by a bacterial (or viral) lung infection. The bronchi and alveoli fill with fluid. Pneumonia can be localized in specific lobules. AIDS patients are subject to a rare form of pneumonia caused by the protozoan *Pneumocystis carinii*.

Cystic fibrosis is a life-threatening genetic disorder that causes excessive mucus production that clogs the lungs, digestive system, and other organs.

Pulmonary tuberculosis (TB) is caused by the bacterium *Mycobacterium tuberculosis* (tubercle bacillus). A TB skin test is a highly diluted extract of the bacilli injected into the patient's skin. If a person has been exposed, the immune response causes inflammation. Bacilli that invade lung tissue are isolated by the lung tissue in tubercles (tiny capsules). If the person is highly resistant, the isolated bacteria die. If the person is not resistant, the bacteria can spread.

A chest X-ray can detect active tubercles. Appropriate drug therapy can ensure localization and the eventual destruction of live bacteria. The resurgence of pulmonary tuberculosis has accompanied the increased incidence of AIDS and is often seen in lower socioeconomic demographics. The new strains of tuberculosis are often resistant to standard antibiotics.

Hypoxia is the deficiency of oxygen at the tissue level.

Four types of hypoxia:

Hypoxic hypoxia, which is characterized by reduced arterial pO_2.

Anemic hypoxia is when the total oxygen content of blood is reduced due to an inadequate number of *erythrocytes* (I.e., red blood cells) and *hemoglobin*.

Ischemic hypoxia is when blood flow to the tissues is low.

Histotoxic hypoxia is when tissues cannot utilize O_2 due to interference from a toxic agent.

Emphysema is a chronic and incurable disorder involving distended and damaged alveoli. It is a disease characterized by increased airway resistance, decreased surface area for ventilation due to alveolar fusion, and ventilation-perfusion inequalities (i.e., the difference in the amount of air reaching the alveoli and the amount of blood sent to the lungs). The lungs often balloon due to trapped air and ineffective alveoli.

Emphysema is often preceded by *chronic bronchitis*. The elastic recoil of the lungs is reduced, and the airways are narrowed, making expiration difficult. Since the surface area for gas exchange is reduced, insufficient O_2 reaches the heart and brain. This triggers the heart to work furiously to force more blood through the lungs, leading to a heart condition. Lack of oxygen in the brain makes the patient feel depressed, sluggish, and irritable.

Exercise, drug therapy, and supplemental oxygen may relieve the symptoms and slow the condition's progress.

Notes for active learning

Lung and Alveoli

Lungs structure

Lungs are two large, lobed organs in the chest.

Thorax is a closed compartment bound at the neck by muscles and separated from the abdomen by the *diaphragm*, a sheet of skeletal muscle.

Thorax wall comprises *ribs*, *sternum* (breastbone), and *intercostal muscles* between ribs.

Lungs are ingrowths of body walls connected to the outside by tubes and small openings.

Pleura (thin sheet of cells) separates the inside of the chest cavity from the lungs' outer surface.

Pleural sac (closed sac) surrounds each lung. The pleural surface coating the lung is the *visceral pleura* attached to the lung by connective tissue.

Parietal pleura (outer layer) is attached to the thoracic wall and diaphragm. A thin layer of intrapleural fluid separates the two layers of the pleura. Changes in the hydrostatic pressure of the intrapleural fluid (the intrapleural pressure P_{ip}, the intra-thoracic pressure) cause the lungs and thoracic wall to move together during breathing.

Lung breathing evolved about 400 million years ago. Lungs are not solely in the domain of vertebrates. Some terrestrial snails have gas exchange structures like those in frogs.

Lungs are composed of alveoli, the air sacs where gas exchange with blood occurs.

Lungs have a non-respiratory function, and biologically active substances are released and removed into the blood. They trap and dissolve small blood clots.

Alveoli as the site of gas exchange

Alveoli are open-ended, hollow sacs that are continuous lumens of airways. Their inner walls are lined with a single layer of flat epithelial cells called *type I alveolar cells*, interspersed by thicker, specialized *type II alveolar cells*.

Alveolar walls contain capillaries and a small interstitial space with interstitial fluid and connective tissue.

Alveolar wall cells secrete a fluid that keeps the inner surface of the alveoli moist, allowing gases to dissolve.

Surfactant, a natural detergent, prevents the alveoli sides from sticking. Blood within an alveolar-capillary wall is separated from the air within an alveolus by a thin barrier of 0.2 μm thick. Pores in the walls permit the flow of air. The extensive surface area and thin barrier permit the rapid exchange of copious quantities of oxygen and carbon dioxide by diffusion.

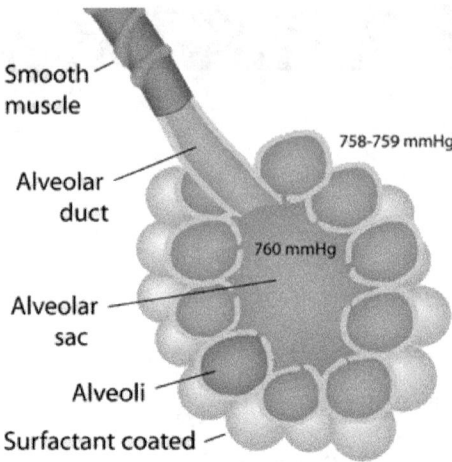

Gas exchange of oxygen and carbon dioxide occurs at the alveoli in the lungs

Mechanisms of Breathing

Measuring respiration rates and lung capacity

Tidal volume is the air entering the lungs during a single, regular inspiration or leaving the lungs in a single expiration.

Inspiratory reserve volume is the air above the tidal volume during deepest inspirations.

Functional residual capacity is the air remaining in the lungs after expiring the tidal volume.

Expiratory reserve volume is the additional air volume after expiring the resting tidal volume. It is the volume expired via active contraction of the expiratory muscles.

Residual volume is the air remaining in the lungs after maximal expiration.

Vital capacity is the maximal volume of air that expires after a maximal inspiration.

Minute ventilation is the volume of gas inhaled (or exhaled) from a person's lungs per minute.

Minute ventilation (ml/min) = Tidal volume (ml/breath) × Respiration rate (breaths/min)

Anatomic dead space is within the airways that do not permit gas exchange with the blood.

Alveolar ventilation is the volume of air entering the alveoli per minute.

Ventilation (ml/min) = [Tidal volume (ml/breath) − anatomic dead space (ml/min)] × respiratory rate (breaths/min)

Since a fixed volume of tidal volume is dead space, increased *depth of breathing* elevates alveolar ventilation *more than* increased breathing rate.

Alveolar dead space is the inspired air not used for gas exchange at the alveoli.

Physiological dead space is the sum of the anatomic and alveolar dead space.

Diaphragm and rib cage

Diaphragm is a muscle that pulls down when contracting, which increases chest volume, decreases air pressure, and stimulates *inspiration*.

Rib cage expands outward during inspiration. *Intercostal muscles* help this expansion.

At rest, the rib cage maintains lung volume, prevents the lungs from collapsing, and forms a cage around the lungs for protection.

Lung volume is dependent on two factors.

Trans-pulmonary pressure is 1) the *pressure difference* between the inside and outside of the lungs, and 2) lung *compliance* is the lung's ability to stretch.

Muscles used in respiration are attached to the chest wall. When they contract (or relax), they change the chest dimensions, changing the transpulmonary pressure, lung volume, and alveolar pressure, causing air to flow in (or out) the lungs.

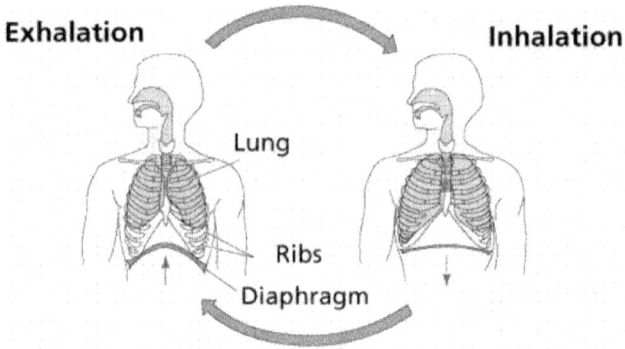

Diaphragm contraction during inspiration and relaxation during expiration

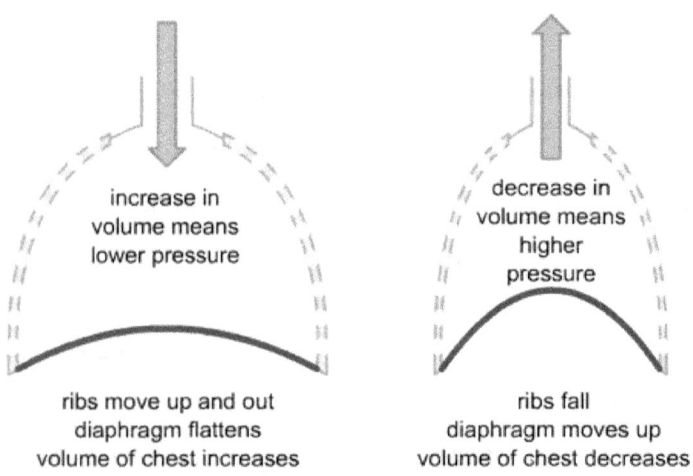

*Inspiration when diaphragm contracts (air in, on the left)
and expiration when the diaphragm relaxes (air out)*

Inhalation causes chest wall muscles to contract, lifting the ribs and pulling them outward. The diaphragm contracts and moves downward, enlarging the chest cavity. The reduced air pressure in the lungs causes air to enter the lungs. Exhaling reverses these steps.

Pressure differences facilitate breathing

Intrapulmonary pressure is atmospheric pressure because the lungs are open to the atmosphere and, therefore, have the same pressure as the environment.

If the intrapleural pressure is less than the atmospheric pressure, it sucks on the lungs and prevents them from collapsing. During inspiration, intrapleural pressure decreases and causes the lungs to expand.

Differential pressure is the difference between intrapulmonary (i.e., inside the lungs) and intrapleural (i.e., outside the lungs) pressure.

Like other mammals, humans breathe through a *negative pressure* mechanism; akin to sucking.

Lowering the diaphragm and raising the ribs during inhalation form negative pressure by increasing thoracic cavity volume. Air, which is under greater outside pressure, enters the lungs.

Increases in $[CO_2]$ and $[H^+]$ in the blood are the primary stimuli that increases breathing rate.

Resiliency and surface tension effects

Lungs are elastic; due to surface tension, they recoil when relaxed after inspiration. If not for the rib cage, the lung would collapse even further.

$$\text{Trans-pulmonary pressure} = P_{alv} - P_{ip}$$

where P_{alv} is alveolar pressure and P_{ip} is intrapleural pressure.

P_{alv} is zero and equal to the atmospheric pressure.

P_{ip} is negative, or less than the atmospheric pressure, because the elastic recoil of the lung inwards and the elastic recoil of the chest wall outwards increases the volume of the intrapleural space between them and decreases the pressure within.

Therefore, the transpulmonary pressure is greater than zero, which creates an expanding force equal to the elastic recoil force of the lung (keeping it from collapsing).

Lung volume is kept stable with air inside the lungs. By a similar phenomenon, the pressure difference across the chest ($P_{atm} - P_{ip}$), which is directed inward, keeps the elastic chest wall from excessively moving outward.

Resistance is determined mainly by radius. Trans-pulmonary pressure exerts a distending force, which keeps the airways from collapsing. This makes the airways larger during expiration and smaller during inspiration.

Lung compliance (LC) is a measure of elasticity (or the magnitude of change) in lung volume (ΔLV) that a given change in transpulmonary pressure can produce.

$$LC = \Delta LV / \Delta(P_{alv} - P_{ip})$$

With low lung compliance, P_{ip} must be made lower to achieve lung expansion. This requires more vigorous contractions of the diaphragm and intercostal muscles.

Since the surface of alveolar cells is moist, surface tension between water molecules resists the stretching of lung tissue.

Type II alveolar cells secrete pulmonary *surfactant* that *decreases surface tension* and *increases lung compliance*, helping the alveoli to stay open.

Respiratory distress syndrome in newborns is a result of *low lung compliance*.

Thermoregulation

Nose and nasal cavity warm and moisten inspired air and retrieve moisture and heat during expiration.

High-water content of the mucus film humidifies inhaled air. A bed of capillaries and thin-walled veins lies under the nasal epithelium: capillaries and thin veins warm incoming air.

If the air is frigid, the *plexus* (i.e., a network of veins and capillaries) fills with blood, and the heat-intensifying process is amplified.

Heat and moisture are exchanged from expired air. Conchae are cooled by inspired cold air. As warm air leaves, it precipitates moisture on the conchae, which extracts heat from the humid air flowing over them.

Surfaces involved in respiratory evaporation must be *moist* as water continuously *evaporates*.

On a chilly day, people see water vapor in their breath; water evaporates from the lungs.

Water is a product of cellular respiration (i.e., glycolysis, Krebs cycle, and electron transport chain), and it, along with carbon dioxide, is expired during breathing.

Thermal panting is caused by a buildup of body heat resulting from increased environmental temperature or additional activity and increased metabolic rates.

Appropriate chemical receptors perceive oxygen (O_2) and carbon dioxide (CO_2) levels.

When oxygen levels are low (or carbon dioxide levels are high), the respiratory system responds by increasing the overall rate of respiration.

Panting rate increases at high altitudes (due to low pO_2 levels).

Alveolar Gas Exchange

Diffusion

Even though alveoli are tiny, their abundance in the lungs results in a large surface area for gas exchange.

Alveoli walls have a single layer of thin cells, creating a short diffusion distance for the gases.

Diffusion is the passive movement of materials from a higher to a lower concentration.

A short diffusion distance allows for rapid gas exchange.

Ventilation is the mechanism of breathing that brings air into the alveoli and removes stale air.

Ventilation maintains the concentration gradient of carbon dioxide and oxygen between the alveoli and capillaries of the blood.

Partial pressures measure the differences between oxygen and carbon dioxide concentrations (i.e., [CO_2]). The greater the difference in partial pressure, the higher the diffusion rate.

The body must expel CO_2, the product of cell respiration.

The body needs to take in oxygen for cellular respiration to make ATP.

There must be a low concentration of carbon dioxide in the alveoli so that it can diffuse out of the blood in the capillaries (where it exists in a high concentration) and into the alveoli.

Differential partial pressures of O_2 and CO_2

There must be a high concentration of O_2 in the alveoli compared to a low concentration of O_2 in the capillaries so that oxygen can diffuse into the blood of the capillaries from the alveoli.

O_2 in the alveoli flows down its partial pressure gradient from the alveoli into the pulmonary capillaries. Here, O_2 binds to hemoglobin for transport.

CO_2 flows down its partial pressure gradient from the capillaries into the alveoli for expiration.

Blood entering pulmonary capillaries is the venous blood of systemic circulation. This blood has high pCO_2 and a low pO_2.

Partial pressure differences of O_2 and CO_2 on the two sides of the alveolar-capillary membrane result in the net diffusion of oxygen from the alveoli to the blood and carbon dioxide from the blood to the alveoli.

With this diffusion, capillary blood pO_2 rises, and pCO_2 falls; net diffusion of gases ceases when the partial pressures in the capillaries equal the alveoli.

Diffusion improves with vascularization (i.e., more blood vessels); O_2 delivery to cells is promoted by erythrocytes (i.e., red blood cells) with the O_2-binding protein hemoglobin.

Diffuse interstitial fibrosis is a disease where the alveolar walls thicken with connective tissue and reduce gas exchange.

Ventilation-perfusion inequality can result from ventilated alveoli with no blood supply or blood flow through the alveoli with no ventilation, resulting in reduced gas exchange.

Steady-state is when the volume of oxygen consumed by cells per unit of time equals the volume of oxygen added to the blood in the lungs.

Rate of expiration is the volume of carbon dioxide produced by cells.

Respiratory quotient (RQ) is ratio of CO_2 produced/O_2 consumed and nutrients used for energy.

Ventilation is the exchange of air between the atmosphere and alveoli.

Air moves by *bulk flow* from high-pressure to low-pressure regions.

Flow rate (F) is:

$$F = (P_{atm} - P_{alv}) / R$$

where P_{atm} is the atmospheric pressure, P_{alv} is the alveolar pressure, and R is airflow resistance.

During ventilation, air moves into the lungs from changing alveolar pressure and size.

Alveolar pO_2 (partial pressure of O_2) is lower than atmospheric pO_2 because oxygen in the alveolar air keeps entering the pulmonary capillaries.

Alveolar pCO_2 is higher than atmospheric pCO_2 because carbon dioxide enters the alveoli from pulmonary capillaries.

pO_2 positively correlates with alveolar ventilation rate and inversely with oxygen consumption.

pCO_2 is inversely correlated with the rate of alveolar ventilation and positively correlated with the rate of oxygen consumption.

Hypoventilation is an increase in the ratio of carbon dioxide production to alveolar ventilation.

Hyperventilation is a decreased ratio of carbon dioxide production to alveolar ventilation.

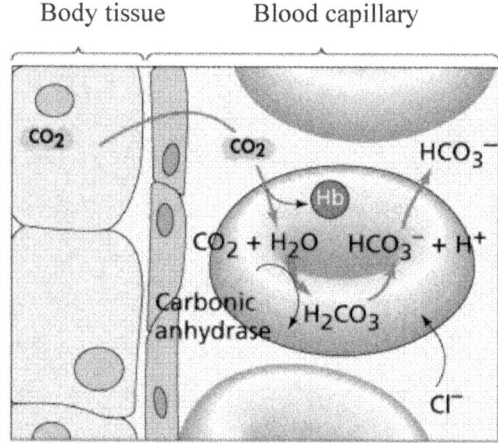

Erythrocyte (red blood cell) and gas exchange of O_2 and CO_2

In the alveoli capillaries, bicarbonate (HCO_3^-) combines with an H^+ ion (a proton) to form carbonic acid (H_2CO_3), which dissociates into carbon dioxide and water. CO_2 then diffuses into the alveoli and out of the body with the next exhalation.

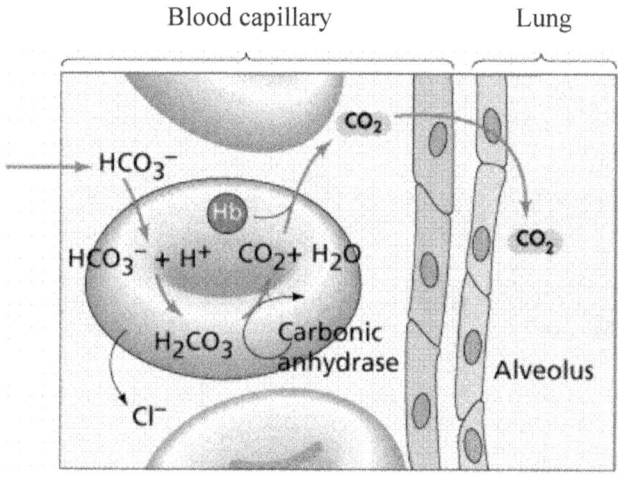

$$CO_2\ (g) + H_2O\ (l) \leftrightarrow H_2CO_3\ (aq) \leftrightarrow HCO_3^- + H^+\ (aq)$$

Henry's Law

Mechanism of gas exchange follows Henry's law, which states that there is an equilibrium concentration of oxygen dissolved in the blood.

Blood that reaches the lungs has less than the equilibrium O_2 concentration that is delivered to tissues. Therefore, oxygen diffuses from the alveoli into the blood.

CO_2 in the blood that reaches the lungs is higher than the equilibrium concentration because the body releases CO_2. Therefore, CO_2 diffuses out of the blood.

Notes for active learning

pH and Neural Regulation

pH control

Ventilation is stimulated by a change in H^+ concentration (e.g., due to lactic acid), input from mechanoreceptors in joints and muscles, an increase in body temperature, and an increase in plasma epinephrine.

Lactic acid in exercising muscles can cause metabolic acidosis or metabolic alkalosis (too much or too little acid), changing H^+ concentration and stimulating peripheral chemoreceptors.

Respiratory regulation refers to the variability in pH due to pCO_2 changes from alterations in ventilation. These changes in ventilation can occur rapidly and significantly affect pH.

Carbon dioxide is lipid-soluble and freely transverse cell membranes rapidly. Therefore, changes in pCO_2 result in rapid changes in [H+] in all body fluid compartments.

Two concepts express the connection between alveolar ventilation and pH by pCO_2.

The relationship between alveolar ventilation (V_A) and pCO_2 is shown.

Changes in alveolar ventilation are inversely related to changes in arterial pCO_2 and directly proportional to total body CO_2 production (V_{CO_2}). The equation uses a constant of 0.863:

$$pCO_2 = 0.863 \times (VCO_2 / V_A)$$

Henderson-Hasselbalch equation

Henderson-Hasselbalch equation states that the changes in pCO_2 cause changes in pH.

$$pH = pK_a + \log (HCO_3) / (0.03 \times pCO_2)$$

During hyperventilating, arterial H^+ concentration rises due to increased pCO_2, which is *respiratory acidosis*.

On the contrary, hyperventilation lowers [H^+], which is respiratory alkalosis.

Deoxyhemoglobin has a higher affinity for H^+ than oxyhemoglobin, binding most H^+ produced. When deoxyhemoglobin is converted to oxyhemoglobin, H+ ions are released in the lungs.

Hemoglobin (Hb) combines with H^+ ions as reduced hemoglobin (HHb). HHb is vital in maintaining blood pH. Blood enters pulmonary capillaries with most CO_2 in plasma as HCO_3^-

$$HbO_2 \rightarrow Hb + O_2$$

Acidic pH levels and warmer temperatures also promote this dissociation.

Nervous system control

Vagus nerve involuntary controls the respiratory system, heart, and viscera, so breathing cannot be consciously stopped for prolonged periods. Breathing occurs when able and needed.

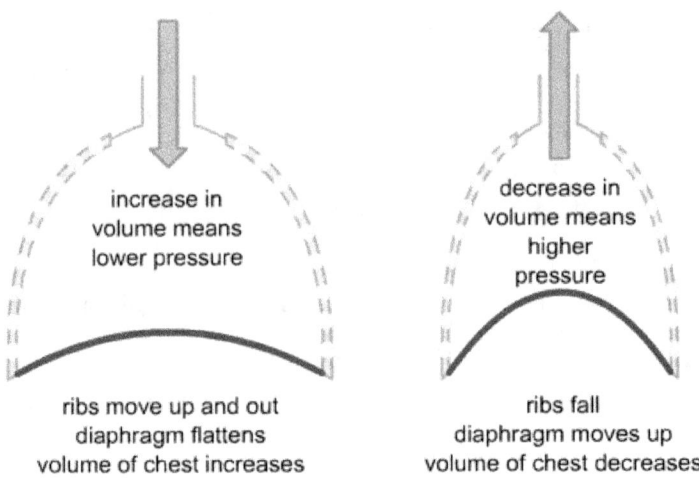

Ventilation with inspiration where diaphragm contracts (air in, on the left) and expiration where diaphragm relaxes (air out)

Diaphragm and *intercostal muscles* are skeletal muscles.

Therefore, breathing depends on the cyclical excitation of these muscles.

Neural activity control resides with *medullary inspiratory neurons* in the medulla oblongata.

Peripheral chemoreceptors (i.e., carotid bodies) and *aortic bodies* in close contact with arterial blood are stimulated by a steep decrease in arterial pO_2 and an increase in H^+ concentration.

Medullary inspiratory neurons receive inputs from apneustic and pneumotaxic centers in pons.

Negative feedback from pulmonary stretch receptors controls respiration, known as the *Hering-Breuer reflex*. This reflex is triggered to prevent over-inflammation of the lung.

Protective reflexes (e.g., coughing, sneezing) protect the respiratory system from irritants.

Receptors for sneezing are in the nose or pharynx, while those for coughing are in the larynx, trachea, and bronchi. These reflexes are characterized by a deep inspiration followed by a violent expiration.

Descending pathways accomplish *voluntary control* of breathing from the *cerebral cortex*. It cannot be maintained when involuntary stimuli are high.

Tachypnea (i.e., rapid breathing) is a reflex effect from the *J receptors* in the lungs. It is stimulated by an increase in interstitial lung pressure due to the occlusion of a pulmonary vessel as a pulmonary embolus.

CO_2 sensitivity

Carbon dioxide concentration in metabolically active cells is much greater than in capillaries. Thus, CO_2 diffuses from the cells into the capillaries.

About 7% of CO_2 dissolves in plasma. Another 23% of the CO_2 binds to the amino groups in hemoglobin to form *carb-amino-hemoglobin*. The remaining 70% is transported in blood as a bicarbonate ion (HCO_3^-).

CO_2 combines with water, forming *carbonic acid* (H_2CO_3), which dissociates H^+, forming bicarbonate ions (HCO_3^-):

$$CO_2 + H_2O \leftrightarrow H_2CO_3 \leftrightarrow H^+ + HCO_3^-$$

Carbonic anhydrase is an enzyme in red blood cells that speeds the reaction to remove carbon dioxide from the blood. Hence, the diffusion of more carbon dioxide from cells into capillaries occurs for expiration out of the body.

Release of H^+ ions could drastically lower blood pH; however, the globin portions of hemoglobin absorb hydrogen ions, and HCO_3^- diffuses out of red blood cells and into plasma.

The remaining CO_2 diffuses out of blood across pulmonary capillary walls and into the alveoli.

Decrease in plasma CO_2 concentration causes the reverse reaction, also catalyzed by carbonic anhydrase for the release of $CO_2 + H_2O$ from the body:

$$H^+ + HCO_3^- \leftrightarrow H_2CO_3 \leftrightarrow CO_2 + H_2O$$

Notes for active learning

CHAPTER 7

Circulatory System

Circulatory System Structure

Blood Pressure and Cardiac Cycle

Circulation Pathways

Arterial and Venous Systems

Arterial and Venous Regulation

Oxygen and Carbon Dioxide Transport

Exchange Mechanisms

Blood

Cardiovascular Diseases

Page intentionally left blank

Circulatory System Structure

Network for transporting gases, nutrients and hormones

Circulatory systems regulate *thermoregulation* (i.e., body temperature), *transport*, *fluid balance*, and *immune system* function. It transports O_2, CO_2, nutrients, waste, and hormones.

Blood components direct fluid *retention* or *excretion* and maintain appropriate blood volume and composition. They affect how materials move out of or into the bloodstream from surrounding tissues.

Gases are taken in or released via respiration, and nutrients are absorbed from the small intestine and distributed to tissues via the bloodstream.

Blood filtration is at the kidneys and liver; waste and poisons are metabolized and removed.

Steroid and peptide hormones are circulated via bloodstream, allowing cellular communication.

Circulatory system protects the body by facilitating the movement of immune system cells.

Role in thermoregulation

Circulatory system maintains core body temperature by redirecting blood flow to the skin and extremities.

When temperatures drop, the body initiates *vasoconstriction* of the blood vessels to the skin, reducing blood flow near the surface and thus limiting heat loss to the air.

Conversely, elevated temperatures cause *vasodilation* of blood vessels, increasing blood flow to the skin and promoting heat loss to the surroundings.

Four-chambered heart structure and function

Heart is a cone-shaped, muscular organ about the size of a fist between the lungs and directly behind the sternum. It circulates blood throughout the body by a rhythmic pumping action.

Heart chambers are lined with epithelial tissue in the *endocardium*.

Epicardium is the outermost tissue.

Myocardium (i.e., cardiac muscle) is the thick middle layer and the bulk of the heart.

Cardiac muscle is entirely under the control of hormones and involuntary control by the autonomic nervous system. Unlike skeletal muscle, it has branching bands of muscle fibers connected by *intercalated disks*.

Intercalated disks allow electrical signals to travel through cardiac muscle, which contracts as a unit.

Unlike the multi-nucleated skeletal muscle cells, cardiac muscle cells have a single nucleus.

Heart is surrounded by a double-layered *pericardium sac*, cushioned by the *pericardial fluid*.

Connective tissue separates the *four chambers* of the heart.

Septum is an internal wall that divides the heart into its right and left halves.

Each half of the heart contains an upper, thin-walled *atrium* and a lower, thick-walled *ventricle*.

Atria and ventricles

Four chambers function as a double-sided pump.

Atria are thinner and weaker than the muscular ventricles but hold the same blood volume.

Each atrium receives blood from the veins (i.e., blood flowing towards the heart) and delivers it to its respective ventricles through a valve.

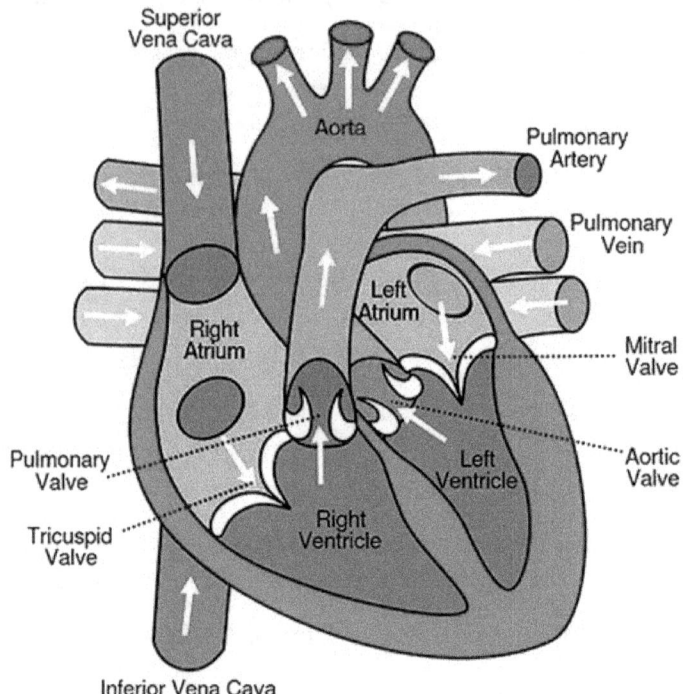

Heart has four chambers, blood vessels, and valves and routes blood through the body

Ventricles pump blood through arteries (i.e., flowing away from the heart), regulated by a valve.

Atrioventricular valve is between the atria and ventricles.

Semilunar valve (half-moon shape when closed) is between the ventricles and arteries.

Heart valves are supported by *chordae tendineae* (i.e., strong fibrous tendons) attached to muscular projections of ventricular walls to prevent valves from inverting.

Deoxygenated blood from the body enters the *right atrium* through two prominent veins:

superior vena cava and the *inferior vena cava.*

Tricuspid and semilunar valves

Right atrium sends blood to right ventricle through right *atrioventricular* (or *tricuspid*) valve.

Tricuspid valve has three flaps, which shut when the *right ventricle contracts,* so blood does not flow back into the right atrium.

Right ventricle ejects blood through the *pulmonary semilunar valve* into the *pulmonary arteries.*

Pulmonary arteries carry *deoxygenated blood*; others carry oxygen-rich blood.

Pulmonary semilunar valve prevents backflow into the right ventricle from pulmonary arteries.

Pulmonary arteries deliver the *deoxygenated blood to the lungs.*

Oxygenated blood returns from the lungs by *pulmonary veins* and is delivered to the *left atrium.*

Left atrium pumps this newly oxygenated blood through the left atrioventricular valve (*bicuspid* or *mitral valve*) to the *left ventricle.*

Blood is ejected into the aorta (i.e., the largest artery) through the aortic semilunar valve in the left ventricle.

Left ventricle is the strongest and thickest chamber of the heart since it must pump blood throughout the body. This blood delivers oxygen to the body tissues and returns deoxygenated blood to the right atrium to restart the cycle.

Right atrium and ventricle are separated from the left atrium and ventricle so that oxygenated blood does not mix with deoxygenated blood.

Blood is pumped out of the heart through one set of vessels and returns to the heart via another. This structure ensures appropriate blood pressure and gas concentrations in different areas of the circulatory system.

Endothelial cells in heart and blood vessels

Heart and blood vessels are lined with *endothelium,* a thin layer of *endothelial cells.* This semi-permeable layer controls the passage of cells and molecules in and out of the bloodstream.

Endothelial cells help prevent *blood clots* and *plaque formation* and facilitate an *inflammation response* to invasive agents and damaged cells.

Basal muscle tone is a muscle's passive baseline resistance to stretching, which varies. Endothelial cells can rapidly change a blood vessel's smooth muscle tone from its basal level. Hormones and nerve signals regulate this *vasoconstriction* and *vasodilation.*

Endothelial cells control blood pressure by producing *nitric oxide* (a potent vasodilator) and *endothelial-1* (i.e., a potent vasoconstrictor). Controlled nitric oxide production is essential to maintaining basal tone and balanced blood pressure.

Endothelial cells are involved in *angiogenesis*, the formation of new capillaries. This process is vital to wound healing and the formation of collateral vessels, which provide alternate routes for blood flow during a circulatory system blockage.

Blood Pressure and Cardiac Cycle

Systolic and diastolic blood pressure

Blood pressure is the pressure blood exerts on the walls of the blood vessels. It is usually measured in the arteries since blood pressure is strongest.

Systolic pressure is measured as ventricles contract, and blood is forcefully ejected from heart.

Diastolic pressure is when blood is not pumped, and the ventricles relax.

Systolic pressure is the maximum and is higher than diastolic blood pressure. Reference blood pressure is 120 (systolic) over 80 (diastolic).

Both measurements of blood pressure represent a stage of a single heartbeat.

Systole is the phase of contraction and blood ejection. When the term systole is used alone, it only refers to the ventricles. During ventricular systole, the atria are relaxed (i.e., in *diastole*).

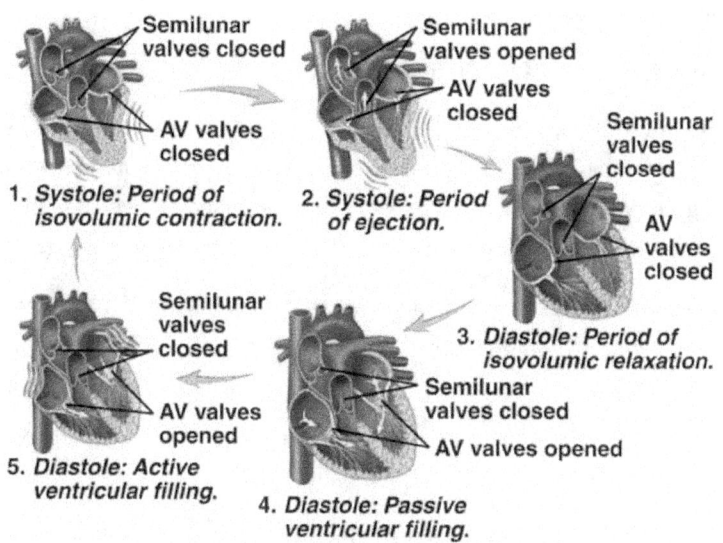

Valves of the heart open and close during rhythmic contractions of the atria and ventricles

Diastole and systole are the *cardiac cycle*, known as a *heartbeat,* and lasts 0.85 seconds.

Systole is 0.30 seconds, and diastole is 0.55 seconds.

The heart beats about 70 times a minute in an average adult and undergoes over 3 billion contraction cycles during the average lifetime.

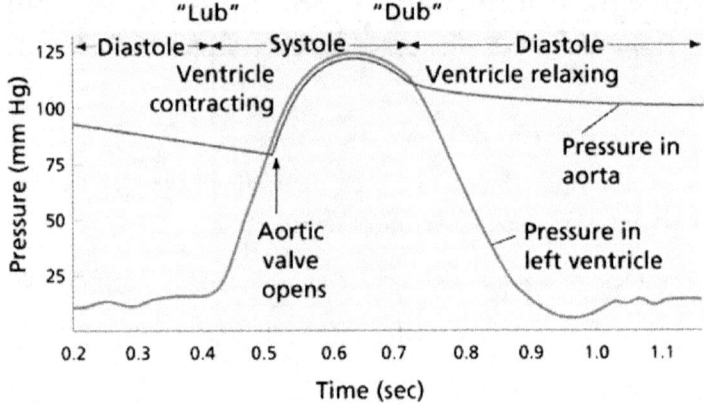

Blood pressure vs. time cardiac cycle

Cardiac cycle

Lub-dub sound is when the heart beats as the heart *valves close*.

"Lub" results from the vibrations of the heart when the atrioventricular valves close.

"Dub" is heard as semilunar valves close.

Lub and dub sounds mark divisions in the cardiac cycle.

At the beginning of systole, *atrioventricular valves* close and cause the *lub* sound. Semilunar valves have already been closed for some time. The ventricles contract while all valves are closed, building up pressure in the ventricles before the blood is ejected. This is *isovolumetric ventricular contraction*, as the blood volume in the heart remains the same (*iso-*).

At 0.10 seconds into systole, semilunar valves open as ventricles contract, expelling blood from the right ventricle into the pulmonary artery and out of the left ventricle into the aorta. This is a *ventricular ejection*.

Blood volume ejected from each ventricle is *stroke volume* (SV), while the amount of blood remaining after ejection is the *end-systolic volume* (ESV).

At the end of an ejection, semilunar valves close and generate the dub sound. This marks the beginning of diastole when all the chambers rest for 0.40 seconds.

The first part of diastole is *isovolumetric ventricular relaxation,* as the semilunar valves close and the ventricles relax. In the next phase, *passive ventricular filling,* the atrioventricular valves open, allowing blood from the atria to fill the ventricles passively. There is still no contraction in either the atria or ventricles.

In the last 0.15 seconds of ventricular diastole, atrial systole occurs; the atria contracts and actively fills the ventricles. This period is *active ventricular filling.*

End-diastolic volume (EDV) is the amount of blood in the ventricle at the end of diastole.

Stroke volume is calculated by subtracting end-systolic volume from end-diastolic volume:

$$SV = EDV - ESV.$$

The atrioventricular valves close, and the cycle repeats as the ventricles re-enter systole.

Contraction strength is not constant but increases in response to greater stretch up to an *optimum length* (OL). A higher volume of blood entering the ventricles (i.e., a greater EDV) stretches the ventricular muscles and stimulates a more forceful contraction. This empties the ventricles more entirely and results in a lower ESV.

Frank-Starling mechanism is whereby a greater EDV produces stronger contraction. The overall effect of a higher EDV and a lower ESV is a higher stroke volume.

Pulse rate

Pulse is measured in arteries far from the heart since it is a wave effect that passes arterial blood vessels' walls. The pulse occurs when the aorta expands and immediately recoils following ventricular systole. Since there is one arterial pulse per ventricular systole, the arterial pulse rate determines the heart rate.

For adults, an average pulse rate (resting heart rate) is between 60 and 100 beats per minute (bpm); children have high resting pulse rates.

Generally, a lower heart rate (i.e., bradycardia) implies an efficient heart function and better cardiovascular fitness (e.g., a well-conditioned athlete may have a pulse rate closer to 40 bpm).

Bradycardia is a low heart rate (less than 60 bpm), while *tachycardia* is greater than 100 bpm.

Cardiac control of heart rate

Intrinsic and extrinsic stimulation controls the circulatory system.

Intrinsic stimulation comes from the *sinoatrial* (SA) node's pulses as the heart's " pacemaker " in the right atrium's upper dorsal wall initiates the heartbeat.

Cardiac muscle cells in the SA node are self-exciting and initiate contraction in nearby cells.

The SA node's capacity for spontaneous, rhythmical self-excitation results from gradual depolarization, the *pacemaker potential*, of the cells.

Depolarization quickly spreads to the left atrium when the node spontaneously generates an excitatory impulse, and the two atria contract simultaneously.

After a slight delay, the action potential spreads through the *atrioventricular* (AV) *node* at the right atrium base close to the septum. The delay in the action potential allows atrial contraction to be completed before the ventricles contract.

AV bundles extend from the node toward the ventricles and carry the signal to the bottom of the heart, branching into *Purkinje fibers*. These fibers cause rapid contraction of the ventricles.

The long refractory period of cardiac muscle cells limits the re-excitation of neurons. It ensures that there is time for the chamber to fill with blood before the next contraction occurs.

Tetanus is when skeletal muscle remains contracted and cannot relax.

The heart may experience many arrhythmias (i.e., abnormal heart rate patterns) due to disruptions in the heart's electrical conduction system.

Tachycardia (i.e., high heart rate) and *bradycardia* (i.e., low heart rate) are two arrhythmias.

EKG and fibrillation

Fibrillation is a rapid, abnormal heartbeat that can affect the atria and ventricles.

Atrial fibrillation is concerning but typically not an emergency, while *ventricular fibrillation* is an emergency that usually accompanies a cardiac arrest.

SA node may reestablish a coordinated beat with a strong electric current.

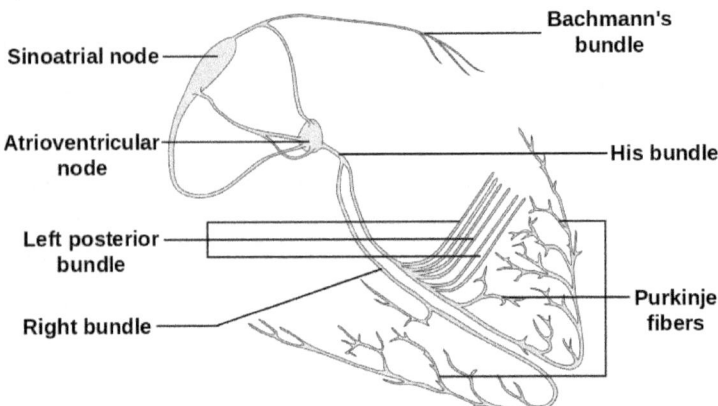

Electrocardiogram monitors electrical charges during cardiac contractions.

Electrocardiograms (ECG or EKG) diagnose arrhythmias and heart abnormalities by recording the electrical changes in the myocardium during a cardiac cycle.

Contraction pulses generate currents in extracellular fluids, recorded at the skin's surface.

EKG typically consists of five deflections:

>P wave, Q wave, R wave, S wave, and T wave.

Heart innervation:

>Heartbeat originates in SA node → AV node → bundle of His → Purkinje fibers for ventricular contraction.

The heart may spontaneously generate electrical impulses, but nervous and endocrine signals control the rate of these impulses.

Heart is innervated by both the parasympathetic and sympathetic nervous systems.

Stimulation of the parasympathetic fibers, such as the *vagus nerve*, decreases heart rate and force of contraction. This may occur in response to rest or hypertension.

Parasympathetic neurons release the neurotransmitter *acetylcholine,* which increases the time required to reach the threshold voltage necessary to initiate an action potential.

During rest, the parasympathetic nervous system dominates and diverts blood flow to the gastrointestinal tract to aid digestion.

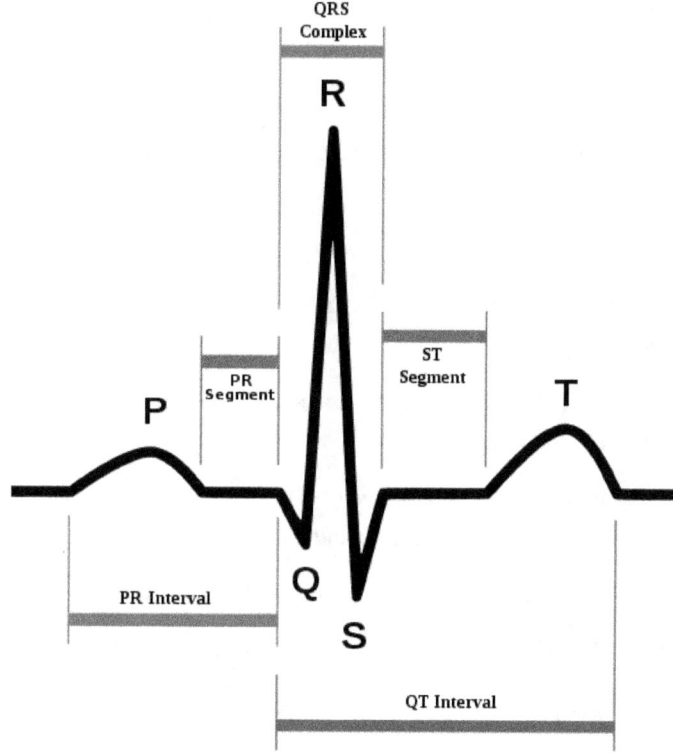

Electrocardiogram illustrates the electrical charges during a cardiac cycle

Cardiac cycle can be recorded by an electrocardiogram (EKG).

P wave represents depolarization of the atria; it occurs during atrial contraction.

QRS complex represents rapid depolarization of the ventricles, signaling that the ventricles are contracting. It has a much larger amplitude than the P wave.

Atrial repolarization occurs at this time but is obscured by the activity of the QRS complex.

T wave represents the repolarization of the ventricles as their muscle fibers recover.

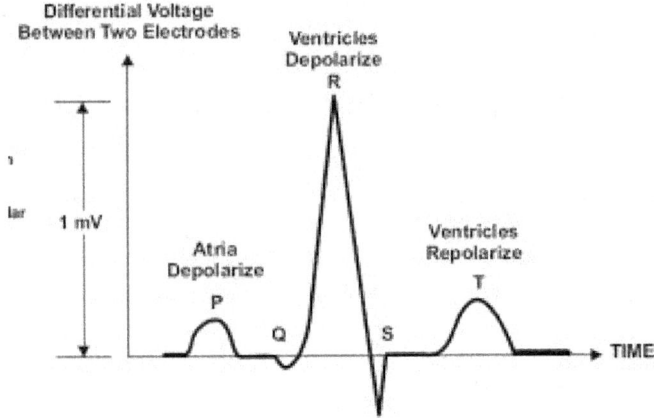

EKG with corresponding atria and ventricular depolarization and repolarization

Neural and hormonal control of heart rate

Stimulation of sympathetic *fibers* increases heart rate and force of contraction.

Sympathetic neurons release *norepinephrine*, which binds to receptors on the SA node's cardiac muscle cells, increasing calcium ion uptake.

Higher intracellular calcium levels allow cells to rapidly reach the threshold voltage, increasing heart rate and contractility.

Sympathetic responses are activated during exercise; blood flow is redirected to muscles, cardiac output increases, and constriction occurs in the veins to help return blood to the heart.

Kidney adrenal medulla releases *epinephrine* (i.e., adrenaline) in response to stress and other stimuli. This acts similarly to norepinephrine and causes a sympathetic heart rate increase.

Circulatory responses occur in the heart and throughout the systemic and pulmonary circulation.

Various receptors monitor conditions throughout the circulatory system.

The receptors may be *peripheral* (in blood vessels) or *central* (in the brain).

Peripheral receptors often transmit the signal to the brain to conduct responses. However, blood vessels can respond to stimuli with a local reflex. For example, the walls of arterioles automatically constrict in response to stretching.

Chemoreceptors and baroreceptors

Chemoreceptors monitor pH, oxygen, and carbon dioxide levels.

Peripheral chemoreceptors are in the aorta and carotid arteries and transmit signals to the *cardiovascular control center* (CVCC) in the *medulla oblongata* of the brain.

Central chemoreceptors are in the *medulla*, measuring gas levels and pH in the brain. If receptors detect that oxygen levels are low, carbon dioxide levels are high, or pH is low, the body attempts to increase gas exchange to compensate. This occurs due to exercise.

Sympathetic nervous system stimulates an increase in heart rate and stroke volume, resulting in higher cardiac output. This causes more rapid blood flow through the lungs, the rapid release of excess carbon dioxide, and oxygen uptake.

Selective vasoconstriction delivers oxygen to the tissues that need it most. In the long term, *angiogenesis* ensures these tissues receive greater oxygen.

Baroreceptors are in the carotid arteries, aorta, and medulla. They work with chemoreceptors to control blood pressure by continually adjusting vasoconstriction and vasodilation.

Arterial pressure drop causes the carotid and aortic baroreceptors to signal the medulla to immediately initiate a *sympathetic* response of *vasoconstriction* and *higher cardiac output*.

In the long term, the kidneys retain fluids to maintain blood volume.

Arterial pressure increase stimulates the carotid baroreceptor reflex to initiate *vasodilation*.

Medulla decreases sympathetic and increases parasympathetic activity, lowering cardiac output to reduce blood pressure.

Over time, the kidneys increase urination to lower blood volume.

Notes for active learning

Circulation Pathways

Pulmonary and systemic circulation

Cardiovascular system has two circulation pathways.

Systemic circulation is the loop between the heart and nearly all arteries, capillaries, and veins.

Pulmonary circulation is the path from the heart to the pulmonary arteries, capillaries, veins, and heart. This is the only part of the circulatory system where arteries transport *deoxygenated* blood, and veins transport *oxygenated* blood.

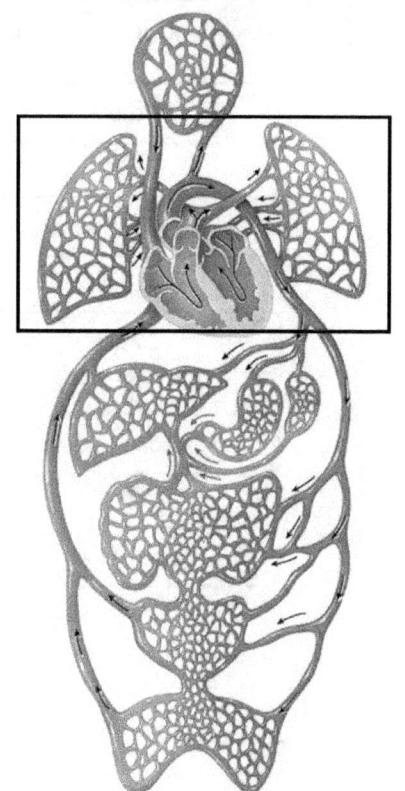

Pulmonary (enlarged) between heart and lungs and systemic circulation between heart and body

Blood pressure is lower in pulmonary circulation since the blood vessels are shorter and have less *vascular resistance* to blood flow.

Pulmonary circulation begins when deoxygenated blood from systemic circulation enters the right atrium and drains to the right ventricle through the right atrioventricular (tricuspid) valve. Blood is ejected through the pulmonary semilunar valve into right and left pulmonary arteries.

Pulmonary arteries branch often into hundreds of thousands of *pulmonary capillaries* in lungs.

Pulmonary capillaries surround *alveoli,* the tiny sacs in which gas exchange occurs.

Carbon dioxide and water from blood diffuse through the alveoli and are exhaled, while oxygen is inhaled and diffuses into the blood.

Oxygenated blood returns to the heart's *left atrium* via the *pulmonary vein.*

Once oxygenated, blood returns to the heart and is delivered through the left atrioventricular (bicuspid or mitral) valve into the left ventricle. It is pumped from the left ventricle into the aorta via the aortic semilunar valve.

Systemic circulation begins as oxygenated blood travels through the body.

Blood flow

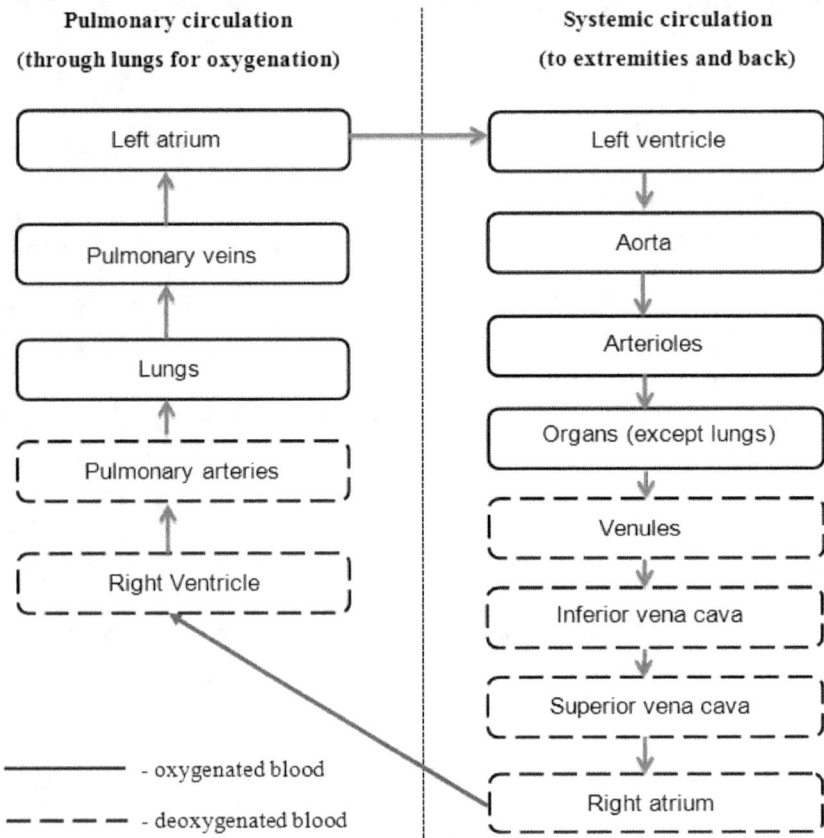

Fetal blood pathway

In a fetus, circulation is more complicated since the fetal lungs are immersed in the fluid and cannot perform gas exchange (O_2 from inspiration and CO_2 released from expiration).

Oxygenated, nutrient-rich blood from the maternal side of the placenta is carried to the fetus via the *umbilical vein*. Most of this blood passes through the liver before entering the inferior vena cava, but some bypass the liver via the *ductus venosus*.

Oxygenated blood ends up in the inferior vena cava and enters the right atrium. From the right atrium, most blood flows directly into the left atrium via the *foramen ovale*, which allows blood to bypass the fetal pulmonary circulation.

Foramen ovale in the fetus is in the septum of the heart, which must close before or shortly after birth to avoid heart abnormalities.

Blood enters the left ventricle from the left atrium and is ejected into the aorta, circulating throughout the body. Once fully deoxygenated, the blood flows back into the placenta via the two *umbilical arteries* to be replenished.

Fetal blood that did not pass through the *foramen ovale* enters the right ventricle and is pumped into the pulmonary artery. This is mixed blood but is mostly deoxygenated.

Ductus arteriosus is a vessel branching from the pulmonary artery and joining the aorta, shunting most deoxygenated blood into the aorta.

Therefore, mixed blood travels from the aorta throughout the fetus' body.

Only some blood in the fetal *pulmonary artery* travels throughout the pulmonary circulation and is returned via the pulmonary veins.

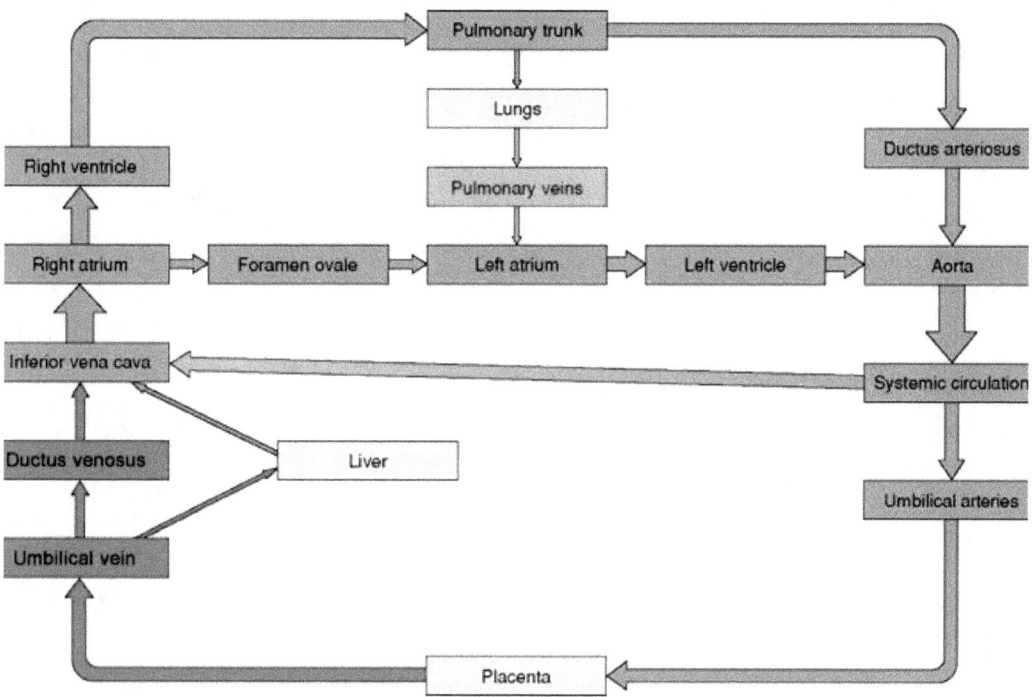

Fetal circulation is the pathway of blood before the lungs function for gas exchange. Note the foramen ovale and ductus arteriosus.

Notes for active learning

Arterial and Venous Systems

Arteries, capillaries and veins

Arteries are the thickest and strongest blood vessels, followed by veins, arterioles, venules, and capillaries.

Sympathetic nervous system innervates the walls of arteries, arterioles, veins, and large venules.

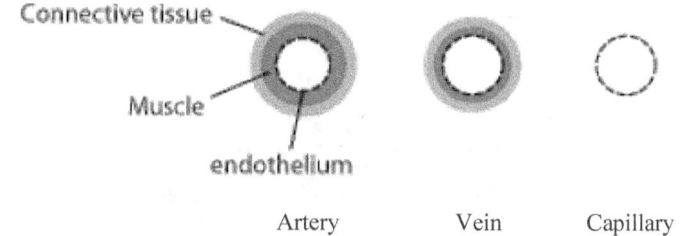

Cross-sectional comparison of the three main vessels of the circulatory system

The aorta is the body's largest and thickest artery. It arches and branches into the upper body's major arteries before descending through the diaphragm, where it branches into arteries supplying the lower parts of the body.

Arteries become capillaries near organs and tissues to exchange gases, nutrients, and waste.

Capillaries merge into venules and veins as blood returns to the heart. Veins of the lower body coalesce into the *inferior vena cava*, while those of the upper body coalesce into the *superior vena cava*.

Superior and *inferior vena cava* empty into the right atrium, so blood may enter pulmonary circulation and be re-oxygenated.

When oxygen levels are low, systemic capillaries that feed tissues needing oxygen undergo vasodilation to deliver more blood to where it is needed most.

By contrast, pulmonary capillaries, which feed low-oxygen alveoli, undergo vasoconstriction so that blood is diverted to alveoli where gas exchange (uptake of O_2) is efficient.

Coronary circulation supplies blood to the heart itself. *Coronary arteries* originate from the aorta and feed into capillaries that cover the heart and nourish myocardial cells.

Deoxygenated blood from the coronary capillaries drains into the *cardiac veins,* which merge directly into the right atrium.

Blocked flow in coronary arteries can result in chest pain and heart attacks.

Structural and functional differences

Circulatory system is divided into arterial, capillary, and venous portions.

Arterial system carries blood away from the heart.

Systemic arteries carry *oxygenated* blood from *the heart to the body*.

Pulmonary arteries carry *deoxygenated* blood from *the heart to the lungs*.

Arteries are large, thick, and elastic, with multi-layered connective tissue walls, smooth muscle, and endothelium. The outermost layer is made of longitudinal collagen and elastic fibers to avoid leaks and bulges (i.e., an aneurysm).

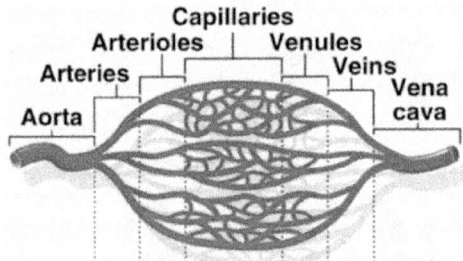

Blood is received from the arteries, and gas exchange occurs at the capillaries before blood returns to the heart through the veins

Within the connective tissue layers are circular smooth muscle and elastic fibers, which maintain muscle tone and contract to force blood through vessels.

An inner layer of endothelium lines the narrow lumen.

The strong, elastic arterial walls can maintain high blood pressure in the arterial system and aid in pumping blood throughout the body.

During *systole*, the contraction of ventricles ejects blood into arteries, distending arterial walls.

During *diastole*, the walls recoil elastically and force blood through.

There is always blood in the arteries to keep them semi-inflated, so diastolic blood pressure is not zero (averages 80 mmHg).

Artery types

Three major arteries are elastic, muscular, and coronary arteries.

Elastic arteries include the aorta and its major branches. They are the largest, thickest, and most elastic of arteries, providing an elastic pipe for blood directly out of the heart. Elastic arteries are *not able* to undergo *vasoconstriction.*

Muscular arteries (distributing arteries) distribute blood to specific organs. They contain a large amount of smooth muscle to direct blood flow and participate in vasoconstriction.

Coronary arteries supply and nourish the heart. They originate from the base of the aorta above the aortic semilunar valve and branch across the heart's outer surface, the epicardium.

Arterioles are smaller vessels that branch from the arteries. They have walls of an endothelium, smooth muscle, and connective tissue, but these layers are thin.

Arterioles are active in vasoconstriction and vasodilation, allowing the body to redirect and control blood flow and pressure.

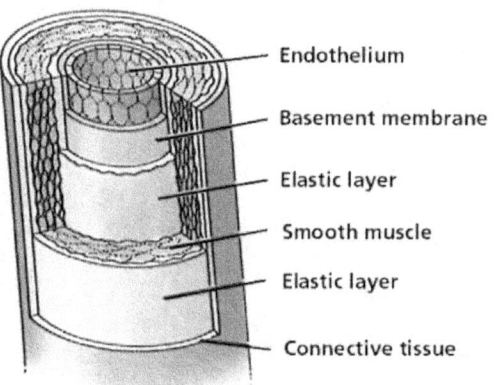

Distributing artery cross section

Capillaries as the site of diffusion

Small arterioles branch into a network of *capillary beds.*

Capillary beds surround organs and tissues and connect the arterial and venous systems.

Capillaries are microscopic blood vessels that contain no muscle or connective tissue, a single layer of endothelial cells across which gases, nutrients, enzymes, hormones, and wastes diffuse.

Capillaries in the body span approximately 60,000 miles in total, permeating every tissue to exchange nutrients, gases, and metabolic byproducts.

Capillaries concentrate around organs such as the liver and intestines, which undergo high metabolic activity levels.

Blood velocity decreases as blood flows through capillaries because the total cross-sectional area of capillaries is relatively large.

Narrow, water-filled spaces often separate endothelial cells of a capillary as *intercellular clefts*.

Three capillaries are continuous capillaries:

fenestrated capillary, and sinusoidal capillary.

Continuous capillaries contain no pores on endothelial cells, but many have clefts at cell boundaries. They exchange materials through their clefts or via endocytosis and exocytosis. Continuous capillaries are predominantly in the skin, muscles, and cranium, where their tight junctions seal the blood-brain barrier.

Fenestrated capillaries contain tiny pores large enough for molecules to leak through but not blood cells. They are predominantly in the small intestine (facilitate nutrient absorption), in the endocrine glands (allow passage of hormones), and in the kidneys (filter blood).

Sinusoidal capillaries contain pores large enough for blood cells to pass through. They are primarily in lymphoid tissues, the liver, and bone marrow. They facilitate lymphocyte travel and blood cell modifications.

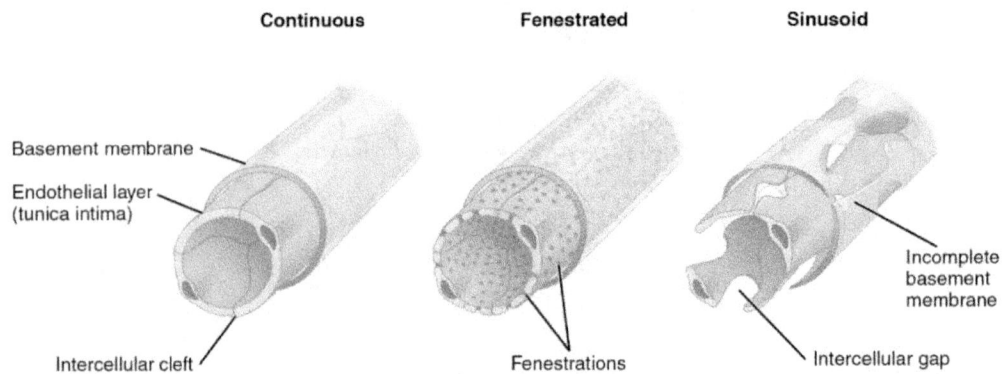

Capillary beds have two kinds of vessels: *true capillaries* (involved in the exchange between cells and blood) and *metarterioles* (which allow some blood to bypass the capillary bed).

Metarterioles directly connect the arteriole and venules on opposite sides of the bed.

Capillaries branch from the arterial side of the metarteriole, connecting as a muscular sphincter.

Contraction of the sphincters shuts blood flow to the bed and causes blood to pass directly to the venule.

During exercise, metarterioles divert blood from the capillary beds of the skin and digestive organs so it is directed to the muscles.

Autoregulation permits constant blood flow in capillary beds because arterioles reflexively stretch and constrict to counteract pressure changes.

Capillary angiogenesis is continuous in response to growth, injury, and changing metabolic activity. This process is activated by growth factors that direct partial digestion of an existing capillary to split in two or "sprout" a new capillary.

Angiogenesis is active in wound repair, muscle development, tumor formation, and fat deposition since these processes require an increased blood supply to the new tissues.

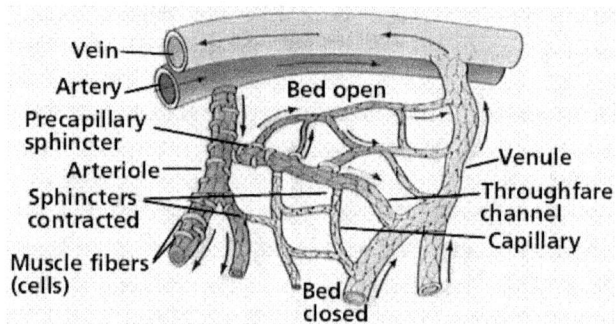

Capillary beds with metarteriole

Venules and veins return blood to the heart

After blood from the systemic arterial system exchanges nutrients and wastes with the capillaries of organs and tissues, deoxygenated blood leaves the capillaries and flows into the systemic *venous system*.

Venous system vessels (e.g., venules, veins) are thinner, porous, and less elastic. They contain an outer layer of *fibrous connective tissue*, a middle layer of *smooth muscle and elastic tissue*, and an *endothelium inner layer*.

Vasoconstriction and dilation occur in the venous system.

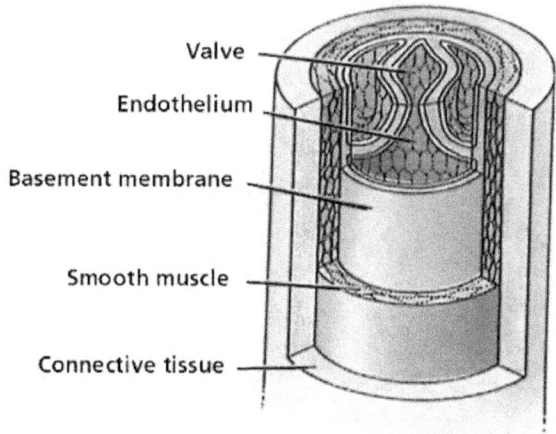

Veins with valves and without a thick layer of smooth muscle, as in arteries

Venules, thin and porous, are analogous to arterioles. They gather blood from capillary beds and merge into larger veins.

Veins have thicker and more resistant walls but are still weaker than arteries: their thin walls and wide lumens lower venous blood pressure than arterial blood pressure.

Unlike arteries, veins collapse when they contain little blood and are compressed by neighboring skeletal muscles. The squeezing of skeletal muscles helps the low-pressure, slow-moving blood travel to the heart.

Veins depend on the action of the diaphragm and its smooth muscle walls to deliver blood to the heart. Larger veins have valves that prevent blood's backflow when moving against gravity.

Not all blood received from the capillaries is immediately delivered to the heart. For example, blood from the gastrointestinal capillary beds is first delivered to the liver to process and filter nutrients via the *hepatic portal vein*.

Hepatic vein leaves the liver and enters the inferior vena cava. Blood below the diaphragm returns through the *inferior vena cava*, while blood from the upper body returns through the *superior vena cava*.

Arterial and Venous Regulation

Cardiac output

Pressure differential between the high-pressure arteries and low-pressure veins facilitate blood flow throughout the circulatory system.

At a basic level, the flow can be calculated by the following equation:

$$F = \Delta P / R$$

where ΔP is the difference in pressure between two points, and R is *resistance to flow*.

Total peripheral resistance (TPR) is resistance throughout the circulatory system. TPR is a function of blood vessel diameter, length, and viscosity.

Cardiac output (CO) is blood flow rate from heart; equals stroke volume (SV) per minute:

$$CO = HR \text{ (heart rate)} \times SV$$

CO is increased by a significant increase in heart rate, resulting from increased sinoatrial node (SA) activity. A slight increase in SV is caused by increased ventricular contractility mediated by sympathetic activity.

Frank-Starling mechanism accounts for an increase in end-diastolic volume.

Blood velocity describes the speed at which blood moves through a vessel.

Since the blood volume flow rate (or *cardiac output*) is approximately constant, blood velocity depends on the total cross-sectional area.

Bernoulli's principle states that velocity is inversely proportional to cross-sectional area and is calculated by dividing cardiac output by the vessel's cross-sectional area.

Blood pressure is highest in arteries and decreases as it travels to arterioles, capillaries, venules, and veins. It depends on cardiac output, resistance to flow, total blood volume, vessel elasticity, and other factors.

Systemic arterial blood pressure is usually measured, but systemic venous blood pressure is of interest. Additionally, the pressure in the pulmonary circulation is measured.

The difference between systolic and diastolic pressure is *pulse pressure* (PP), while the average is *mean arterial pressure* (MAP).

MAP is calculated by multiplying cardiac output by *total peripheral resistance* (TPR).

$$MAP = CO \times TPR$$

Blood pressure is highest in the arteries for several reasons: arteries are closest to the heart's forceful ejections, have a small cross-sectional area, and have high resistance. Arterioles have the greatest resistance to flow since they are most capable of vasoconstriction, but the aorta has the highest pressure since it is closest to the heart.

Valves regulate blood flow in veins

Veins have the lowest blood pressure because the force of cardiac output diminishes over time, and a larger cross-sectional area provides less resistance.

Veins require *skeletal muscle pump* (i.e., *skeletal muscle contraction*), *respiratory pump* (diaphragm), and *valve* action to maintain flow.

Blood volume is an essential determinant of venous pressure. At any given time, most of the blood is in veins. Walls of veins are less elastic; they can stretch to accommodate large volumes of blood without recoiling (i.e., resisting flow).

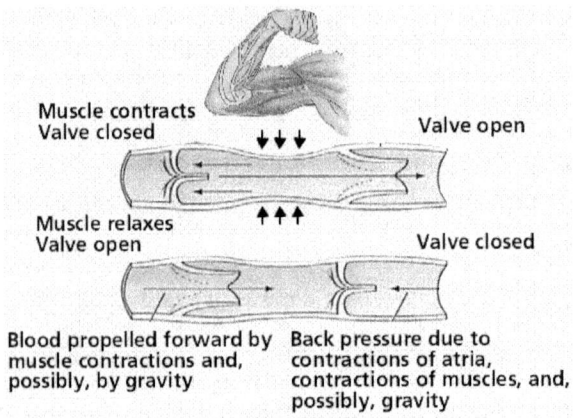

Venous blood system used values for unidirectional blood flow towards the heart

Consequently, veins have low blood pressure, and vasoconstriction is necessary to increase blood pressure and drive blood towards the heart.

Varicose veins are abnormal distention developing when veins' valves become weak and ineffective. Commonly, they are in the back of the legs and pool blood under gravity pressure.

Capillaries have slow and even blood flow due to their high total cross-sectional area. Capillaries are the narrowest vessels, but the total cross-sectional area is higher than other vessels.

There is a decrease in the effective systemic circulating blood volume during a transition from horizontal to vertical body positioning.

Blood vessels are at same level in a horizontal position, and all pressure is due to cardiac output.

In a vertical position, there is additional pressure at every point below the heart, equal to the weight of the blood column above. This results in distension of blood vessels due to the pooling of blood (e.g., varicose veins) and increased capillary filtration in the lower parts of the body.

The contraction of skeletal muscles in the legs can offset gravity's effect on pooling blood. People can faint when standing for extended periods because of blood pooling in the lower extremities and less blood flow to the brain.

Systemic circulation is a high-pressure system, while pulmonary circulation is low-pressure. Therefore, the right ventricle is weaker than left ventricle since it does not need to work as hard.

Pulmonary circulation has shorter blood vessels and requires less force to work against gravity. The elasticity and lack of smooth muscle in pulmonary vessels decrease resistance.

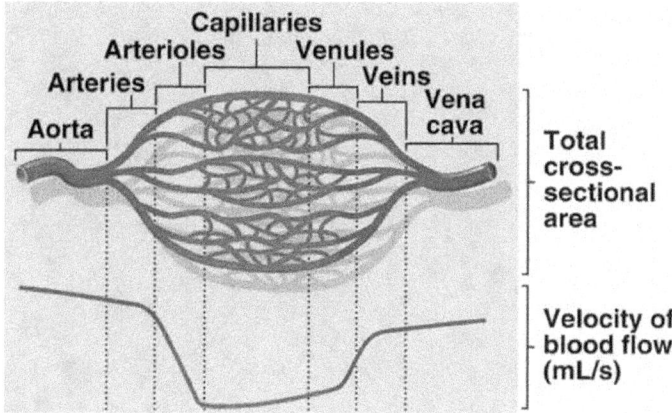

Relationship between total cross-sectional area and velocity of blood flow

Blood volume and pressure

Human blood pressure is usually measured at the upper arm's brachial artery, reflecting systemic arterial pressure due to the contraction and relaxation of the right ventricle.

Sphygmomanometer uses a pressure cuff to measure blood pressure. Healthy young adults have a systolic pressure of about 120 mmHg and a diastolic pressure of 80 mmHg (mm of mercury).

Hypotension is low blood pressure due to low blood volume, excessive vasodilation, anemia, or heart conditions. If prolonged, hypotension can lead to *arrhythmia* (irregular heartbeat), dizziness, and fainting.

Shock is severe hypotension that may cause tissues or organ damage due to reduced blood flow.

Hypovolemic shock, in which blood volume is reduced, may be caused by severe external bleeding (i.e., hemorrhage), dehydration, diarrhea, or vomiting.

Blood volume refers to the dissolved substances in the blood and not the fluid itself; therefore, a person can have a healthy 5 liters of blood but be hypovolemia due to a lack of electrolytes.

Low-resistance shock is a consequence of excessive vasodilation, which may occur due to endocrine or nervous system malfunction, weakened blood vessels, and various drugs.

Cardiogenic shock is when heart conditions reduce cardiac output to dangerous levels. Severe cardiogenic shock may be due to a heart attack and cardiac arrest.

When the body detects hypotension, it activates the sympathetic nervous system, promptly increasing stroke volume, heart rate, and total peripheral resistance to raise mean arterial pressure. Interstitial fluid enters the bloodstream due to reduced capillary pressure.

Over time, fluid ingestion and kidney excretion are altered, and erythropoiesis (i.e., red blood cell production) is stimulated to replace blood volume.

Usually, the body can rapidly offset hypotension, but it is fatal if it is severe and long-lasting.

Oxygen and Carbon Dioxide Transport

Hemoglobin and hematocrit

Vertebrates use red-colored pigment hemoglobin to increase blood's oxygen-carrying capacity.

Hemoglobin includes a tetrameric *globin* protein that surrounds a *heme* group. Heme is an iron-containing molecule that loosely binds to a single O_2 molecule.

Hematocrit is the percentage of blood volume made of erythrocytes. It is a valuable measure of a person's ability to transport oxygen.

Low hematocrit indicates *anemia,* which is a reduced ability to carry oxygen in the blood.

Anemia causes fatigue and weakness due to decreased O_2 circulation. It may be due to an abnormally low concentration of healthy, functional erythrocytes, insufficient hemoglobin, or a combination.

Anemia can occur due to blood loss, iron, vitamin B12 deficiency, abnormal erythrocytes, insufficient erythrocyte production, or excessive erythrocyte destruction.

Sickle cell anemia

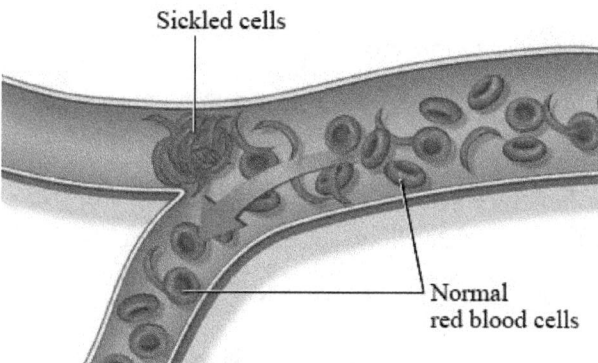

In sickle cell anemia, the red blood cells are shaped like sickles (a crescent moon) and become rigid and sticky. Due to their irregular shape, these cells can get stuck in small blood vessels (capillaries), slowing or blocking blood flow to the body.

Oxygen content of blood

Hemoglobin is a *tetramer* with *four heme groups* per hemoglobin and *four O_2 binding sites.*

With millions of hemoglobin molecules per erythrocyte, the blood can carry 70 times more oxygen than if dissolved in plasma.

It is more difficult for animals to obtain O_2 from water than from the air.

Water fully saturated with air contains only a fraction of the O_2 as the same air volume, and water is denser than air; therefore, aquatic animals must use more energy to breathe.

Fish use up to 25% of their energy to breathe, while land mammals use only 1–2%. The tradeoff is that air dries out wet respiratory surfaces, and as a result, humans lose 350 ml of water per day at 50% relative humidity.

Oxygen in the blood is measured by *partial pressure* (i.e., pO_2), *saturation*, or *total content*.

Partial pressure describes oxygen's contribution to the total pressure of gases in the blood.

Saturation refers to how many heme-binding sites are bound to oxygen in the blood.

Content is calculated by saturation, partial pressure, and hemoglobin concentration to determine the number of oxygen molecules in the blood.

Oxygen consumption increases proportionately to the magnitude of physical exercise up to maximal oxygen consumption – *VO_2 max*.

After VO_2 max is reached, an increase in exertion is sustained briefly by anaerobic metabolism.

Typically, VO_2 max is determined by cardiac output. It may be limited by carbon monoxide content, the respiratory system's ability to deliver oxygen to blood, and muscle oxygen use.

Oxygen affinity and dissociation curves

Inhaled oxygen diffuses into alveolar capillaries and binds to hemoglobin in erythrocytes. Oxygen is transported to tissues for cellular respiration.

A small amount of blood oxygen is carried as dissolved O_2 in plasma, but the majority is reversibly combined with hemoglobin molecules in erythrocytes.

Hemoglobin with no bonded oxygen is *deoxyhemoglobin* (Hb).

Hemoglobin bonded to oxygen is *oxyhemoglobin* (HbO_2).

The fraction of Hb as HbO_2 is the *percent of hemoglobin saturation*.

$$\% \text{ hemoglobin saturation} = \frac{O_2 \text{ bound to Hb} \times 100}{\text{Maximal capacity of Hb to bind } O_2}$$

When pO_2 is high, hemoglobin binds to oxygen to form oxyhemoglobin. Blood is fully saturated with oxygen when erythrocytes contain oxyhemoglobin. This occurs in the lungs, where oxygen content is highest.

In body tissues deprived of oxygen, pO_2 is low, and erythrocytes release oxygen from oxyhemoglobin, so oxygen diffuses into the plasma and tissue cells.

Oxygen dissociation curve shows the percent of oxyhemoglobin and non-bonded hemoglobin at various partial pressures of oxygen. Usually, a curve is labeled with the value at which the erythrocytes are fifty percent saturated with oxygen, the *p50 value.*

Hemoglobin has a sigmoidal oxygen dissociation curve because oxygen binding to one subunit somewhat relaxes the other subunits' conformation, resulting in easier binding for additional oxygen. This is *cooperative binding.*

When one O_2 molecule binds, the others bind with less difficulty.

Likewise, when one O_2 is released, the remaining O_2 is easily released.

Thus, oxygen has the highest affinity to hemoglobin when three of its four polypeptide chains are already bound to oxygen.

Myoglobin is a single-chain protein subunit similar to hemoglobin, responsible for carrying oxygen in muscle tissue. It saturates quickly and is released in emergencies of low oxygen when a burst of muscle movement is needed under reduced pO_2 conditions (e.g., swimming to the surface of a body of water after being submerged).

Myoglobin binds to oxygen tighter than hemoglobin, as it has a greater affinity towards oxygen but can bind only one O_2 molecule. This does not allow cooperative binding, giving myoglobin a *hyperbolic oxygen dissociation curve.*

Myoglobin curve does not change over a wide range of pH.

Myoglobin in bloodstream after muscle injury must be removed since it is toxic to the kidneys.

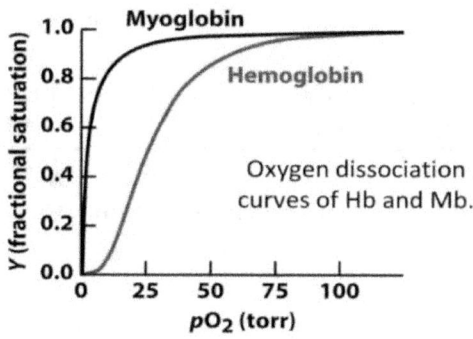

Myoglobin (hyperbolic) and hemoglobin (sigmoidal) dissociation curves

Bohr effects on the oxygen dissociation curves

Oxygen dissociation curve is not static and can *shift* to the right or left.

Right shift means that for a given pO_2, *less* O_2 is bound to hemoglobin.

Several conditions produce a right-shifted dissociation curve, including increased temperature, increased pCO_2, or decreased pH. Increasing temperature denatures the bond between oxygen and hemoglobin, naturally decreasing oxyhemoglobin concentration.

Bohr Effect describes how the oxygen dissociation curve is altered by pH and CO_2. It was proposed in 1904 to explain how H^+ and CO_2 affect the affinity of O_2 for hemoglobin.

Affinity of O_2 for hemoglobin is *inversely related* to acidity ($\uparrow H^+$) and pCO_2 levels.

Although CO_2 does not directly compete with O_2 for hemoglobin binding sites, it binds to specific areas of hemoglobin molecules and encourages the release of O_2 molecules.

Decreased pH increases H^+ molecules, which bind to hemoglobin and promote the O_2 release.

Both factors result in a Bohr shift, in which the O_2 dissociation curve shifts to the right.

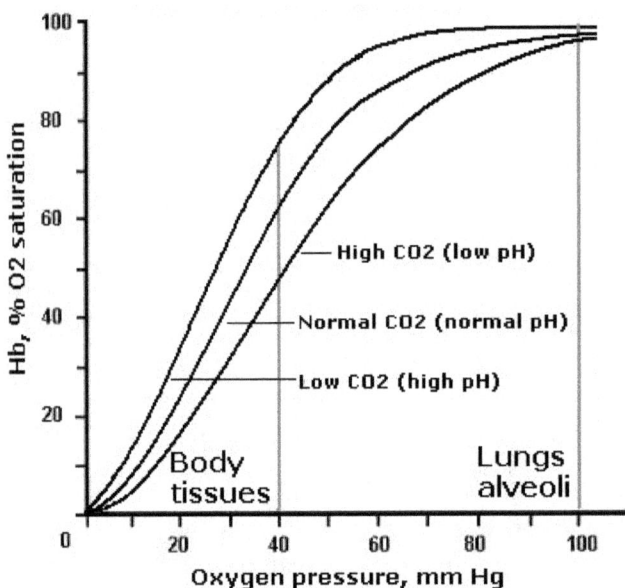

Bohr effect shifts the hemoglobin dissociation curve to the right

Elevated temperature, high CO_2, and low pH are observed during exercise since temperature and CO_2 levels rise due to increased metabolism, and pH is decreased due to lactic acid buildup.

2,3-Diphosphoglycerate (2,3-DPG), also known as 2,3-Bisphosphoglycerate (2,3-BPG), is the primary organic phosphate in erythrocytes.

Like CO_2 and H^+, 2,3-DPG is an allosteric effector that binds to hemoglobin to change conformation with decreased oxygen affinity.

2,3-DPG shifts the curve to the right (i.e., *Bohr effect*) to facilitate oxygen release near the tissues that need it most.

Under normal physiology, the oxygen dissociation curve predictably shifts to the left in the lungs to maximize O_2 loading.

Oxygen loads in the lungs and dissociates at the tissue

As seen in the curve, as pO_2 increases, the O_2 saturation of hemoglobin increases.

Lung alveoli is O_2 rich, causing hemoglobin of deoxygenated blood to be saturated with O_2.

Diffusion gradient favoring oxygen movement from alveoli to blood is maintained because oxygen binds to Hb and keeps plasma pO_2 low since only dissolved oxygen contributes to pO_2.

In tissues, the procedure is reversed.

Low pO_2 and high pCO_2 in tissues cause hemoglobin in the bloodstream to release O_2.

There is a net diffusion of O_2 from blood into cells and CO_2 from cells into the blood.

Fetal hemoglobin binds O_2 more tightly than adult hemoglobin to attract O_2 from maternal blood.

Fetal hemoglobin curve shifts to the *left* of the adult curve due to its higher binding affinity.

Carbon monoxide binds hemoglobin with high affinity

Carbon monoxide (CO) is lethal since it can bind to hemoglobin around 200 times more tightly than oxygen.

Carbon monoxide interferes with O_2 transport in blood by combining with Hb to form *carboxyhemoglobin* (COHb).

Due to high binding affinity, lesser amounts of CO occupy a sizable proportion of Hb in blood, making it unavailable to transport O_2.

Blood Hb concentration and dissolved O_2 are typical, but $[O_2]$ is dangerously reduced.

COHb shifts the O_2 dissociation curve left, interfering with the unloading of O_2 into oxygen-deprived tissues.

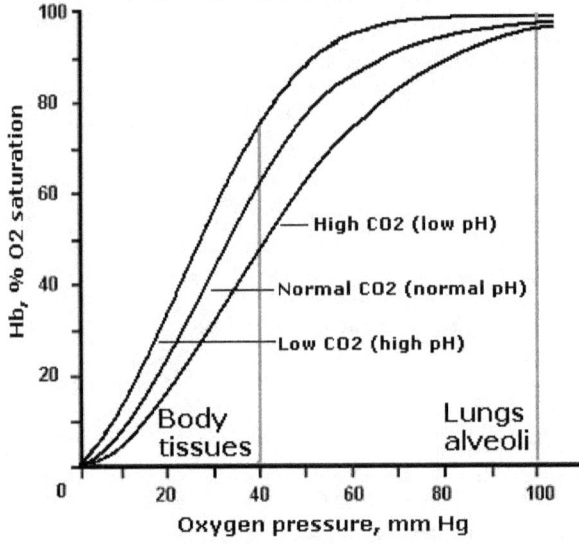

Bohr effect shifts hemoglobin dissociation curve to the right

Carbon dioxide levels and transport by the blood

Carbon dioxide is transported in the blood in three forms:

1) dissolved in plasma as CO_2,

2) dissolved in plasma as the bicarbonate ion (HCO_3^-), and

3) combined with hemoglobin.

As CO_2 diffuses from the tissues into the blood, about 5% remains dissolved in plasma as CO_2.

10–20% combines with hemoglobin as *carbaminohemoglobin* ($HbCO_2$).

As with oxygen, this complex can be unbound so that CO_2 is released into plasma.

Unlike O_2, CO_2 binds to amino groups on hemoglobin rather than the iron heme group.

$$CO_2 + Hb \leftrightarrow HbCO_2$$

75 to 85% of CO_2 enters erythrocytes and combines with H_2O to form carbonic acid (H_2CO_3), dissociating into HCO_3^- and H^+. This reaction is catalyzed by *carbonic anhydrase* (enzymes end with ~*ase*).

Ions are released into the plasma to continue transport.

Bicarbonate and *hydrogen ions* create a *bicarbonate buffer system* that maintains blood pH.

$$CO_2 + H_2O \leftrightarrow H_2CO_3 \leftrightarrow HCO_3^- + H^+$$

Some H^+ remains in erythrocytes and binds oxyhemoglobin, releasing oxygen. This is a critical process for O_2 transport and prevents fluctuations in pH since excess H^+ is removed from blood.

Exchange Mechanisms

Gas and solute exchange mechanisms

Capillaries are so narrow that only single red blood cells can pass.

Some capillaries have tiny pores between the capillary wall cells, allowing white blood cells and other substances to flow in and out of capillaries by *paracellular* transport.

Substance movement across capillary walls to enter or leave the interstitial fluid uses:

diffusion, vesicle transport, and bulk flow.

Diffusion is the passive movement of substances through a plasma membrane. Small molecules such as glucose and oxygen leave the capillaries and diffuse into tissues, while carbon dioxide and small waste leaves tissue and enter the capillaries.

Vesicle transport allows for the passage of materials via endocytosis and exocytosis. Larger, hydrophobic molecules typically travel through capillary walls by vesicle transport.

Bulk flow results from *hydrostatic pressure* and causes fluid to move from capillaries to tissue fluids. It is higher in sinusoidal and fenestrated capillaries and lower in continuous capillaries.

Bulk flow is opposed by *osmotic pressure*, which moves fluid from tissues to the capillaries due to differences in protein concentration.

Hydrostatic and *osmotic pressure* are described in the *Starling equation*, which explains how fluid and dissolved solutes leave the capillaries (filtrate) or enter the capillaries (reabsorbs).

Net filtration pressure (NFP) can be calculated using four forces, the *Starling Forces*.

P_c is the hydrostatic capillary pressure, which favors fluid movement out of the capillary.

P_{IF} is the interstitial fluid hydrostatic pressure, which favors fluid movement into the capillary.

π_P is osmotic pressure due to plasma protein (e.g., albumin) concentration, favoring fluid movement into the capillary.

π_{IF} is osmotic pressure due to interstitial fluid protein concentration, favoring fluid movement out of the capillary.

Net hydrostatic pressure is the difference between P_c and P_{IF}, while the net osmotic pressure is between π_P and π_{IF}. Together, the difference is the net filtration pressure.

A positive NFP indicates movement out of the capillary (i.e., filtration), while a negative NFP indicates movement into the capillary (i.e., reabsorption).

Net filtration pressure equation:

$$NFP = Pc - PIF - \pi P + \pi IF$$

Hydrostatic pressure is higher than the *osmotic pressure* at the *arterial end* of a capillary, so water leaves the capillary and enters the tissues.

Midway along a capillary, there is no net movement of water. Oxygen and nutrients diffuse into the tissue fluid, while carbon dioxide and other metabolic wastes diffuse into the capillaries.

At the venous end of a capillary, *osmotic pressure is higher than hydrostatic pressure*, so water is reabsorbed in the bloodstream.

Heat exchange mechanisms

Hypothalamus is responsible for monitoring *blood temperature* at about 37 °C.

If significant fluctuations occur from this set point, the hypothalamus sends nerve signals to the blood vessels to restore proper body temperature.

When external conditions are hot, vasodilation allows blood to flow near skin surfaces so that heat dissipates through convection and radiation.

When external conditions are cold, vasoconstriction shunts blood from skin surfaces. Blood flow is most reduced in the extremities, where the high surface-area-to-volume ratio causes heat to dissipate rapidly.

Humans use *countercurrent heat exchange* to conserve heat. Major veins and arteries run parallel deep in the arms and legs' muscles, with blood flowing in opposite directions.

When heat loss is not a concern, most blood returns from the skin through surface veins not parallel to the deep arteries.

However, blood returns through deep veins to exchange heat with the arteries when cold.

Blood moving through the warm arteries cools as it travels toward the extremities. When it reaches the body's surface, it is closer to the outside air temperature, minimizing the temperature gradient and reducing heat loss.

As cold blood returns through the deep veins, it is reheated by the nearby warm arterial blood.

Peripheral resistance impedes blood flow

Resistance to flow (i.e., peripheral resistance) is the impedance of arterial blood flow caused by blood entering arteries faster than it leaves, resulting in *vessels stretching by increased pressure*.

Elastic walls of the arteries contract during diastole, but the heart contracts before enough blood flows into the arterioles to relieve pressure in arteries.

Peripheral resistance is a function of *blood viscosity, vessel length,* and *vessel diameter.*

Higher concentration of blood cells and plasma proteins increases viscosity and creates a higher resistance to flow.

Diseases that cause an increase in the number of blood cells are problematic due to increased resistance, which forces the heart to work harder.

Blood vessel length may impact flow resistance. For example, an overweight individual with additional blood vessels to service fat cells has greater resistance, increasing heart problems.

Vasoconstriction and vasodilation

Blood *vessel diameter* is critical for resistance to flow.

>   *Vasoconstriction* increases resistance.

>   *Vasodilation* decreases resistance.

Plaque obstruction (i.e., atherosclerosis) inside blood vessels increases resistance by reducing blood flow diameter.

Total peripheral resistance (TPR) is the sum of resistance to flow by systemic blood vessels, although the primary determinant is resistance in the arterioles.

TPR affects blood pressure; deviations from normal blood pressure elicit homeostatic reflexes that alter TPR to offset the difference.

>   *Hypertension* causes blood vessels to vasodilation (i.e., *dilate*) to relieve resistance.

>   *Hypotension* causes *vasoconstriction* (i.e., *narrowing*) to increase resistance.

Notes for active learning

Blood

Blood composition

There is an average of 4 to 6 liters of blood in humans.

Blood is connective tissue; mammalian blood contains up to 60% *plasma* (a liquid matrix) and 40% *cellular components* suspended in the plasma.

Plasma is 90% water and 10% dissolved organic and inorganic substances such as salts, gases, metabolic wastes, nutrients, proteins, and hormones. Salts and proteins in plasma act as buffers, maintaining the blood to a pH of 7.35. They maintain blood osmotic pressure to regulate osmosis into and out of the bloodstream.

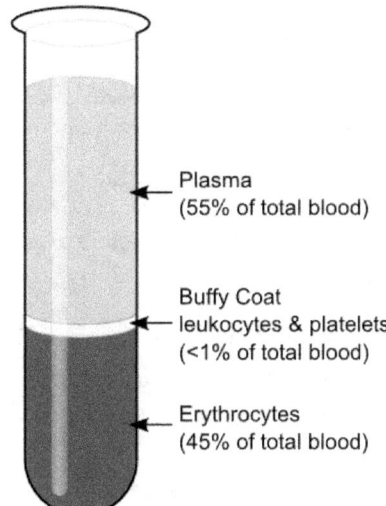

Albumin is the primary protein in plasma, partially responsible for maintaining osmotic pressure and carrying steroid hormones and fatty acids.

Fibrinogen and its derivative, *fibrin,* are other essential plasma proteins that form blood clots. Plasma contains *bilirubin*, a hemoglobin breakdown product in bile, urine, and feces.

Globulins are another class of plasma protein with various functions; *immunoglobulins* are antibodies the immune system produces.

Serum is the plasma from which fibrinogens and other clotting factors have been removed, an essential non-clotting fluid in medicine.

Erythrocytes (i.e., red blood cells) are flattened biconcave cells about 7 μm in diameter. The disk shape of mature erythrocytes is due to a lack of nucleus. They are the most abundant blood cells, with 4 to 6 million in 1 cubic millimeter of blood.

Each cell contains about 200 million red-colored hemoglobin molecules that transport O_2 and CO_2. Erythrocytes catalyze the conversion of CO_2 and H_2O to H_2CO_3.

Leukocytes and cells of the immune system

Leukocytes (white blood cells) are larger, have irregularly shaped nuclei, and lack hemoglobin. They make up less than 1% of the blood's volume.

Leukocytes are essential immune system components and, like erythrocytes, are generated from stem cells in the bone marrow. They may be in the bloodstream, lymphatic system, body tissues, or stored in the spleen.

Five types of leukocytes have specific functions.

Neutrophils are the most abundant leukocytes, which travel throughout the bloodstream. Neutrophils and other white blood cells enter interstitial fluid tissues by slipping through capillary walls by *diapedesis.*

Neutrophils engulf pathogens such as bacteria and fungi, making them *phagocytes.* They are the first responders to infection and initiate the early inflammation response.

Eosinophils respond to parasites, cancer cells, and allergic irritants.

Basophils participate in allergies, releasing chemical histamine to promote vasodilation, part of the inflammation response. Both leukocytes are in the blood and the tissues.

Monocytes in the bloodstream differentiate and become *macrophages,* upon which they enter the tissues and consume dead cells, damaged cells, and pathogenic agents. Monocytes regulate the chemical signals, which other leukocytes respond to inflammation.

Lymphocytes and platelets

Lymphocytes are white blood cells primarily in the lymphatic system rather than the blood.

B lymphocytes differentiate in the bone marrow and produce antibodies in response to antigens. They are stored after infection for future use if the same pathogen recurs.

T lymphocytes mature in the thymus and have a variety of roles.

Some T cells directly attack virus-infected and cancerous cells, while others assist other leukocytes in their functions. An important group of T cells inhibits an immunological response when it is no longer needed.

Platelets are enucleated cell fragments budding from bone marrow cells as *megakaryocytes.*

Platelets carry clotting factors and adhere to damaged tissues and blood vessels to stop uncontrolled bleeding. They survive for ten days before being removed by the liver and spleen.

Erythrocytes, spleen and bone marrow

In children, most bones produce blood cells, while in adults, only bones of the upper body do.

Blood cells descend from a single bone marrow cell population, the *pluripotent hematopoietic stem cells.*

Pluripotent hematopoietic stem cells divide into two lineages:

> *lymphoid stem cells,* which give rise to lymphocytes and
>
> *myeloid stem cells,* which give rise to other leukocytes and erythrocytes.

Protein hormones and paracrine agents regulate cell division and differentiation, collectively the *hematopoietic growth factors* (HGF).

Erythropoiesis (i.e., erythrocyte production) is stimulated by the *erythropoietin* hormone, secreted mainly by the kidneys. Erythrocytes are continuously manufactured from stem cells in the bone marrow of the long bones, ribs, skull, and vertebrae.

Iron, folic acid, and vitamin B_{12} are essential constituents of the blood absorbed in the small intestine from food. Folic acid and vitamin B_{12} stimulate the process of erythropoiesis, and iron is necessary for the structure and function of hemoglobin.

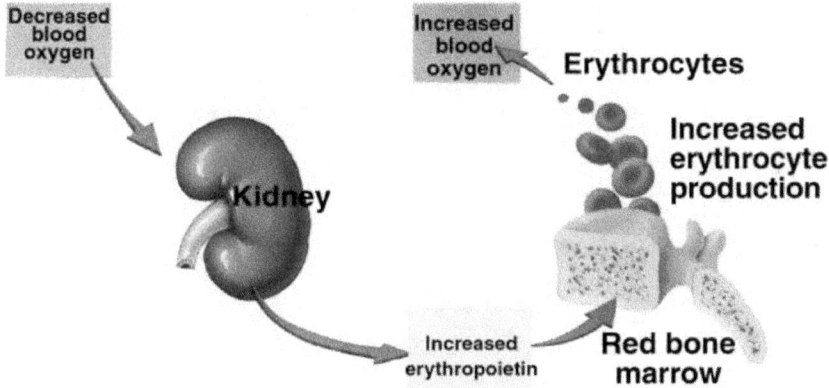

Erythrocyte production in response to blood oxygen levels

Polycythemia results from excess erythrocyte production, leading to a condition with extra erythrocytes, which results in sluggish blood flow through the capillaries.

Anemia results from insufficient production (or excessive degradation) of erythrocytes.

Erythrocytes have no nucleus; they cannot generate proteins and gradually degrade over time.

After 120 days, erythrocytes are destroyed by phagocytes in the liver, spleen, and bone marrow.

Heme, the iron-containing cofactor of hemoglobin, undergoes chemical degradation by the liver and becomes bilirubin, secreted as the pigment in bile.

Globin is the protein component of hemoglobin and is degraded into amino acids.

Two million erythrocytes are produced each second to replace those taken out of circulation.

Iron released from degraded erythrocytes may be incorporated into the hemoglobin of new erythrocytes or stored for later use in the liver and spleen as *ferritin*.

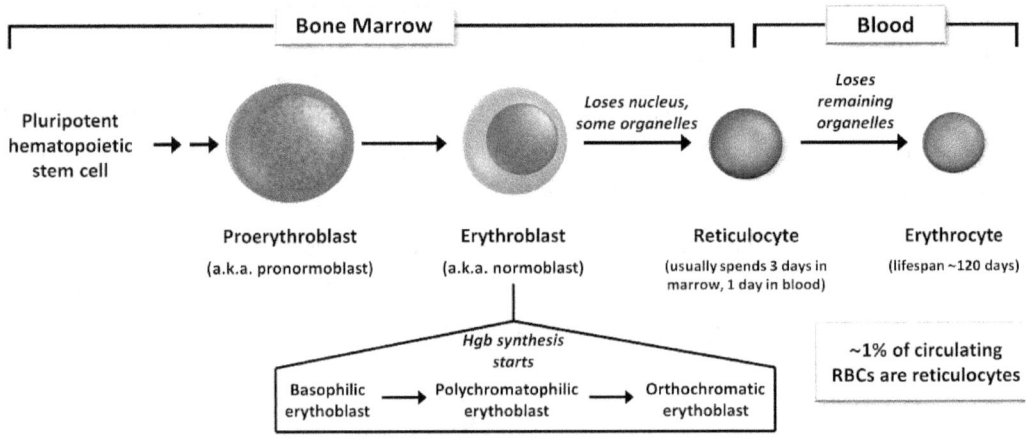

Erythropoiesis for red blood cell production

Regulation of plasma volume

Fluid volume is regulated by *blood osmolality*, the number of moles of a dissolved substance per kilogram.

Osmolality affects blood viscosity; the concentration decreases, and various materials travel in or out of the bloodstream.

When there is a higher blood osmolality, water travels into the blood via osmosis, increasing the blood volume and diluting the blood.

During lower blood osmolality, water leaves blood and enters tissues, lowering blood volume.

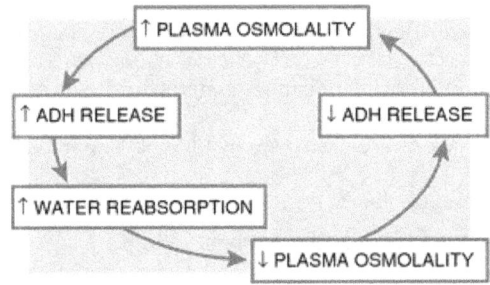

Fluid balance homeostasis by ADH as stimulated by changes in blood osmolality

Reductions in plasma volume (or increases in plasma osmolality) stimulate the secretion of *vasoconstrictors* to *increase blood pressure*.

Pituitary gland releases *vasopressin*, (*or antidiuretic hormone* (*ADH*), to inhibit urination and increase the kidneys' water reabsorption, thereby maintaining blood volume.

Supraoptic nucleus of the hypothalamus synthesizes ADH.

Vasopressin (or ADH) causes *vasoconstriction*, raising blood pressure to compensate for lower fluid levels.

Vasopressin also stimulates the secretion of *angiotensinogen* from the liver, which is then converted to angiotensin II by renin.

Angiotensin II further stimulates *aldosterone* secretion, which increases salt retention and promotes fluid reabsorption in the kidneys.

Norepinephrine and *epinephrine* (or adrenaline) are vasoconstrictors secreted by the adrenal medulla in response to stress.

Atrial natriuretic peptides (ANP) respond to high blood volume or decreased blood osmolality by increasing water filtration and urination. This counteracts ADH and aldosterone to reduce blood volume and pressure.

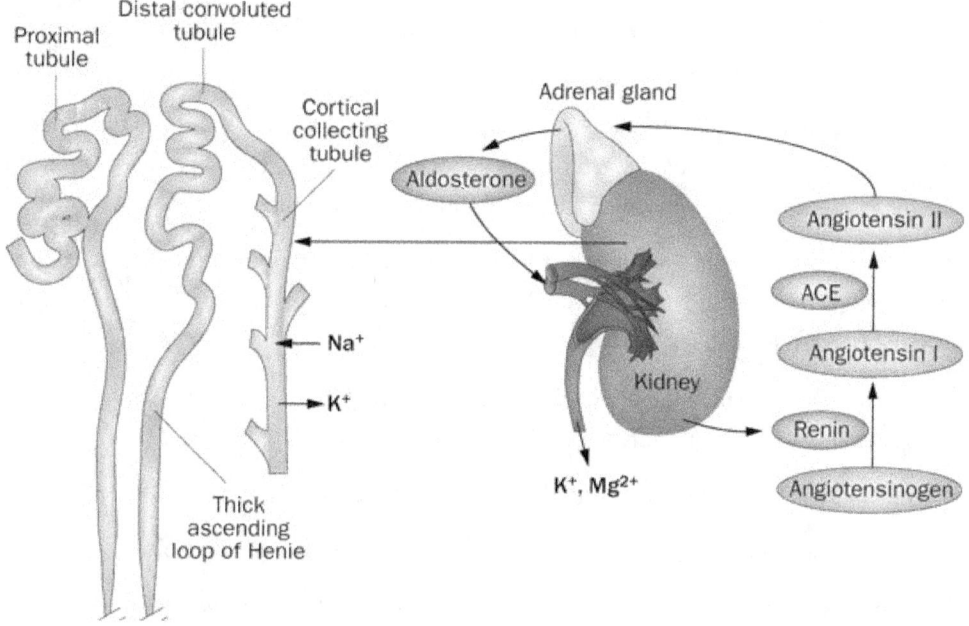

Angiotensin stimulates aldosterone to increase blood pressure

Clotting factors and wound healing

Hemostasis is the stoppage of bleeding from blood vessels. Venous bleeding leads to less rapid blood loss because veins have lower blood pressure.

Hematoma (bruise) is the accumulation of blood in tissue from bleeding. When a blood vessel is severed, it constricts, and the opposite endothelial surfaces of the vessel stick to slow the outflow. Other processes, such as *clotting*, follow this.

Coagulation (i.e., clotting) occurs when liquid blood becomes gel-like to repair an injury. Platelets contain enzymes and chemicals involved in the clotting process.

The liver produces clotting factors (e.g., fibrinogen) circulating in the plasma.

Platelets sense blood vessel abnormalities (usually a tear) and bind to exposed connective tissue. They partially seal the leak via an intermediary called the *von Willebrand factor* (vWF), a plasma protein secreted by endothelial cells and platelets.

Platelet binding to collagen triggers them to secrete substances that change the surface platelet proteins' shape for *platelet activation*. Activation attracts other platelets to form an aggregation as a *platelet plug*.

Fibrinogen binds to the platelets and forms crosslinks, further strengthening the plug.

Platelet plugs are a primary sealer of the injury; this is *primary hemostasis*.

Intact endothelial cells synthesize and release *prostacyclin* to inhibit platelet activation and keep the growth of the plug in check.

Clotting cascade of proteins initiates *secondary hemostasis*. Platelets and damaged tissue cells release the *prothrombin activator* clotting factor. Along with calcium ions, prothrombin activator catalyzes a reaction, converting prothrombin to *thrombin*.

Thrombin binds to receptors on the platelet surfaces and severs two amino acid chains from each fibrinogen molecule. These activated fragments join end-to-end, forming long threads of *fibrin*, the fibrous mesh that seals the clot.

Fibrin threads wind around the platelet plug and provides a framework for a clot. Erythrocyte cells are trapped within fibrin threads, making the clot appear red.

Anticoagulant *plasmin* degrades fibrin to prevent excess fibrin formation.

Clots contract and become compact as the wounded blood vessel repairs itself.

When repair is complete, the clot is dissolved by the *fibrinolytic* or *thrombolytic* system, which activates plasmin to digest the fibrin network.

Hemorrhagic disorders are primarily hereditary and nonhereditary diseases in which the affected individual's blood cannot clot.

Minor cuts and bumps cause uncontrolled external and internal bleeding, which can be deadly.

Hemophilia is a hereditary disorder in which the liver cannot produce one of the clotting factors.

Liver disease or *vitamin K deficiency* can cause non-genetic forms of hemorrhagic disorders.

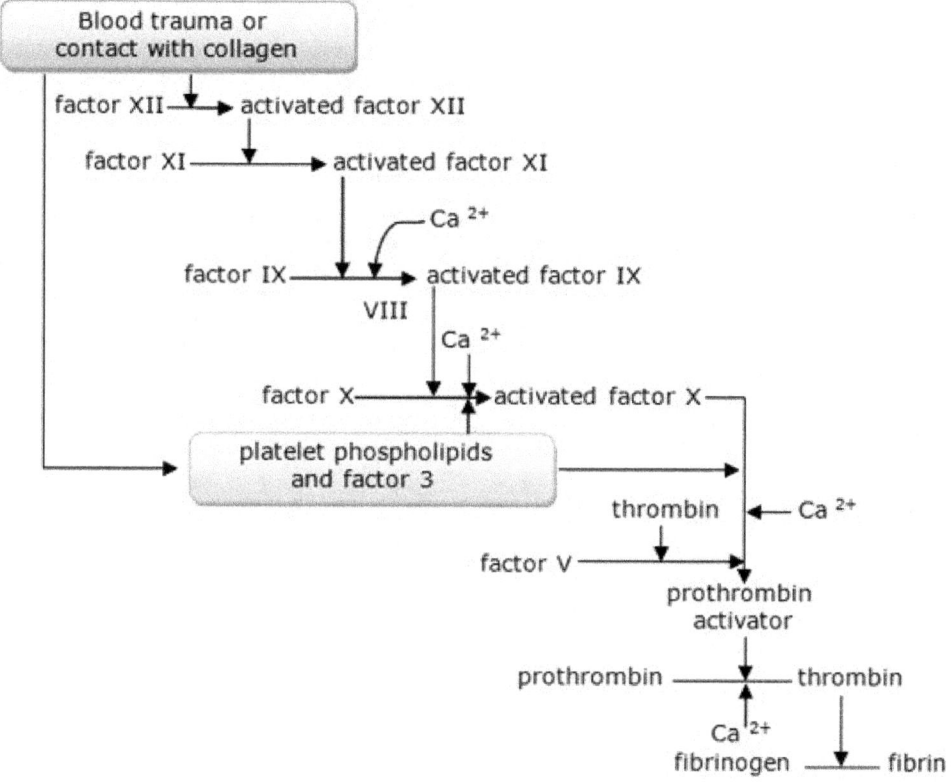

Blood clotting cascade

Notes for active learning

Cardiovascular Diseases

Heart failure

Heart issues can be diagnosed by observing irregularities in the cardiac cycle.

Heart failure is when the heart does not pump an adequate blood volume.

Heart failure may be due to *diastolic dysfunction* when a ventricle wall has *reduced compliance* and cannot fill adequately, resulting in reduced EDV and SV.

Heart failure may be caused by *systolic dysfunction*, which results from myocardial damage that impairs cardiac contractility and, therefore, decreases SV.

Adaptive reflexes to counter the reduced SV strive to maintain blood pressure by retaining fluid to increase blood volume or constrict vessels.

Excess fluid retention can impair respiration, and vasoconstriction makes it difficult for the heart to pump. It becomes weaker if the heart does not quickly recover from heart failure.

Hypertension

Hypertension occurs when arterial pressure increases, due to an increased peripheral resistance from the reduced arteriolar radius.

Renal hypertension results from renin's increased secretion, generating *angiotensin II* vasoconstrictor.

Prolonged hypertension increases the left ventricle's muscle since it pumps against increased arterial pressure. This could decrease contractility and lead to heart failure.

Hypertension may be caused by stress, obesity, high salt intake, or smoking, along with a genetic predisposition.

Two genes are involved in hypertension for some individuals; they produce angiotensin. People with this form of hypertension may be treated by gene therapy in the future.

Hypertension is often not detected until a stroke or heart attack occurs; however, it is monitored by blood pressure.

Pressure above 160 / 95 mmHg in women or 130 / 95 mmHg in men indicates hypertension.

Hypertension is seen in people with *atherosclerosis* (or *arteriosclerosis*). This condition occurs when soft masses of fatty materials, mainly cholesterol, accumulate beneath the inner linings of arteries. As *plaque* accumulates, it protrudes into a vessel and interferes with blood flow. The thickened wall reduces blood flow and releases vasoconstrictors, exacerbating the problem.

Platelets may detect the plaque as a vascular irregularity and adhere to it, forming a *clot*.

Blood clots, myocardial infarction and stroke

Thrombus is a clot that remains stationary.

Embolus is a dislodged clot in the bloodstream, which is deadly if it reaches the heart or brain.

Atherosclerosis can develop in early adulthood, but symptoms may not appear until age 50.

In families, atherosclerosis is inherited as *familial hypercholesterolemia*.

Atherosclerosis of a coronary artery may cause occasional chest pain (i.e., *angina pectoris*), which flares during stress or physical exertion.

Angina indicates oxygen demands are greater than the capacity to deliver it and is a warning sign of heart disease.

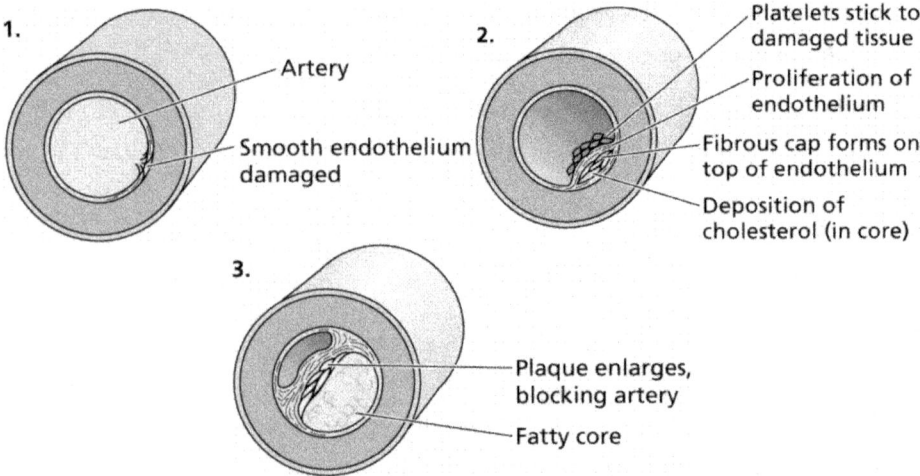

Progressive degeneration of the arterial lumen due to atherosclerosis and obstruction by cholesterol plaque

Nitroglycerin and related drugs *dilate blood vessels* and relieve pain.

Hypertension and atherosclerosis are significant contributors to heart disease, the leading cause of death in the US.

If atherosclerosis and clotting in the coronary arteries create insufficient blood flow (i.e., *ischemia*), some heart muscles may die due to the lack of oxygen. This leads to *myocardial infarction* (MI), a *heart attack*.

Damaged myocardial cells may create abnormal impulses that cause *ventricular fibrillation* (i.e., uncoordinated ventricular contractions).

If ventricular fibrillation severely impairs the heart's ability to deliver blood to the systemic circulation, it results in *cardiac arrest*.

Stroke is insufficient blood flow to the brain, which may occur if an embolus blocks a small cranial arteriole or bursts; it can result in paralysis, severe neurological impairment, or death.

A stroke is a *cardiovascular accident* (CVA).

Warning symptoms that foretell stroke include numbness in the hands or face, difficulty speaking, and blindness in one eye.

If a cerebral artery is partially blocked, it is a temporary and less severe impairment as a *transient ischemic attack*.

Notes for active learning

CHAPTER 8

Lymphatic & Immune System

Lymphatic System

Lymphatic Fluid

Lymph Nodes

Non-Specific and Specific Immunity

Innate Immune System

Adaptive Immune System

Immune System Tissues and Organs

Antigen and Antibody

Blood Types and Rh Factor

Page intentionally left blank

Lymphatic System

Lymph nodes, lymphatic vessels and capillaries

Lymphatic system is an open, unidirectional, secondary circulatory system. It contains a network of *lymph nodes*, *lymphatic vessels*, and *lymphatic capillaries*.

Lymphatic system usually transports excess *interstitial fluids* known as *lymph*. However, lymph can be moved by autonomic, smooth muscle contraction in larger lymph vessels.

Lymph returns proteins to the bloodstream, redistributes body fluid, removes foreign bodies, and maintains tissues' structural and functional integrity.

Lymph monitors blood for bacterial or viral infection.

Lymph system is associated with the cardiovascular system and has three main functions.

Lymphatic system equalizes fluid distribution

Lymph vessel opens if the interstitial fluid pressure exceeds the lymphatic pressure. When the lymph vessel opens, interstitial fluid enters the lymphatic capillaries.

Lymphatic circulation merges with venous circulation, returning the lymph fluid to the blood.

However, if the interstitial fluid pressure is less than the lymphatic pressure, the lymph vessel closes, preventing lymph from leaking.

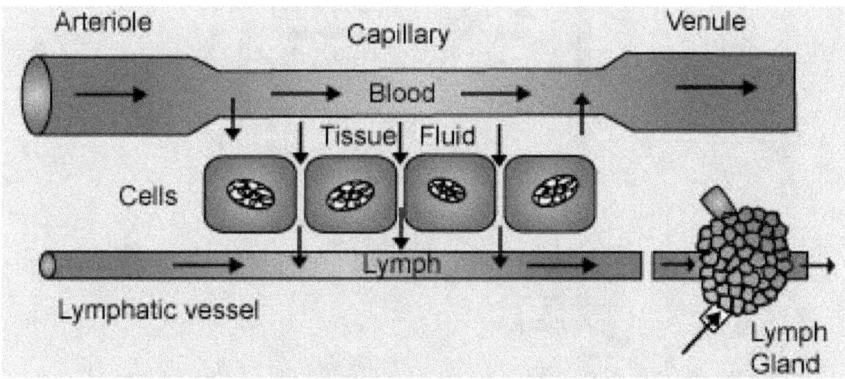

Fluid exchange between the circulatory and lymphatic systems

Fluid movement is dependent upon skeletal muscle contraction. When muscles contract, fluid is squeezed past a valve that closes, preventing backflow.

Transport of proteins and large glycerides

Lymphatic system is a pathway for *fat* absorbed in the gastrointestinal tract to reach the blood.

Fats are absorbed into small intestine *lacteals* (i.e., lymphatic capillaries in small intestine).

Lacteals receive lipoproteins *at intestinal villi*. Lymphatic vessels transport absorbed fats into the bloodstream.

Lymph in the lacteals (i.e., chyle) has a milky appearance due to its high-fat content.

Proteins and large particles that capillaries cannot absorb are removed by lymph.

Lymph returns substances to the blood

Lymphatic system takes up fluid that has diffused from capillaries and has not been reabsorbed.

Lymphatic vessels carry interstitial fluid to the cardiovascular system to compensate for the net filtration out of the blood capillaries.

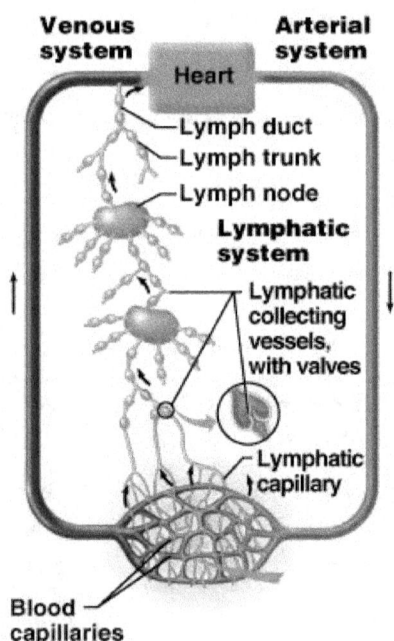

Interstitial fluid moves from the lymphatic to the cardiovascular system

Lymphatic capillaries collect cells and plasma proteins that leak out of the blood capillaries and transport them to the veins.

Lymph

Composition of lymph

Lymph is fluid that enters lymphatic capillaries. Lymph, derived from interstitial fluid, runs through the lymphatic vessels, lymph nodes, and other lymphatic organs.

Lymph contains *lymphocytes* (cells in immune response), which clean and filter the fluid.

Peristalsis propels lymph by rhythmical contractions of smooth muscle lining the larger lymphatic vessels. Contractions are triggered by stretching of the walls when lymph enters.

Lymphatic vessels have *valves* that produce a *unidirectional flow*. The vessels are innervated by *sympathetic neurons* and are influenced by skeletal muscles and the respiratory pump.

Lymph is a clear, colorless liquid with a similar composition to blood plasma; however, lymph has a higher protein content (e.g., lymphocytes) than blood plasma.

Blood hydrostatic pressure forces plasma fluid out of capillary walls and into surrounding tissues, forming *interstitial fluid*.

Some interstitial fluid re-enters capillaries, and some enter the lymphatic vessels to form lymph.

Lymph transports substances

Lymph is mostly water, plasma proteins, chemicals, and white blood cells.

Lymphatic system is responsible for transporting oxygen, carbon dioxide gas, and chemical substances such as amino acids, glucose, and fats.

Lymphatic system transports other nutrients and cellular compounds.

Lymph contains various clotting factors, including fibrinogen, globulin, chemical elements (e.g., calcium and iron), and some waste (e.g., uric acid).

Diffusion of lymph from capillaries by differential pressure

Lymphatic capillaries have a single layer of endothelial cells resting on a basement membrane with water channels permeable to interstitial fluid components, including protein molecules. Interstitial fluid enters these capillaries by bulk flow.

Fluid flows through the lymph nodes into two lymphatic ducts that drain into *subclavian veins* in the lower neck.

Lymph flows through blood plasma from the capillaries into the interstitial fluid, where it becomes lymph and is returned to the blood.

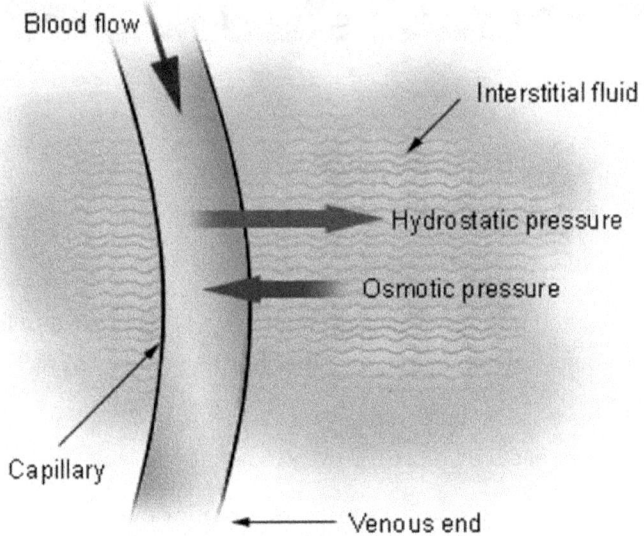

Blood becomes lymph due to higher hydrostatic pressure forcing plasma into the interstitial space

Lymph Nodes

Lymph nodes anatomy and function

Lymph nodes are tiny (about 1–25 mm), ovoid or spherical masses of lymphoid tissue located along lymphatic vessels.

Lymph nodes filter the lymph before it is returned to the blood.

Lymph nodes are concentrated with phagocytic white blood cells.

Lymph nodes are absent in the central nervous system.

Lymph nodes have two regions:

>   *outer cortex* and *inner medulla*.

Typical lymph nodes are surrounded by connective tissue compartments as *lymph nodules*.

Cortex contains nodules where lymphocytes and macrophages congregate to fight pathogens.

Macrophages are concentrated in the medulla and cleanse the lymph.

Lymph sinuses separate the macrophages and lymphocytes.

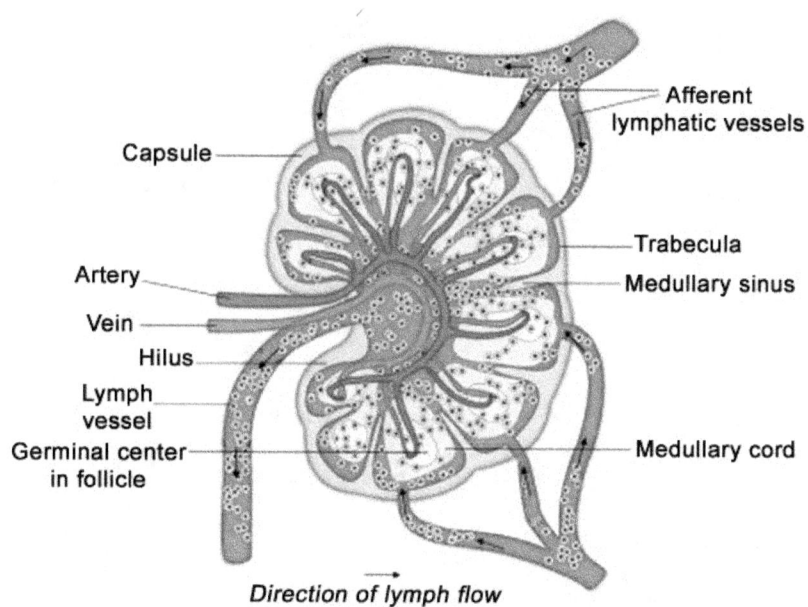

Afferent lymphatic vessels deliver lymph to lymph nodes

Afferent and efferent lymphatic vessels

Afferent lymphatic vessels (only in the lymph nodes) enter the lymph nodes periphery.

Afferent lymphatic vessels open into the cortical lymph sinuses after branching and forming a dense plexus in the capsule's substance.

Many afferent lymphatic vessels carrying lymph to the nodes enter via the convex side.

Lymph travels through the sinuses and eventually enters an *efferent lymphatic vessel*.

Efferent lymphatic vessels (in lymph nodes, spleen, and tonsils) carry lymph away from nodes.

Efferent lymphatic vessels begin at the *medullary* part of the node's lymph sinuses in the lymph node and leave the nodes for the veins or greater nodes.

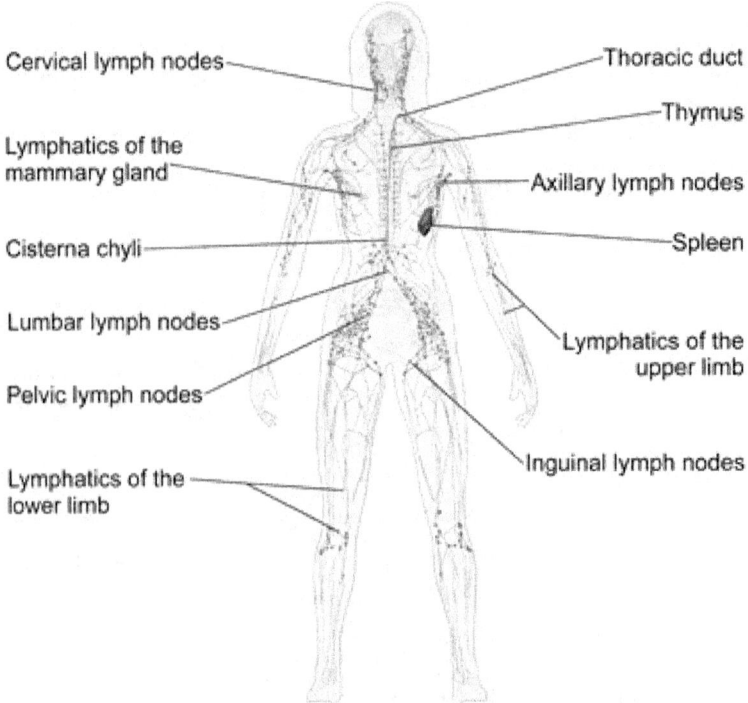

Lymphatic nodes and associated glands

Lymph nodes and lymphocytes

Lymph nodes cluster in some areas of the body, including the inguinal nodes in the groin, the axillary nodes in the armpits, and the cervical nodes in the neck.

Lymphatic capillaries join as *lymphatic vessels* that merge before entering one of two ducts.

Larger lymphatic vessels resemble veins, including the presence of valves.

Thoracic duct is larger than the right lymphatic duct, serving the lower extremities, abdomen, left arm, the left side of the head and neck, and the left thoracic region.

Thoracic duct delivers lymph to the left subclavian vein of the cardiovascular system.

Right lymphatic duct serves the right arm, the right side of the head and neck, and the right thoracic region. It delivers lymph to the *right subclavian vein* of the cardiovascular system.

Activation of lymphocytes

Lymphocytes produced in the red bone marrow by differentiating progenitor cells are the primary immune response agents.

When pathogens (or foreign antigens) enter a lymph node, local lymphocytes are released into the bloodstream towards the invasion site.

Once the lymphocytes are activated, they release chemicals that stimulate an immune response for proliferation, antibody production, and cytokine release.

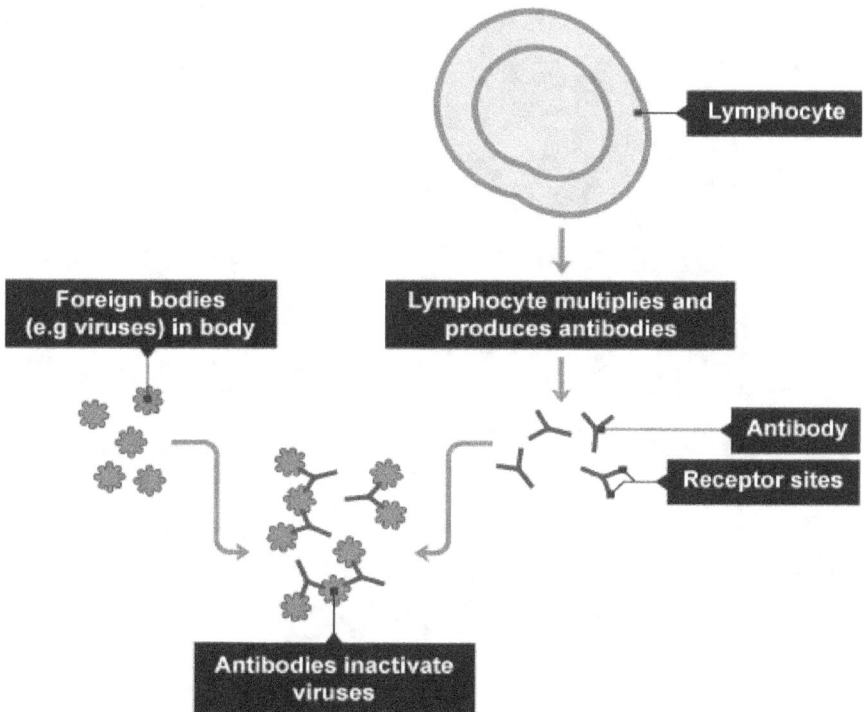

Immune response from pathogen to antibody production specific to the antigen

Notes for active learning

Non-Specific and Specific Immunity

Active and passive immunity

Immunity defends against infectious agents, foreign cells, and abnormal cancer cells. Immunity usually lasts for some time, and individuals do not ordinarily get the same illness twice. Immunity is acquired naturally through infection or artificially by medical intervention (e.g., vaccination).

Induced immunity includes:

    active immunity and *passive immunity*.

Active immunity is when an individual produces antibodies.

Passive immunity is when an individual receives prepared antibodies.

Active immunity can develop naturally after infection, induced when a person is healthy to prevent future infection. For example, a vaccine induces active immunity.

Vaccination and antibody titer

Vaccinations are used to expose bodies to a particular antigen. These antigens are usually destroyed or severely weakened before they are administered to decrease their potency.

After vaccination, serum antibody levels, known as *antibody titer*, measure immune response.

At first exposure, a *primary response* occurs, going from no antibodies present to a slow rise in titer. After a brief plateau, a gradual decline follows as antibodies bind to antigens or degrade.

A secondary response occurs at the second exposure to the antigen, and the antibody titer rises rapidly to a level much greater than before; this is a *booster*.

High antibody titer is expected to prevent disease symptoms if the individual is infected.

Active immunity depends on *memory B* and *T cell* responses (i.e., adaptive immunity section).

Active immunity is usually long-lasting, although a booster may be required every few years.

For example, an infant receives antibodies through the placenta or the mother's breast milk, rendering the child immune to a specific pathogen.

If in immediate danger of an infectious agent, a patient can receive antibodies from another as a medical intervention.

However, the effects of this passive immunity are short-lived because antibodies are not made by an individual's B cells.

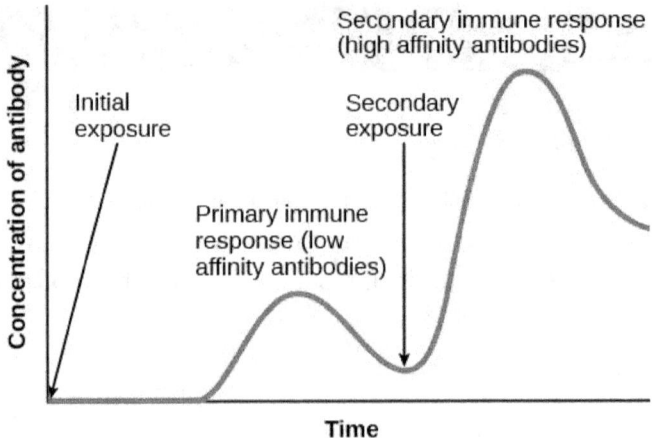

Antibody production profile comparing primary and secondary responses

Passive immunity defends against antigens by using antibodies from a foreign source.

For example, a patient receives a gamma globulin injection (a serum containing antibodies against the agent) taken from another animal previously exposed to the antigen.

If antibodies are derived from animals, individuals may become ill with *serum sickness*, an inflammatory response from the individual's hypersensitivity to animal proteins due to detecting the animal's proteins as potentially harmful antigens.

Immunity includes both *non-specific* and *specific* defenses (detailed below).

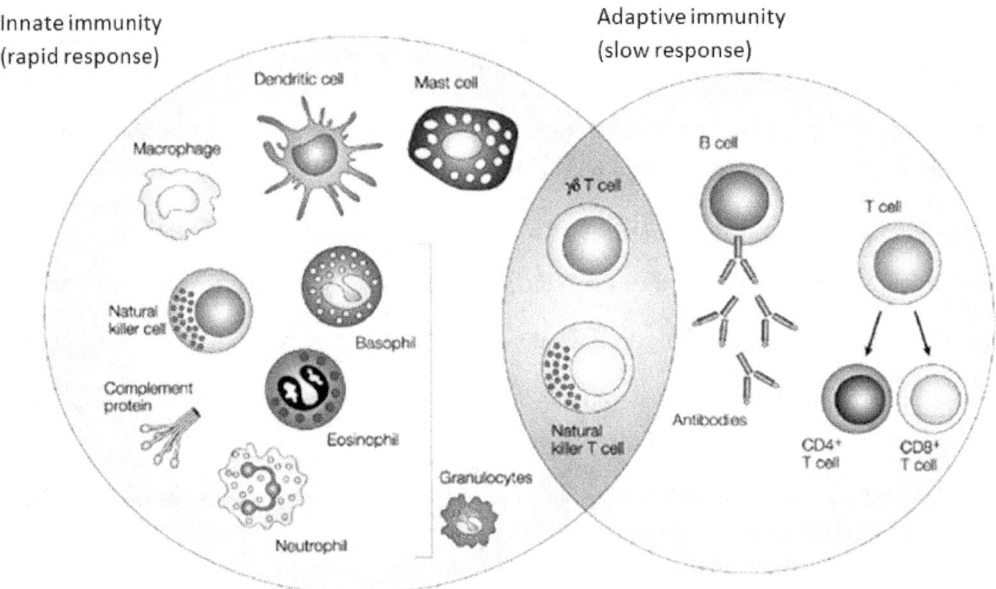

Innate immunity (rapid response) compared to adaptive immunity (slow response)

Major histocompatibility complex

Major histocompatibility complex (MHC) comprises genes that encode cell surface proteins. These complexes, which are in highly evolved vertebrates, help the immune system recognize foreign substances.

Cell surface proteins are layered in human genes, clustered on the same chromosome region.

Human MHC proteins are the HLA (human leukocyte antigens).

Two major classes of MHC molecules.

> Class one MHC molecules are along the membranes of all cell types.
>
> Class two MHC molecules are only in immune cells, *macrophages*, and *lymphocytes*.

Individuals do not have the same MHC molecules because genes have many alleles (i.e., alternative gene forms).

These molecules are collectively the *tissue type*.

MHC molecules contain genes that encode for other proteins, including *complement proteins*, chemical messengers of *cytokines*, and *enzymes* (i.e., a third class of MHC molecules).

MHC molecules were recognized as antigens stimulating an organism's immunological response to transplanted organs and tissues. After skin graft experiments on mice in the 1950s, graft rejection was an immune reaction mounted by the host organism against foreign tissue.

Host organisms recognize MHC molecules as foreign and attack them. The importance of the major histocompatibility complex (MHC) proteins was recognized to contribute to the difficulty of transplanting tissues from one organism (or person) to another.

Recognition of self *vs.* non-self

Each virus, bacteria, or foreign body has unique molecular markers. Host lymphocytes recognize and differentiate *self-molecules* that belong to the body and are not foreign.

Lymphocytes target *non-self-molecul*es. An example of a non-self-molecule is an antigen, which triggers B and T lymphocytes' mitotic activity.

When a pathogen invades a body, MHC markers on the cells' plasma membranes distinguish between self and non-self-cells.

Pathogens display a combination of self and non-self-markers; T cells interpret this as non-self.

T cells often recognize cancer cells or tissue transplant cells as non-self.

When T cells encounter non-self-cells, they divide and produce four kinds of cells:

> *cytotoxic T cells*, *helper T cells*, *suppressor T cells*, and *memory T cells*.

MHC molecules are vital to the immune system because they allow T lymphocytes to detect macrophages that have ingested a foreign microorganism. The partially digested microorganism displays a distinctive peptide bound to an MHC complex on the macrophage's surface.

T lymphocytes recognize fragments attached to MHC molecules and begin immune responses.

In adaptive immunity, an antigen-specific response is initiated. This requires the identification and recognition of *non-self-antigens* during antigen presentation.

Autoimmune disease

Autoimmune diseases are when cytotoxic T cells (or antibodies) attack body cells as a foreign antigen. Under these conditions, the differentiation between self and non-self-molecules is lost.

Autoimmune diseases may be genetic or caused by bacteria, viruses, drugs, or chemicals.

Examples of autoimmune diseases include:

myasthenia gravis, multiple sclerosis, systemic lupus erythematosus, rheumatic fever, and *type I diabetes.*

Typical Immune Response	**Autoimmune disease**
Antigens invade ↓ Antibodies form ↓ Antibodies remove invading antigens ↓ Antibodies remain and protect	Immune system forms antibodies to self-antigens ↓ Antibodies attack self-antigens ↓ Inflammation and tissue damage

In *myasthenia gravis*, neuromuscular junctions do not function, and muscular weakness results.

In *multiple sclerosis* (MS), the myelin sheaths of nerve fibers are attacked.

In *systemic lupus erythematosus*, symptoms are elicited before dying from kidney damage. Many symptoms are elicited in systemic lupus erythematosus, resulting in further disease.

While there are no cures for autoimmune diseases, they are managed by therapeutics.

Innate Immune System

Nonspecific immune responses

First line of defense in the body is *surface coverage*. Skin and mucous membranes protect the body from pathogens.

Skin is a dry, acidic, dead cellular layer, allowing optimal, non-specific surface protection.

Mucous membranes contain *lysozymes*, which are enzymes that break down bacteria. Other cells in the mucous membranes contain *cilia* that filter the pathogens and particulates.

Nonspecific responses are generalized responses to pathogen infection and do not target cell types. Individuals do not ordinarily become immune to their cells; the immune system can distinguish self from non-self-cells. In this manner, the immune system aids, rather than counters, homeostasis.

Lymphocytes recognize antigens because they have antigen receptors; the protein shape allows the receptors and antigens to combine like a *lock and key*.

During maturation, differentiation occurs, so there is a lymphocyte for various antigens.

Non-specific response comprises white blood cells (WBCs) and plasma proteins.

Four nonspecific defenses include *barrier to entry*, *inflammatory reaction*, *natural killer cells*, and *protective proteins*.

Barrier to entry is the first non-specific response. Skin and the mucous membrane lining the respiratory, digestive, and urinary tracts are mechanical barriers. Oil gland secretions inhibit the growth of bacteria on the skin.

Ciliated cells line the upper respiratory tract to sweep mucus and particles into the throat to be swallowed. The stomach has a low pH (between 1.2 and 3) that inhibits bacteria's growth.

Harmless bacteria in the intestines and vagina inhibit pathogens from colonizing.

Inflammatory reaction is the second non-specific response, which occurs from tissue damage. Inflamed areas often have four symptoms: redness, pain, swelling, and heat. For example, aspirin, ibuprofen, and cortisone are anti-inflammatory agents that counter the chemical mediators of inflammation.

Natural killer cells are the third non-specific response. Natural killer cells are a class of lymphocytes that recognize abnormal cells (e.g., cancerous cells), attach to abnormal cells, and release chemicals that eventually destroy them.

Protective proteins are the fourth non-specific response; proteins protect cells nonspecifically.

Complement proteins

Complement proteins are plasma proteins involved in non-specific and specific defenses.

Complement system contains plasma proteins and is designated by the letter C and a subscript.

One activated complement protein activates another protein in a cascade reaction. In this way, a limited number of proteins can activate other proteins, "*complementing*" immune responses.

Complement amplifies an inflammatory reaction by attracting phagocytic cells to injury site.

Complement proteins bind to antibodies on the surface of pathogens, increasing the probability of neutrophil or macrophage phagocytizing pathogens.

Complement proteins form a *membrane attack complex* that produces holes in bacterial cell walls and plasma membranes; from osmotic pressure, fluids and salts enter the bacterium to the point where the cell bursts.

Lymphocytes produce antibodies

Lymphocytes are leukocytes that produce antibodies.

Lymphocytes are any of three subtypes of white blood cells in a vertebrate's immune system.

White blood cells include:

> natural killer, T, and B cells.

Each lymphocyte makes one specific antibody. Different lymphocytes are needed so the body can produce specific antibodies.

Antibodies are on the surface of the plasma membrane of lymphocytes, with the antigen-combining site projecting outwards.

Pathogens have surface antigens, which bind to specific lymphocyte antibodies at the antigen-combining site (i.e., the *epitope* of the antigen for antibody binding).

When this happens, the lymphocyte becomes active and makes *clones* by dividing via *mitosis*.

Clones synthesize antibodies to defend the body against the pathogen.

Macrophages digest foreign material

In general, *macrophages* participate in engulfing foreign objects. A macrophage engulfs a pathogen and acts as an antigen-presenting cell.

Monocytes enter tissues and differentiate into macrophages to ingest pathogens. Connective and lymphoid tissues have resident macrophages that devour old blood cells and debris.

Macrophages trigger an explosive increase in leukocytes by releasing colony-stimulating factors; these chemicals diffuse into the blood and are transported to the red bone marrow to stimulate the production of white blood cells (WBC).

Inflammation promotes macrophage (i.e., phagocytic white blood cell) activity.

Macrophages secrete *interleukins*, communication proteins among WBCs.

Interleukin-1 increases body temperature, causing fever. Fever causes drowsiness and reduces the body's energy usage and stress, enhancing the WBC's ability to protect against infection.

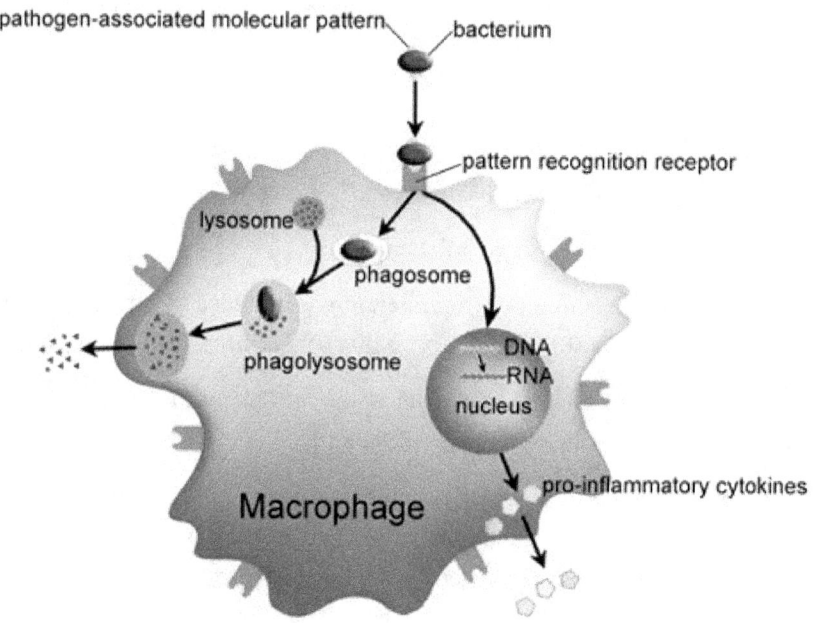

Mast cells are an example of a macrophage.

Mast cells *resemble basophils* and reside in the *connective tissue* and *mucous membranes*.

During an allergic response, they release histamine, bringing about inflammation.

With tissue damage, tissue and mast cells release chemical mediators (e.g., histamine, kinins).

Histamine and kinins cause *vasodilation* and *increased capillary permeability* to white blood cells. Enlarged capillaries produce redness and a local increase in temperature. The swollen area and the kinins stimulate free nerve endings, causing pain.

Phagocytes

Phagocytes are formed from *stem* (i.e., undifferentiated) bone marrow cells and digest foreign material. They do this by recognizing pathogens and engulfing them by *endocytosis*.

Enzymes (lysosomes) within the phagocytes digest the pathogens.

Phagocytes can ingest pathogens in the blood and body tissue since they can pass through the pores of capillaries and into these tissues.

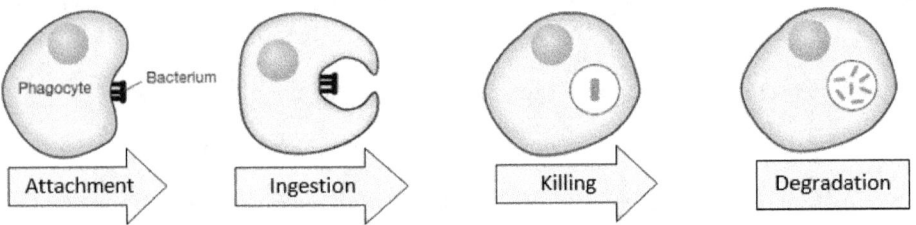

Stages of phagocytosis from attachment to degradation

Neutrophils

Neutrophils phagocytize bacteria.

Eosinophils are phagocytes that secrete enzymes to kill parasitic worms.

Basophils secrete histamine to enhance inflammation.

Neutrophils are granulocytes due to cytoplasmic granules. Because of unique, lobed nuclei, they are polymorpho-nuclear (PMN) leukocytes that phagocytize and destroy pathogens.

Neutrophils and monocytes migrate by the amoeboid movement to the injury site and escape from the blood by squeezing through the capillary wall.

They contain toxic substances that kill or inhibit various bacteria and fungi growth. Like macrophages, they activate a respiratory burst. Respiratory burst products are potent oxidizing agents like hydrogen peroxide, free oxygen radicals, and hypochlorite.

Neutrophils are the abundant phagocytes and are usually the first cells recruited to the infection.

Pus is the accumulation of dead neutrophils and tissue, cells, bacteria, and living WBC.

Dendritic cells are phagocytic cells present in tissues in contact with the external environment, mainly the skin, the nose's inner mucosal linings, the small intestine, the lungs, and the stomach.

Dendritic cells are essential in antigen presentation and serve as the connection between innate and adaptive immunity systems.

Plasma cells secrete antibodies

Plasma cells (a type of B cell) secrete antibodies.

Plasma cells originate in *bone marrow* but leave the bone marrow to differentiate into plasma cells in the *lymph nodes*.

Blood plasma and the lymphatic system transport plasma cells.

When a B cell in a lymph node of the spleen encounters an appropriate antigen (i.e., foreign substance), it is activated to divide.

B cells act as antigen-presenting cells and internalize various offending antigens taken by the B cell through receptor-mediated endocytosis and processing.

Antigenic peptides (i.e., fragments of the antigen) are on the surface of various MHC molecules and are presented to the T cells.

T cells bind to MHC antigen molecules and activate B cells, usually in spleen and lymph nodes.

B cell starts differentiating into specialized cells. For example, *germinal center B cells* differentiate into memory or plasma cells.

Differentiation for B cells is affinity maturation; they become plasmablasts (immature plasma).

Eventually, they produce large volumes of antibodies in the lymph nodes and spleen. Once the threat of infection has passed, new plasma cell development ceases, while those present die.

Inflammatory response to infection

There is an inflammatory response during an infection's initial stages, which is a nonspecific attack. Phagocytes become active and digest the pathogen. It causes localized redness, swelling, heat, and pain.

White blood cells are more active at higher temperatures, and inflammation recruits white blood cells to the infection site by sending chemical signals.

Capillary wall structure changes (i.e., higher permeability) allow more interstitial fluid and white blood cells to leak into tissues.

Neutrophils, lymphocytes, and monocytes are the cells involved in the inflammatory response.

Neutrophils are the first white blood cells that enter the injury site during acute inflammation. Anti-bacterial cells break down bacterial cells by releasing various lysosomal enzymes.

Neutrophils recognize bacterial cells as foreign agents by antibody molecules attached to the bacteria's surface. Antibody molecules are in blood plasma and interstitial fluid. Here, they bind to one specific antigen (or foreign agent) the body has seen before.

Lymphocytes start to accumulate during the inflammatory response process.

If their presence is prolonged or is large in number, it may suggest that the antigen is still present and an infection has formed.

Lymphocytes produce large numbers of antibodies, which are unique to each lymphocyte. Antibodies recognize foreign molecules and differentiate between self and non-self.

Monocytes are phagocytic cells that circulate in the blood along with macrophages. They are in the connective tissue.

Monocytes and macrophages engulf and digest foreign microorganisms, tissue debris, and dead cells. With lymphocytes, they recognize and destroy foreign substances.

Allergies

Allergic reaction is a hypersensitive immune response (e.g., itching, inflammation).

Allergies are hypersensitivities to foreign substances (e.g., pollen). Response to these antigens, *allergens*, usually involves tissue damage.

Immediate and delayed allergic responses are two of the four responses.

Immediate allergic response occurs within seconds of allergen contact; cold-like symptoms are common.

Delayed allergic responses are initiated by sensitized memory T cells at the allergen site.

Tuberculin skin test is an example: a positive test shows prior exposure to TB bacilli but requires time to develop tissue reddening.

Natural killer cells use cell-to-cell contact

Natural killer cells use cell-to-cell contact to destroy virus-infected and tumor cells; they lack specificity or memory. They do not directly attack the invading microbes but destroy the host cells, such as the tumor cells.

This concept is predominantly related to cells with abnormally low major histocompatibility complex markers, resulting in viral infections of various host cells.

Natural killer cells are activated when the MHC markers are altered, have the condition of "missing self," and are involved in the adaptive immune system.

Experiments show that natural killer cells readily adjust to the immediate environment and form an antigen-specific immunological memory vital for secondary infections with same antigen.

Natural killer cells innate, and adaptive immunity is essential in cancer therapy research.

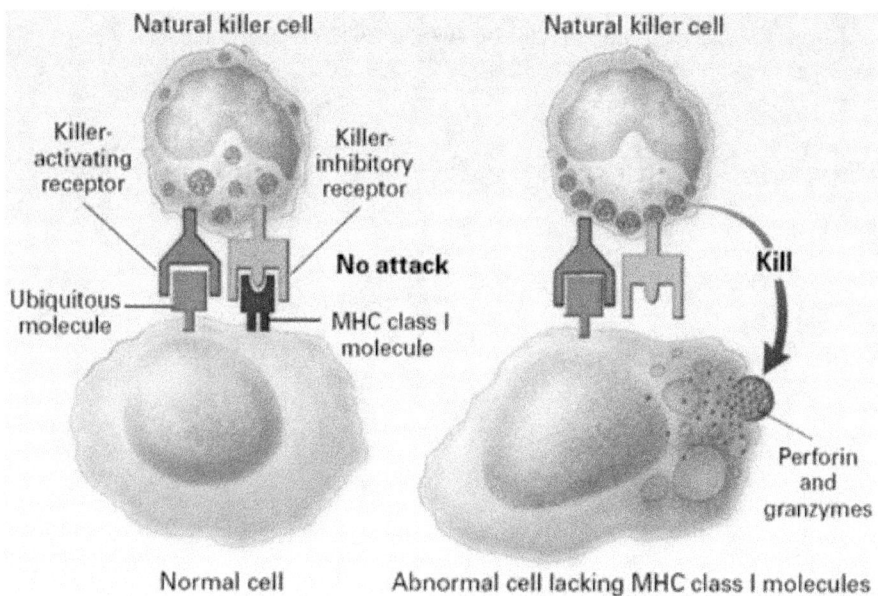

Natural killer cells' mode of activation with action by killer-inhibitory receptor

Notes for active learning

Adaptive Immune System

Specific immune responses

Adaptive immunity is specified for a pathogen (or antigen).

Antigen-presenting cells have foreign antigens on their surface, which *T and B cells recognize*.

Dendritic cells are an example of an antigen-presenting cell.

Specific defenses are physical, chemical, and cellular defenses against viruses, bacteria, and disease agents. Pathogens have antigens that can be components of foreign or cancer cells.

Specific response is activated when insufficient nonspecific methods and the infection spreads.

Specific immune response reacts to unique antigens and is primarily the result of the B and T lymphocytes. Some lymphocytes entrap antigens on their surface.

B lymphocytes (B cells) produce and *release antibodies*.

T lymphocytes (T cells) produce *antibodies* on their surface.

When lymphocytes attach to antigens, they encode unique antibodies that recognize antigens.

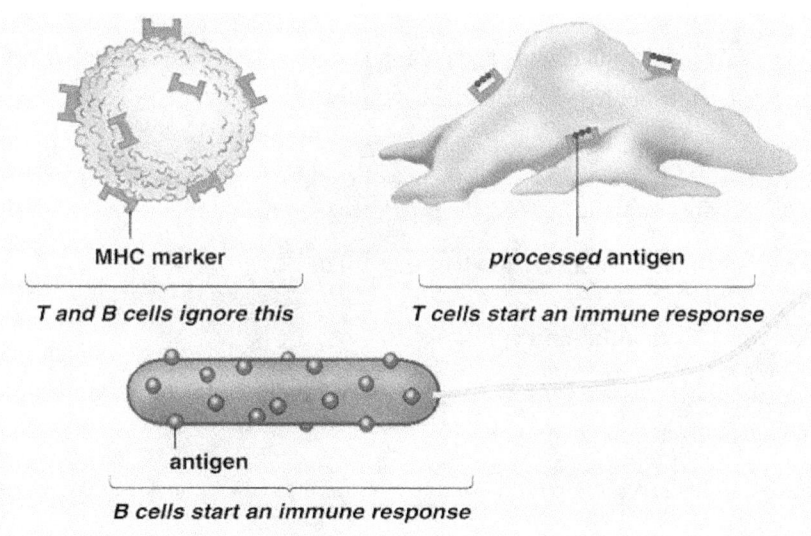

Molecular cues stimulate lymphocytes to create an immune response

Humoral response (antibody-mediated) involves antigens circulating in lymph or blood (e.g., bacteria, fungi, parasites, viruses, and blood toxins).

Humoral response is a form of *adaptive immunity*. For example, humoral response is a bacterial infection. Initially, inflammation persists, and macrophages and neutrophils engulf the bacteria.

Interstitial fluid flushes into the lymphatic system, where *lymphocytes* are in *lymph nodes*.

Macrophages process foreign organisms and present the bacterial antigen to the B lymphocytes.

With assistance from helper T cells, B cells differentiate into plasma and memory cells.

Plasma cells produce *antibodies* released into the blood to attack the antigen, while *memory cells* prepare for the same event if the antigen attacks again (i.e., elicits a secondary response).

Clonal selection initiated by specific antigens

Clonal selection is the response of *lymphocytes* to specific antigens.

Clonal selection theory states that the antigen selects the B cell to produce many clones of the corresponding plasma cells.

Selection is made by B cell lymphocytes activating specific antigens.

B cells are produced from lymphoid stem cells in blood and lymphoid tissues. The clonal portion involves the multiplication of antibodies occurring in particular cells.

B cells present a specific antibody on the surface. The appropriate antigen forms a complex with the antibody on the cell, thereby activating the cell's development.

Cells not meeting specific criteria are not activated.

Antigen-antibody interaction occurs, and complexes populate on the surface. These complexes are internalized and begin to swell and divide rapidly.

B cells differentiate into *plasma* and *memory cells*.

Plasma cells produce specific antibodies.

Memory cells circulate but actively produce no antibodies.

T lymphocytes, interleukins and cytokines

T cells (T lymphocytes) arise from *bone marrow stem cells*, which travel to the thymus, where they differentiate and mature.

T cells have antigen receptors but do not make antibodies; they check molecules displayed by non-self-cells.

At maturity, T cells acquire receptors for self-markers, such as the major histocompatibility complex (MHC) molecules and antigen-specific receptors. They are released into the blood as "*maiden*" T cells.

T cells ignore cells with MHC molecules, as well as free-floating antigens. Antigens must be presented to T cells by an *antigen-presenting cell* (APC).

When an antigen-presenting cell presents a viral or cancer cell antigen, the antigen is linked to an MHC protein; together, they are presented to a T cell. This binding promotes rapid cell division and differentiation into effectors and memory cells (all with receptors for the antigen).

Cytotoxic T cells and *helper T cells* are responsible for *cell-mediated immunity*.

Effector cytotoxic T cells recognize infected cells with the MHC-antigen complex and destroy the cell with perforans (enzymes that perforate the cell membrane, allowing cytoplasm to leak out) and other toxins, which attack organelles and DNA.

Once a cytotoxic T cell is activated, it undergoes *clonal expansion* and destroys cells that possess the antigen if the cell bears the correct HLA antigen. As the infection disappears, the immune reaction wanes, and few cytokines are produced.

Apoptosis is programmed cell death; it is critical to maintaining tissue homeostasis. Apoptosis occurs in the *thymus* if the T cell bears a receptor to recognize a self-antigen; if apoptosis does not occur, T cell cancers result (i.e., *lymphomas* and *leukemias*).

The few T cells that do not undergo apoptosis survive as *memory cells*.

Cytokines secreted by T cells and macrophages regulate the allergic response.

When a donor and recipient are histocompatible, a transplant is likely successful.

Interleukins improve T cells' ability to counter cancer. Interleukin antagonists prevent skin or organ rejection, autoimmune diseases, and allergies to vaccine adjuncts (e.g., suspension solution).

Cancer cells with altered proteins on their cell surface should be attacked by cytotoxic T cells.

Cytokines (e.g., interleukins, interferon, growth factors) may awaken the immune system and destroy cancer. Clinicians withdraw T cells from patients and culture them with interleukin. T cells are re-injected into the patient. The remainder of the interleukins maintains killer activity of the T cells.

T cells have storage vacuoles containing *perforin molecules*, which perforate plasma membranes and cause water and salt to enter, causing the cell to burst.

Effector helper T cells secrete *interleukins* that stimulate T and B cells to divide and differentiate.

Helper T cells stimulate the activation of B cells, cytotoxic and suppressor T cells. They improve response to other immune cells.

When exposed to an antigen, helper T cells enlarge and secrete cytokines.

Cytokines stimulate helper T cells to clone and for immune cells to perform their functions.

Cytokines stimulate the *macrophages* to perform *phagocytosis* and stimulate *B cells* to become antibody-producing plasma cells. For example, the human immunodeficiency virus (HIV), which causes an autoimmune deficiency syndrome (AIDS), infects helper T cells primarily and inactivates the immune response.

Memory T cells remain in the body after encountering an antigen and save time for an immune response to the same antigen. Like B cells, memory T cells have unique antigen receptors.

Suppressor T cells (*regulatory T cells*) use negative feedback in the immune system. They generally suppress the proliferation of effector T cells.

Cell-mediated response is effective against infected cells, mainly using *T cells* to respond to a non-self cell, including cells invaded by pathogens.

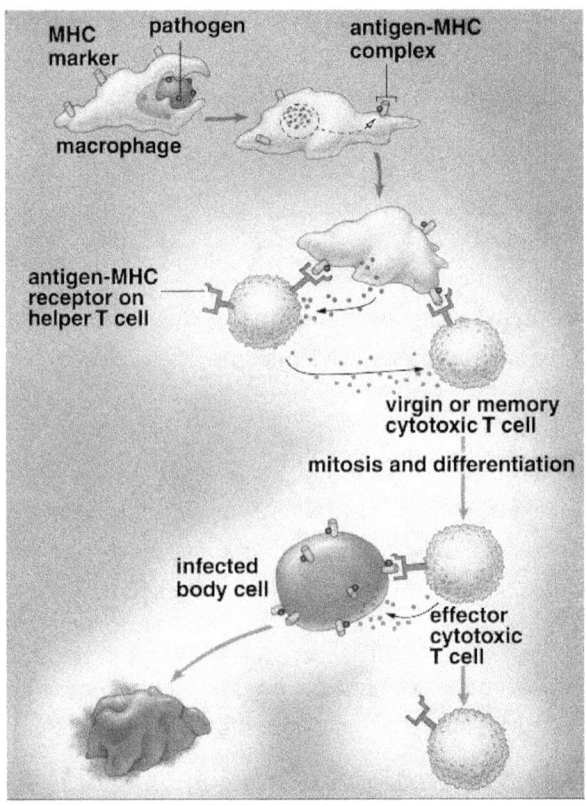

Cell-mediated immune response showing macrophages, antigen-MHC complex, helper T cells, and effector cytotoxic T cells

A non-self-cell binds to a T cell, which starts clonal selection. This initiates a series of events, including the production of cytotoxic T cells and helper T cells, the binding of helper T cells to macrophages that engulf pathogens, and the production of interleukins by the helper T cells, which stimulates the proliferation of T cells, B cells, and macrophages.

Tissue rejection occurs when cytotoxic T cells cause the disintegration of foreign tissue. This is a correct differentiation between self and non-self.

Clinically, the selection of compatible organs and the administration of immunosuppressive drugs prevent tissue rejection. Transplanted organs should have the same type of HLA antigens as the recipient.

Cyclosporine and *tacrolimus* are immunosuppressants that inhibit T-cell responses to cytokines.

Roles of B cells and T cells in immunity

B lymphocytes (B cells) arise from bone marrow stem cells and mature in the spleen. They give rise to plasma cells that produce and secrete antibodies.

Antibodies are released from plasma cells and are antigen specific. Each B lymphocyte produces one antibody type.

Memory B cells are long-lived B cells that do not release antibodies in response to antigen invasion; instead, they circulate in the body, proliferate, and respond quickly (via antibody synthesis) to eliminate a subsequent invasion by the same antigen.

Memory B cells have a similar function to memory T cells.

Antibody-mediated immunity is the defense by B cells. It is *humoral immunity* because antibodies are present in the *humor* and bodily fluids (i.e., blood and lymph).

B cell plasma membranes contain *antigen receptor-antibodies* (i.e., immunoglobulins).

Immunoglobulins are proteins specific to each antigen.

There are five classes (IgA, IgD, IgE, IgG, and IgM) of immunoglobulins based on variation in the Y-shaped protein-constant region and variable regions of the antibody protein.

Each B cell has its antibody as a membrane-bound receptor on its surface. B cells do not clone until its antigen is present, recognizing the antigen directly. *Helper T cell secretions* stimulate them to *clone*.

Some cloned B cells do not produce antibodies but remain in the blood as memory B cells.

Antibodies are proteins that recognize antigens (i.e., foreign substances).

Undifferentiated B cells produce antibodies that move to the cell surface and protrude.

B cell circulates in the blood and becomes primed for replication when it encounters the antigen.

B cells must receive an *interleukin signal* from a helper T cell, which has already been activated by a macrophage with an MHC-antigen complex, promoting rapid cell division.

B cell population differentiates into *effector* and *memory B cells*.

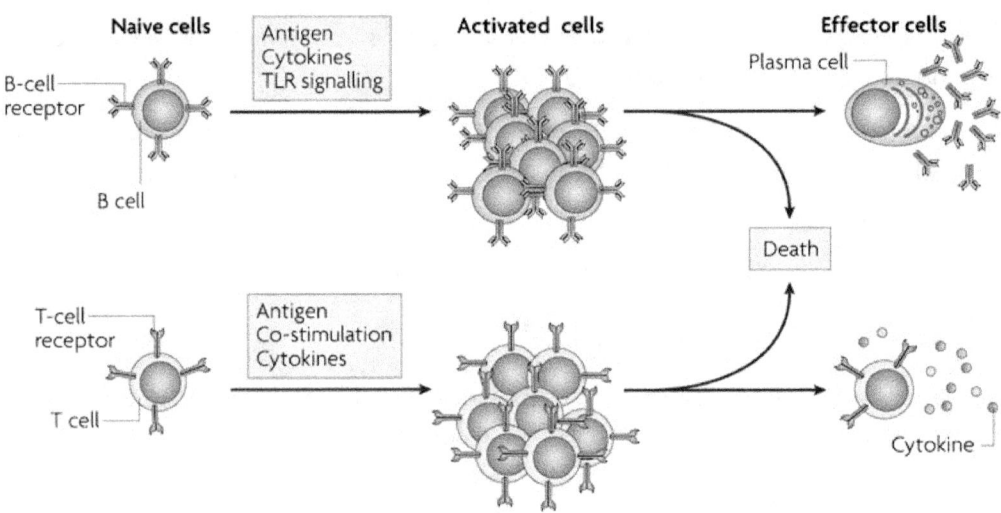

Roles of B cells and T cells in immunity

Effector B cells produce a staggering number of *free-floating antibodies*. When free-floating antibodies encounter an antigen, they tag it for destruction by *phagocytes* and *complementary proteins*.

These responses occur for *extracellular toxins* and *pathogens*; antibodies *cannot* detect pathogens or toxins inside cells.

When mitosis occurs, the daughter populations become subdivided.

Effector cells (or plasma cells), when fully differentiated, *seek and destroy foreign cells*.

Memory cells are efficient because they do not necessitate T cells' activation in proliferating antibodies if the same antigen is present.

Memory cells allow magnified, sustained response against the same pathogen during secondary response. Thus, a secondary response usually takes less time.

Immunological specificity and memory involve three events: recognizing an invader, repeated cell division that forms huge lymphocyte populations, and differentiation into subpopulations of effector and memory cells.

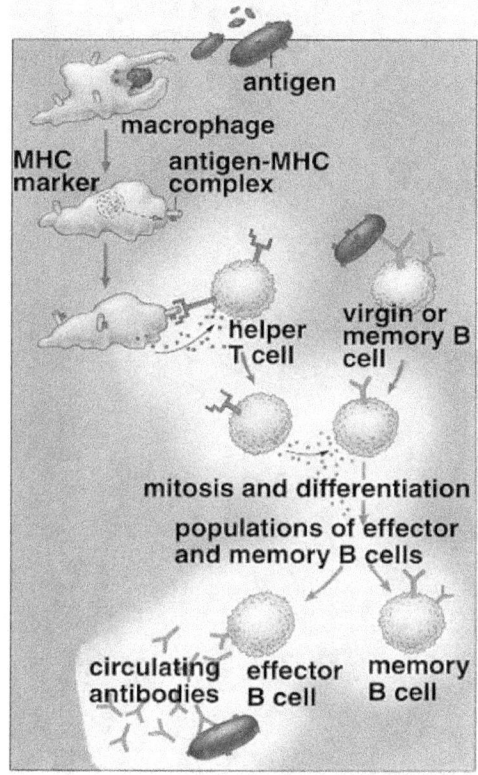

Antigen stimulates B cells to produce circulating antibodies

Interferons

Interferon is a protein produced by a virus-infected animal cell.

Interferons bind non-infected cell receptors, producing substances interfering with viral reproduction.

Interferons are specific to species (e.g., human interferons for humans).

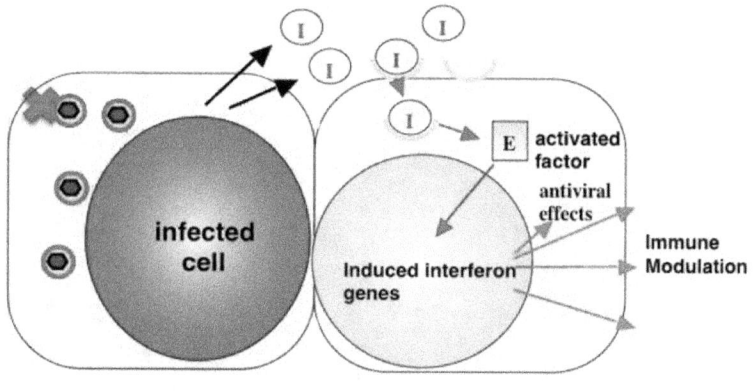

Interferons

Notes for active learning

Immune System Tissues and Organs

Lymphocytes originate from lymphoid tissue

Lymphoid tissue is in the lymph nodes, thymus, and various organs. It is where lymphocytes reside, proliferate, and differentiate.

Lymphoid tissues are where white blood cells (WBC) reside and proliferate.

Bone marrow and blood cell production

Human bone marrow consists of red marrow and yellow marrow.

Red marrow contains mostly hematopoietic tissue; yellow bone marrow primarily fat cells.

Red and yellow marrows contain blood vessels and capillaries.

Red marrow is the origin of blood cells, including leukocytes, platelets, and red blood cells.

At birth, bone marrow is red. However, with age, a portion of the red marrow is converted to yellow; by adulthood, about half of the bone marrow is red.

In adults, red marrow is in the flat bones, including the skull, sternum, ribs, clavicle, pelvic bones, vertebrae, and cancellous (i.e., mesh-like structure with pores) material at the *epiphyseal* ends of long bones (e.g., femur and humerus).

Red marrow has reticular fibers made by *reticular cells* packed around thinly-walled sinuses.

Differentiated blood cells enter the bloodstream at *bone sinuses*.

Yellow bone marrow is in the medullary cavity (i.e., hollow interior in the center of long bones).

When exposed to trauma, such as extreme blood loss, the body converts yellow bone marrow into red bone marrow to increase red blood cell (i.e., erythrocyte) production.

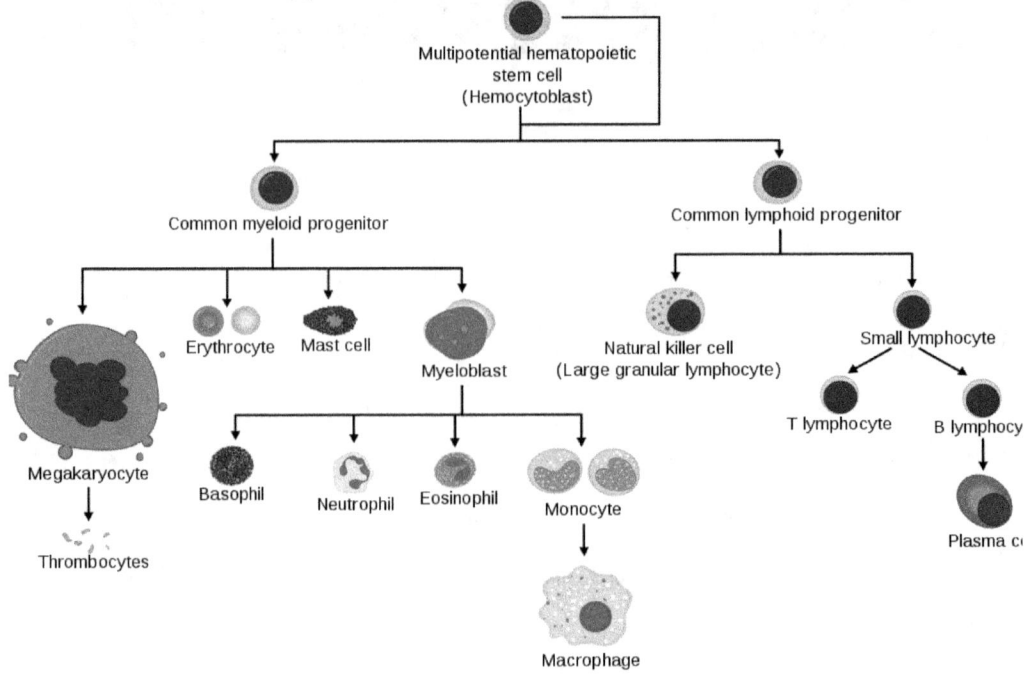

Blood stem cells give rise to cells of the immune system

Spleen filters the blood

Spleen is in the upper left abdominal cavity below the diaphragm.

Spleen is similar to a lymph node but is larger (nearly the size of a fist).

Lymph nodes cleanse the lymph, while the spleen cleanses the blood.

Capsule divides the spleen into nodules containing sinuses filled with blood.

Spleen nodules have red pulp and white pulp.

Red pulp contains *red blood cells*, *lymphocytes*, and *macrophages*. It purifies blood that passes through by removing microorganisms and worn-out or damaged red blood cells.

White pulp mainly contains *lymphocytes*.

If the spleen ruptures due to injury, it can be removed, as other organs assume its functions. However, someone without a spleen may be susceptible to infections and require antibiotic therapy.

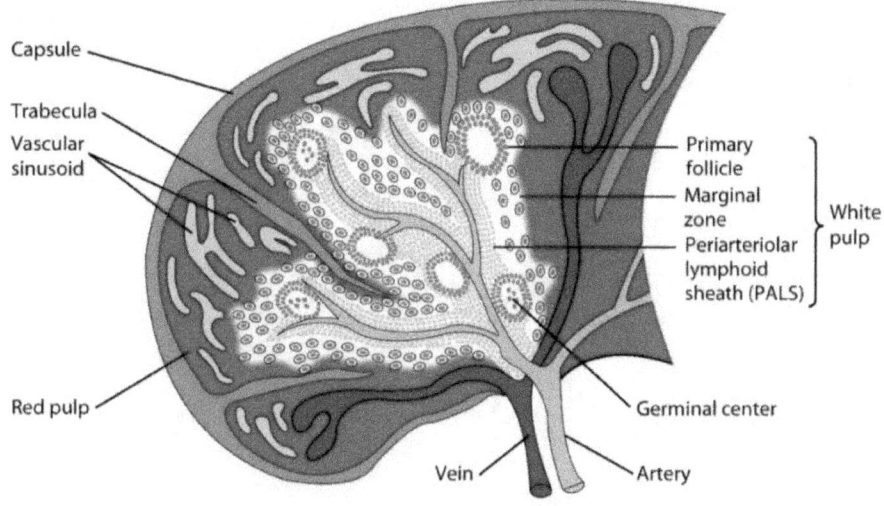

Spleen with regions of red pulp and white pulp

Thymus produces T cells

Thymus is involved in the immune response.

Thymus gland is along the trachea behind the sternum in the upper thoracic cavity. It is larger in children than adults and may disappear in old age.

Thymus is divided into *lobules* by connective tissue, the site of *T lymphocyte maturation*.

Each lobule's *medulla* (i.e., the inner region of an organ or tissue) consists mainly of epithelial cells producing and secreting thymic hormones (i.e., thymosin).

Thymosins stimulate lymphocytes to differentiate into T cells, identifying and destroying infected body cells.

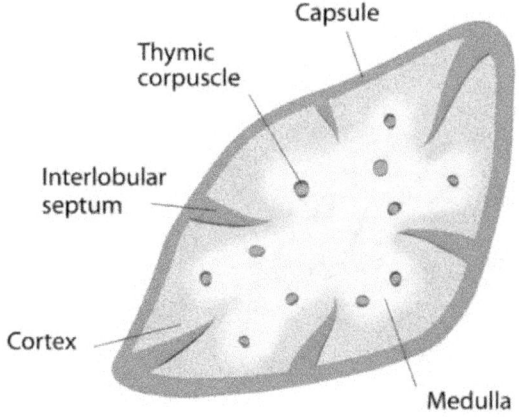

Thymus with outer cortex and inner medulla

Notes for active learning

Antigen and Antibody

Antigen-antibody complex

Antigen is a non-self-molecule that triggers an immune response. Antigens are foreign substances, usually proteins or polysaccharides, stimulating *antibody production*.

Antibodies are molecules that bind to antigens so that *lymphocytes* recognize the antigens. The antigen binds with a specific antibody at the *antigen-binding site*.

Antigen-antibody (or *immune complex*) marks antigens for destruction via neutrophils, macrophages, or complement activation via phagocytosis. Antibodies binding to antigens bring about neutralization, where a pathogen cannot adhere to the host cell.

Opsonization (i.e., a pathogen targeted for destruction by phagocytes) enhances phagocytosis-complement activation, where antibodies destroy infected cells by creating membrane holes.

Additionally, antibodies mark macrophage or natural killer cell phagocytosis by complement proteins, agglutination of antigenic substances, or chemical inactivation (if a toxin).

Structure of the antibody molecule

Antibodies are large globular proteins that defend the body against pathogens by binding to antigens on the pathogen's surface and destroying them.

Antibodies are secreted into blood, lymph, and bodily fluids and bind to specific antigens.

Antibodies are Y-shaped proteins, with each tip of the "Y" binding to an antigen. "Y" tips are *hypervariable regions* because they are unique for antigen-specific antibodies.

Antibodies consist of *two light chains* and *two heavy chains* linked by *disulfide bonds*.

Heavy chains have constant regions and variable regions.

Light chains have constant and variable domains.

Constant regions have amino acid sequences that remain constant but differ among antibodies.

Variable regions have portions of polypeptide chains with amino acid sequences that change, allowing for *antigen specificity*.

Variable region forms the *antigen-binding sites* of antibodies (i.e., tips of the "Y"), where their shape is specific to an antigen.

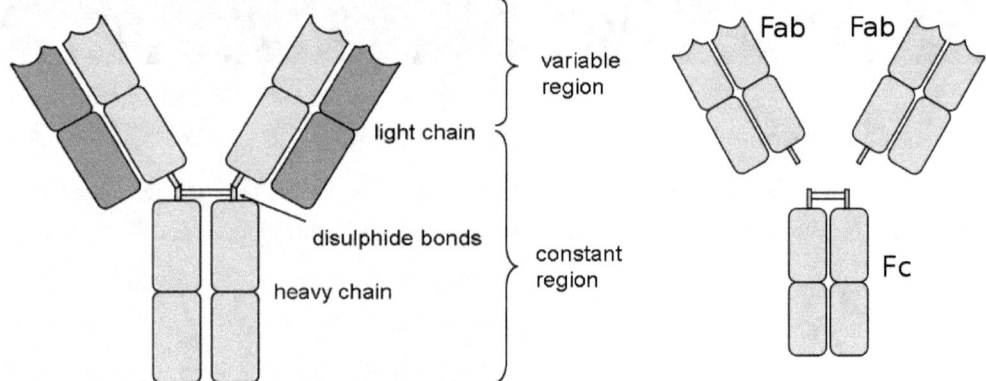

Antibody Fab (fragment antigen-binding) region binds to antigens. Fc (fragment crystallizable) region interacts with cell surface receptors, activating antibodies

Five classes of immunoglobulins

There are five classes of circulating antibodies, or immunoglobulins (Igs):

- *IgG antibodies* contain two Y-shaped structures: the primary antibodies in the blood and extracellular fluids.

  They are not common in the lymph and tissue fluid.

  IgG antibodies protect the body from infection by binding many pathogens and toxins.

- *IgM antibodies* are pentamers (i.e., five Y-shaped structures).

  They appear in blood soon after infection and disappear before it is over.

  They are useful activators of the complement system.

- *IgA antibodies* contain two Y-shaped structures that attack pathogens before reaching the blood.

  They are the primary antibody in *bodily secretions*.

- *IgD antibodies* contain two Y-shaped structures that are receptors for antigens on immature B cells.

- *IgE antibodies* contain two Y-shaped structures and participate in immediate allergic reactions.

  They are attached to mast cell's plasma membrane (in tissues) and basophils (blood).

When an *allergen* attaches to IgE antibodies on mast cells, they release large amounts of histamine and other substances, causing cold symptoms or anaphylactic shock.

Anaphylactic shock

Anaphylactic shock is a severe systemic reaction causing throat swelling, itchy rash, and a sudden drop in blood pressure.

Allergy shots may prevent the onset of allergic symptoms.

Injections of an allergen cause the body to build up high quantities of IgG antibodies because they do not cause allergy.

IgG antibodies combine with allergens received from the environment before reaching IgE antibodies on mast cells and basophils plasma membranes.

Monoclonal antibodies

Every plasma cell derived from the same B cell secretes the same antibody against the same antigen, *monoclonal antibodies*.

Monoclonal antibodies can be produced in vitro. B lymphocytes (usually harvested from mice) are exposed to a particular antigen.

Activated B lymphocytes fuse with *myeloma cells* (malignant plasma cells divide indefinitely).

Hybridomas are two different cells fused—hybrid cells and cancerous cells (suffix *-oma*).

Monoclonal antibodies give rapid, reliable diagnoses of various conditions (e.g., pregnancy). For example, monoclonal antibodies identify infections, distinguish cancerous cells from normal cells, and transport radioisotopes or toxic drugs to target tumors.

Antigen presentation stimulates antibodies

Pathogens enter an antigen-presenting cell (APC) with pieces of the pathogen displayed at the surface of APCs.

T cell receptors recognize the presented antigen and activate various immune responses.

When a macrophage engulfs an extracellular pathogen, pieces of the pathogen become antigen, and they are presented at the macrophage's cell surface.

Helper T cells recognize presented antigens and activate macrophages to destroy pathogens.

Helper T cells activate B cells to produce antibodies against the pathogen.

When an intracellular pathogen enters a host cell, pathogen pieces are presented on cell surface.

Cytotoxic T cells recognize the presented antigen and signal the infected cell to self-destruct.

Notes for active learning

Blood Types and Rh Factor

Rh factor antigen on red blood cells

Rh factor is an antigen in human blood types. Rh-positive (Rh⁺) has the Rh factor on red blood cells (RBC); Rh negative (Rh⁻) lacks the Rh antigen on the RBC.

Rh-negative persons do not have antibodies to the Rh factor but begin to make them when exposed to Rh-positive blood. Rh-positive is a genetically dominant trait.

Hemolytic disease may occur if a mother is Rh-negative and father is Rh-positive. During pregnancy, the Rh factor is important; a Rh-negative mother and an Rh-positive father pose an Rh conflict. The child's Rh-positive RBC can leak across the placenta into the mother's circulatory system when the placenta breaks down.

Presence of the "foreign" Rh-positive antigens causes the mother to produce anti-Rh antibodies.

Anti-Rh antibodies pass across the placenta and destroy the RBC of the Rh-positive child.

The Rh issue has been solved by giving Rh-negative women an Rh immunoglobulin injection (Rho-Gam) either during the first pregnancy or within about 72 hours after the birth of an Rh-positive newborn.

The injection includes anti-Rh antibodies that attack a child's RBCs before they trigger the mother's immune system. The injection is ineffective if the mother has already produced antibodies; hence, timing is essential.

Blood types and transfusions

Blood types (blood groups) are classified by inherited antigens' presence (or absence) on erythrocytes. Antigens include proteins, carbohydrates, glycolipids, or glycoproteins.

There are no O antigens.

Type A⁻ (A negative) blood has A antigens on the erythrocyte but no Rh factor (Rh⁻) and no B antigens. Type A⁻ blood produces anti-B antibodies that bind to B antigens, and antibodies bind to the Rh antigen.

Type B⁻ (B negative) blood has B antigens on erythrocytes but no Rh factor (Rh⁻) nor A antigens. Type B⁻ blood produces anti-A antibodies that bind to A antigens, and antibodies bind to the Rh antigen.

RBC with a particular antigen agglutinate when exposed to corresponding antibodies.

Agglutination is clumping red blood cells due to a reaction between antigens on red blood cells. The recipient's plasma must not have an antibody that causes donor cells to agglutinate during blood transfusions.

Patients with type AB blood can receive any blood; they are universal recipients.

Patients with type O blood cannot receive A, B, or AB but are universal donors.

Patients with type A blood cannot receive B or AB blood.

Patients with type B blood cannot receive A or AB blood.

	Group A	Group B	Group AB	Group O
RBC Antigens	A antigen	B antigen	A and B antigens	None
Plasma Antibodies	Anti-B	Anti-A	None	Anti-A and Anti-B

Blood types with associated antigens and corresponding antibodies

Notes for active learning

Notes for active learning

CHAPTER 9

Digestive System

Digestive System Overview

Ingestion

Stomach

Liver

Bile

Pancreas

Small Intestine

Large Intestine

Muscular Control

Gastrointestinal Tract Summary

Endocrine Control

Neural Control by Enteric Nervous System

Human Nutrition

Page intentionally left blank

Digestive System Overview

Six processes of the digestive tract

Digestion provides energy needed for routine metabolic activities and to maintain homeostasis.

Digestive tract ingests food, breaks it into small molecules, crosses plasma membranes, absorbs the nutrients, and eliminates indigestible remains.

Human digestive system is a coiled, muscular tube (6-9 meters long when fully extended), beginning at the mouth and ending at the anus.

Specialized compartments occur along this length:

> mouth, pharynx, esophagus, stomach, small intestine, large intestine, and anus.

Accessory digestive organs are connected to the central system by a series of ducts: salivary glands, parts of the pancreas, the liver, and the gallbladder (*biliary system*).

Digestive tract performs six processes:

1. *Ingestion* – bringing food into the system
2. *Movement (peristalsis)* – moving food along the system
3. *Digestion* – breaking down food using mechanical and chemical processes
4. *Secretion* – releasing enzymes and bile into the digestive tract
5. *Absorption* – moving food molecules from the digestive tract into the blood
6. *Defecation* – eliminating solid waste from the large intestine

Four macromolecules in the digestive tract

Four groups of macromolecules are digested and absorbed by the digestive tract.

Macromolecules include:

> starch, protein, triacylglycerol (fats), and nucleic acids.

Starches are broken down (i.e., catabolism) into glucose monomers.

Proteins are catabolized (i.e., broken down) into amino acid monomers.

Triacylglycerols (fats) are catabolized (i.e., broken down) into fatty acids and glycerol.

Nucleic acids are catabolized (i.e., broken down) into nucleotide monomers.

Gastrointestinal structures

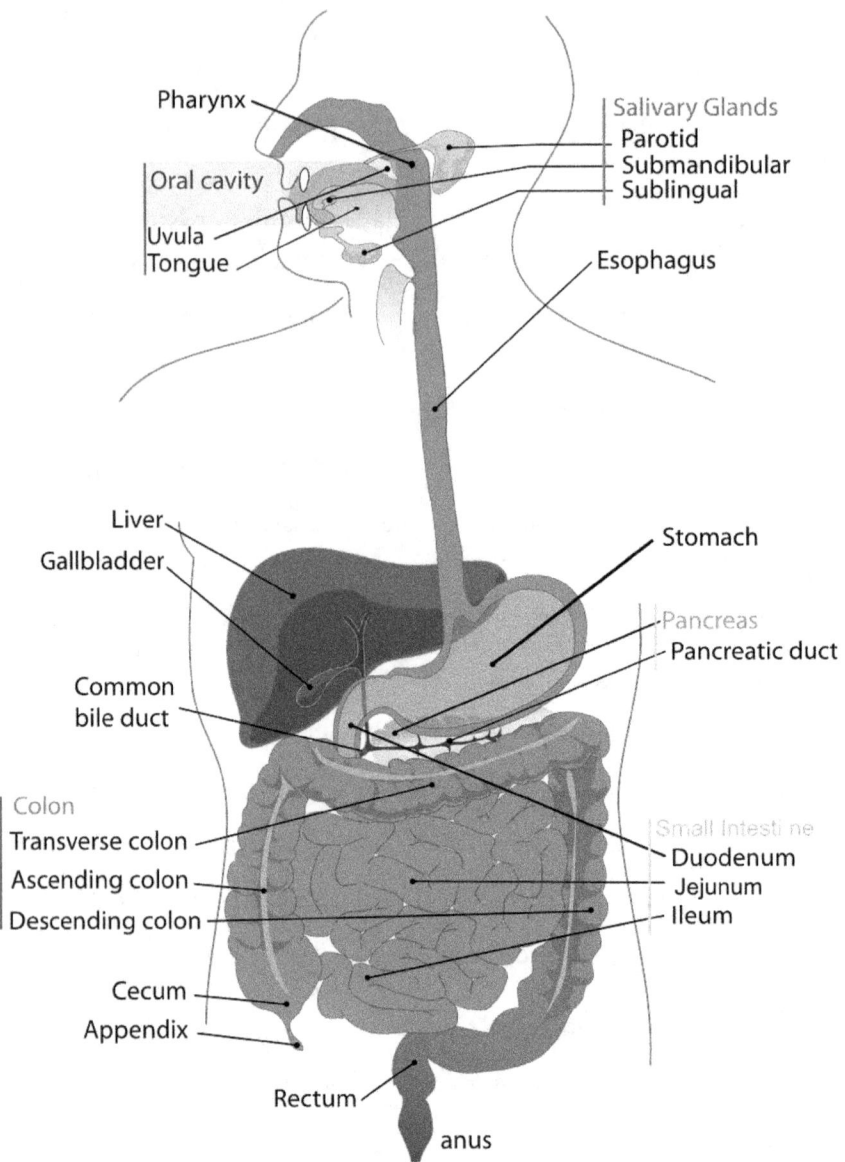

Gastrointestinal tract and associated organs

Ingestion

Saliva and digestive enzymes

Gastrointestinal (GI) tract begins at the mouth, where a mechanical form of digestion begins (i.e., chewing or *mastication*).

Saliva, a form of chemical digestion, contains mucus and amylase (enzymes end with ~*ase*). Saliva is secreted from 3 pairs of salivary glands around the oral cavity. Mucus moistens the food, and amylase partially digests polysaccharides (starches).

Salivary glands secrete saliva into the mouth by ducts. Saliva is a form of lubrication and a source of enzymes that dissolve food and contain *mucin*.

Mucin is a protein that lubricates the bolus. Saliva contains *amylase*, an enzyme that breaks down polysaccharides (starch and glycogen), antibodies, and lysozymes that kill pathogens.

Swallowing moves food (i.e., bolus) from the mouth through the pharynx into the esophagus, past the esophageal sphincter, and into the stomach.

Dentition (i.e., teeth structure) has specializations because humans are *omnivores* (i.e., a diet of plants and animals).

Food is *masticated* (i.e., chewed) in the mouth and mixed with saliva. It is manipulated in the mouth by a muscular tongue containing touch and pressure receptors.

Taste buds, receptors stimulated by the chemical composition of food, are primarily on the tongue but on the mouth's surface.

Mucus (composed of mucin) moistens food and lubricates the esophagus.

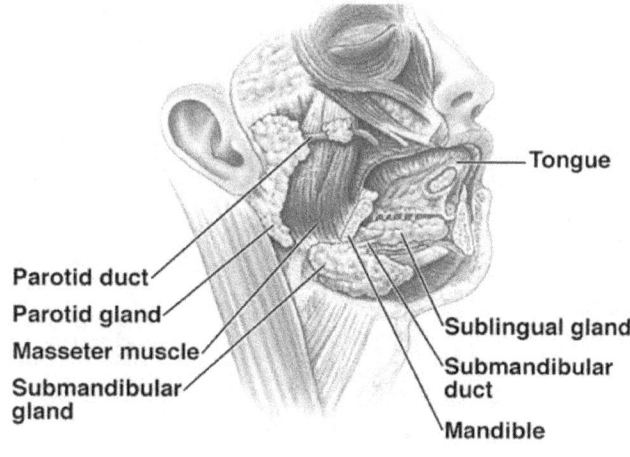

Salivary glands

Salivary amylase (enzymes end with *~ase*) begins digesting starch (α-linked glucose polysaccharide). It breaks down the complex carbohydrates into the simple sugar maltose (a disaccharide of two glucose monomers).

Bicarbonate ions in saliva neutralize the acids in foods.

$$\text{Starch} + H_2O \xrightarrow{\textit{Salivara Amylase Mechanism}} \text{maltose}$$

Pharynx, epiglottis and peristalsis

Pharynx (i.e., throat) is between the mouth and esophagus, where the food and air passage cross. A muscular tube squeezes and routes food to the *esophagus* when swallowing.

Pharynx closes pathways to the nasal cavity and airway to prevent choking.

In the pharynx, *bolus* (i.e., ingested food substance) triggers an involuntary swallowing reflex that prevents food from entering the trachea (directed to the lungs). It moves the bolus into the esophagus (directed to the stomach).

Digestive and respiratory passages join the pharynx and separate as air moves into the *rigid trachea* while food descends the *flexible esophagus* into the stomach.

Peristalsis is the involuntary muscle contractions that move food *via* the esophagus past the esophageal sphincter into the stomach, then the small intestine, large intestine, and rectum.

Epiglottal action

While swallowing, the tongue moves bolus to the back of the mouth.

If food were to enter the trachea, the pathway of air to the lungs could be blocked.

Epiglottis is a flap of cartilage that closes off the airway during swallowing. It covers the opening into the trachea as muscles move bolus through the pharynx into the esophagus.

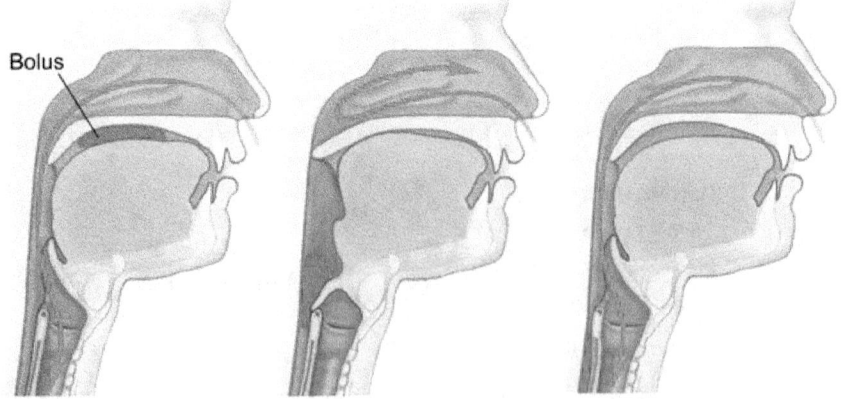

Swallowing where the epiglottis blocks food from entering the trachea

Stomach

Stomach anatomy and function

Stomach is an elastic, muscular sac that stretches to store food.

Bolus (food) passes through the *gastroesophageal sphincter* (or *lower esophageal* or *cardiac sphincter*), a ring of smooth muscle fibers connecting the esophagus and stomach.

Stomach secretes *hydrochloric acid* (HCl), which destroys bacteria and harmful organisms, preventing most food poisonings.

Gastric (i.e., stomach) *juices* may leak through the cardiac sphincter, and irritation of the esophagus causes *acid reflux* or *heartburn*.

Stomach secretes *pepsin*, which digests proteins into smaller polypeptides and amino acids.

Stomach's acidic environment (pH 1.5–3.0) creates optimum conditions for pepsin to function.

Villi (i.e., tiny finger-like projections) absorbs amino acid molecules that protrude from the small intestine's epithelial layer.

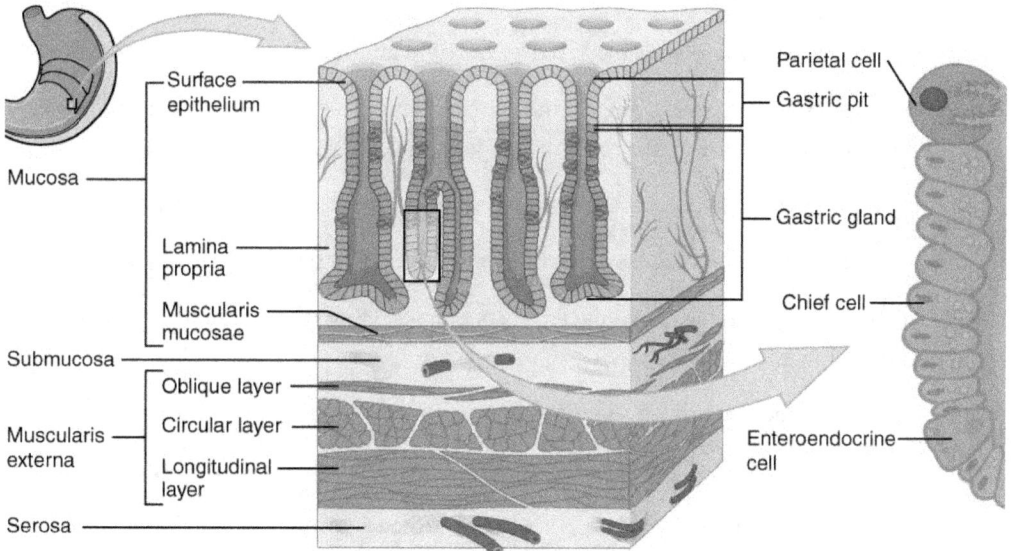

Stomach cross-section with mucosa, submucosa, muscularis externa, and serosa

Mechanical digestion, storage and churning of chyme

The stomach stores partially digested food (i.e., bolus in the stomach), freeing humans from continually eating for energy.

During a meal, the stomach gradually fills from an empty capacity of 50-100 ml (i.e., milliliters) to 1,000 ml (1 liter); with discomfort, the stomach distends to 2,000 ml (2 liters) or more.

Stomach muscles are responsible for the mechanical breakdown of food. This process is churning, where food is mechanically digested and mixed. Walls of the stomach contract vigorously, mixing food with juices secreted when the food enters.

Mixing food with water and gastric juice generates a creamy medium called *chyme*.

Food is mixed in the lower part of the stomach by peristaltic waves that propel the acid-chyme mixture against the pyloric sphincter.

During 1 to 2 hours, increased contractions (i.e., *peristalsis*) of stomach muscles push chyme through the pyloric sphincter and into the small intestine's *duodenum* (first of three sections).

High-fat diets offer satiation by increasing the period for food to remain in the stomach.

Mucus, low pH and gastric juice

Gastric glands are *exocrine glands* (secreted by ducts) within gastric pits.

Gastric pits are indentations in the stomach that denote entrances to the gastric glands, containing secreting epithelial cells (chief cells, parietal cells, and mucous cells).

Epithelial cells line the stomach's inner surface, secreting about 2 liters of gastric juice daily.

Gastric juice contains several digestion components (e.g., HCl, pepsinogen, and mucus).

Chief cells secrete *pepsinogen,* a zymogen (i.e., precursor) to pepsin. Pepsinogen is activated to form *pepsin* by low pH in the stomach.

Once active, pepsin begins protein digestion.

Parietal cells secrete HCl and intrinsic factor, important in vitamin B-12 absorption.

G cells secrete *gastrin*, a large peptide hormone absorbed into the blood, stimulating parietal cells to secrete HCl.

Acetylcholine increases all secretions, while *gastrin* and *histamine* increase *HCl secretion.*

Mucous cells (Goblet cells) secrete mucus that lubricates and protects the stomach's epithelial lining from the acidic environment. *Mucus* forms a *protective barrier* between cells and stomach acids.

Pepsin is inactivated (i.e., pepsinogen) when it contacts mucus.

Bicarbonate ions reduce acidity near the cells lining the stomach by increasing the pH. For protection, tight junctions link the epithelial, stomach-lining cells, preventing stomach acids from affecting other structures.

Stomach with mucus cells and bicarbonate

Ulcers

Peptic ulcers result from the failure of the mucosal lining to protect the stomach. Ulcers are eroded areas of the gastric surface or breaks in the mucosal barrier. Ulcers expose the underlying gastric muscle tissue to acid and pepsin's corrosive action.

Bleeding ulcers result when tissue damage is so severe that blood enters the stomach. Perforated ulcers are life-threatening emergencies when a hole forms in the stomach wall.

About 90% of peptic ulcers are caused by *Helicobacter pylori*, a strain of bacteria that burrows into the stomach's mucous lining, exposing the underlying epithelial cells to the stomach's acidic environment. Other factors contributing to ulcers are stress, excess HCl, and aspirin.

Production of digestive enzymes and site of digestion

Carbohydrate digestion begins with salivary amylase in the mouth and continues as the bolus passes into the stomach.

Bolus becomes *acid chyme* as it is broken down in the *lower third of the stomach.*

Hydrochloric acid does not directly function for digestion, but it lowers the pH of the gastric (stomach) contents to about 2.

Low pH stops salivary amylase activity and promotes pepsin activity; protein digestion begins.

Pepsin is an enzyme that controls the hydrolysis of proteins into peptides.

Chyme leaves the stomach and enters the *small intestine*.

$$\text{protein} + H_2O \xrightarrow{pepsin} \text{peptides (i.e., small chains of amino acids)}$$

Cardiac and pyloric sphincters of the stomach

Stomach has an inner membrane of dense folds as *rugae*, allowing it to accommodate stretching.

Stomach is sealed off at the top by the *cardiac* (or *gastroesophageal*) sphincter.

At the bottom, the stomach is sealed by the *pyloric sphincter*, a circular muscle that controls the release of the acid chyme into the small intestine.

When the pyloric sphincter relaxes, a portion of chyme exits the stomach and enters the duodenum (i.e., the first section of the small intestine).

A neural reflex causes the sphincter to contract, closing off the opening.

The slow, rhythmic pace with which chyme exits the stomach allows for thorough digestion.

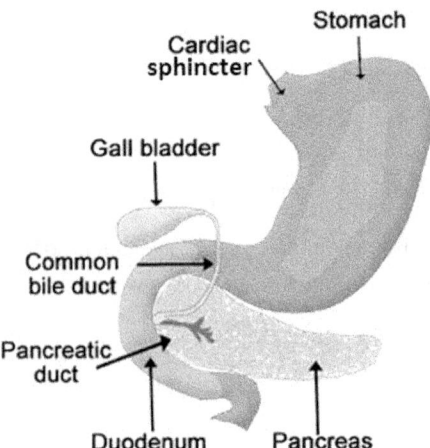

Stomach and duodenum with accessory organs for digestion

Liver

Glandular organ

The liver is a large glandular organ that occupies the top of the abdominal cavity below the diaphragm. The largest gland in the body spans both sides of the abdomen (the right side occupies more space) and has ducts that drain into the duodenum and gallbladder.

The liver is responsible for the detoxification of blood (metabolizing and removing poisonous substances), synthesis of blood proteins (making plasma proteins such as albumin and fibrinogen), production of bile, destruction of old erythrocytes, storage and regulation of blood glucose, and the production of urea from amino acids and ammonia.

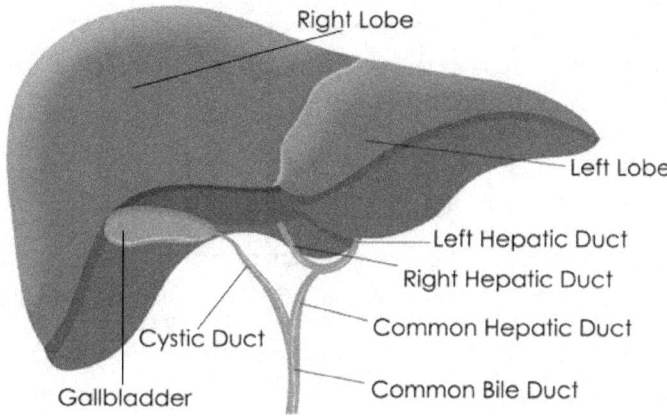

Liver with lobes and ducts that connect the liver to accessory glands

Nutrient metabolism and vitamin storage

Liver stores glucose as glycogen and catabolizes (i.e., breaks down) glycogen to maintain a constant blood glucose concentration.

Blood vessels from the large and small intestines lead to the liver as the *hepatic portal vein*.

Liver maintains the blood glucose level at 0.1% by removing glucose from the hepatic portal vein to store it as glycogen. As needed, glycogen is catabolized, and glucose monomers reenter the hepatic portal vein.

Amino acids are converted to glucose by the liver, but *deamination* (i.e., removal of ammonia from amino groups) must occur first.

Liver produces *urea* from amino groups and ammonia. By complex metabolic pathways, the liver converts amino groups to urea. Urea is the common human nitrogenous waste; the blood transports it to the kidneys (i.e., excretory system).

Liver stores essential nutrients, vitamins (A, D, E, K and B_{12}), and minerals (e.g., iron, copper), releasing them to tissues as needed. These compounds are absorbed from the blood through the hepatic portal system.

Glucose is stored in the liver in its polysaccharide form, glycogen. Under the influence of insulin, glucose is transported to the liver cells (i.e., *hepatocytes*).

Hepatocytes absorb and store fatty acids in the form of digested triglycerides. The storage of nutrients allows the liver to maintain homeostasis of blood glucose levels.

Blood glucose regulation and cellular detoxification

Liver is a storehouse for glycogen, the storage form of glucose. The liver regulates glucose levels in the blood through *gluconeogenesis*, *glycogenolysis*, and *glycogenesis*.

When blood sugar is low, the liver performs *gluconeogenesis* (i.e., synthesizing glucose and increasing blood glucose count) and *glycogenolysis* (i.e., breaking down stored glycogen and increasing blood glucose levels).

When blood glucose is too high, the liver engages in *glycogenesis*, converting the extra glucose into glycogen as a form of storage.

Insulin, an essential hormone in glucose regulation, increases glucose levels. Therefore, insulin promotes glucose conversion into glycogen, storing excess glucose in the liver for later use.

Glucagon, a hormone antagonist to insulin, is released in response to decreased glucose levels, promoting glycogen conversion into glucose. Low glucose is compensated for by the glucose supply by glycogen.

Liver detoxifies the body. It metabolizes alcohol with *alcohol dehydrogenase* (enzymes end with *~ase*), removes blood ammonia, and inactivates drugs and toxins.

Liver excretes detoxified chemicals as part of bile (or polarized to be excreted by the kidneys).

Kupffer cells are liver macrophages that phagocytize the intestines' bacteria.

Most red blood cells are destroyed in the spleen; Kupffer cells destroy irregular erythrocytes.

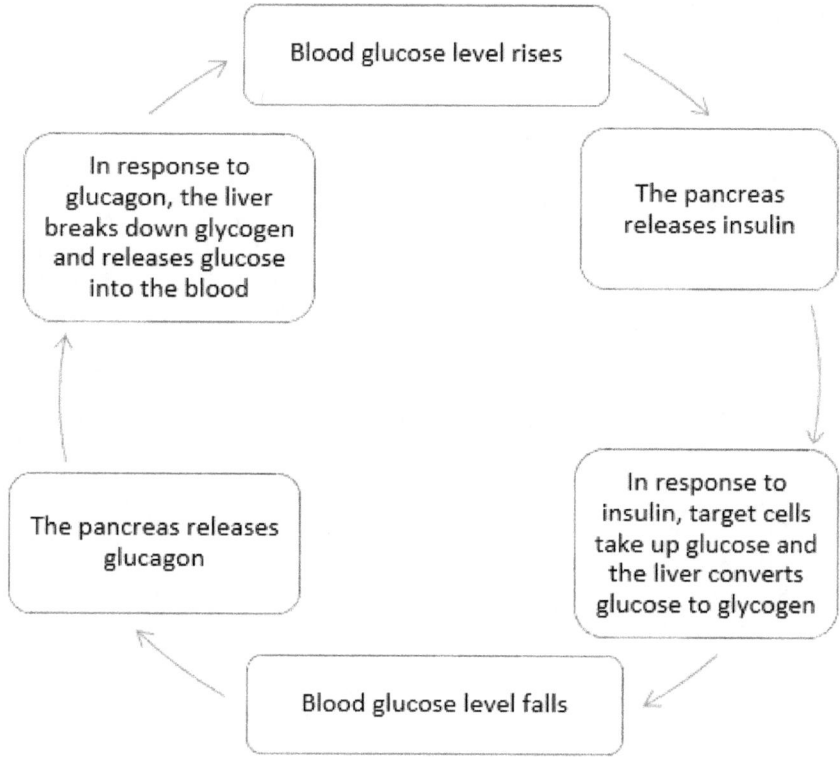

Homeostasis of glucose by the antagonistic actions of insulin and glucagon

Notes for active learning

Bile

Bile production

Liver makes bile from cholesterol and stores it in the gallbladder. To produce bile, *hepatocytes* in the liver destroy old red blood cells.

Bile is a green byproduct resulting from *hemoglobin breakdown*, converted into the two critical components of bile, *bilirubin* and *biliverdin*.

Bile subsequently enters the duodenum from the gallbladder to emulsify fats.

Gallbladder stores bile

Bile reaches the gallbladder through hepatic ducts and is stored for later use. Bile flows through the cystic duct when needed, merging with *pancreatic duct* to form the *common bile duct*.

Sphincter of Oddi is a muscular valve that controls the entry of digestive juices (bile and pancreatic juice) from the liver and pancreas into the duodenum of the small intestine. When the sphincter is *closed*, secreted bile is *shunted into the gallbladder*.

Dietary fats in the intestine release CCK, relaxing the sphincter to discharge bile salts into the duodenum.

Excess, unused bile is concentrated, stored in the gallbladder, and secreted when needed. For example, bile is secreted from the gland during a meal by smooth muscle contraction. Bile reaches the duodenum of the small intestine by the *common bile duct*.

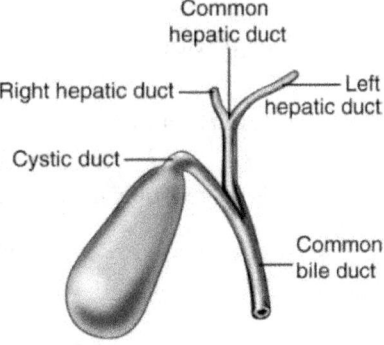

Gallbladder and associated ducts

Bile emulsifies fats during digestion

Bile salts solubilize fats, while bicarbonate ions neutralize stomach acids.

Emulsification breaks fat globules into microscopic droplets.

Bile salts, secreted by *hepatocytes* (i.e., liver cells), enter the GI tract, are reabsorbed by transporters in the intestine, and are returned to the liver via the *portal vein*.

Entero-hepatic circulation recycling pathway.

$$\text{fat} \xrightarrow{\text{bile salts}} \text{fat droplets (by emulsification)}$$

This process increases fat digestion by increasing the surface area of fat globules exposed to lipase (enzymes end with ~*ase*).

Bile *emulsifies fats*, facilitating their breakdown into progressively smaller fat globules until lipases act upon them. Bile contains cholesterol, phospholipids, bilirubin, and a mix of salts.

Unlike carbohydrates (i.e., by salivary amylase in the mouth), fats are digested in the small intestine, and proteins (predigested in the acidic stomach).

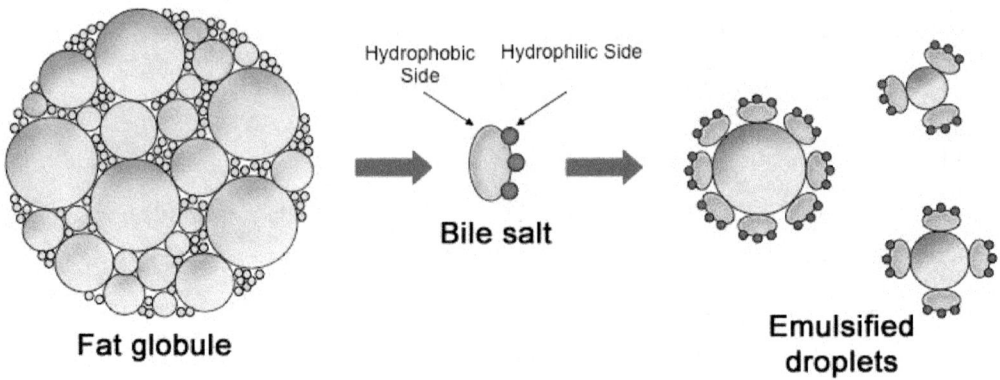

Bile salts emulsify fat into smaller goblets for absorption in the small intestine.

Due to their hydrophobic nature, digested fats are not soluble.

Bile salts surround fats, forming micelles that pass into the epithelial cells to compensate for insolubility. Afterward, bile salts are recycled into the lumen to repeat the process.

Fat digestion is usually completed when food reaches the small intestine's ileum (lower third).

Bile salts are absorbed in the ileum and are recycled by the liver and gallbladder.

Fats pass from the epithelial cells to the small lymph vessels that run through the villi.

Gallstones and jaundice

Excessive secretion of water-insoluble cholesterol in bile results in crystals called *gallstones*. Gallstones can obstruct the opening of the gallbladder or the bile duct.

Fat digestion and absorption decrease if a *gallstone prevents bile* from entering the intestine.

If a gallstone blocks the pancreatic duct's entry, pancreatic enzymes cannot enter the intestine, preventing the digestion of other nutrients.

Blocked bile secretions result in the accumulation of *bilirubin* in tissues.

Elevated levels of *bilirubin* produce a yellowish coloration as *jaundice*.

Jaundice is common in newborns and patients with liver disease.

Pancreas

Endocrine and exocrine functions

Pancreas, an elongated, tadpole-shaped organ, lies deep within the abdominal cavity. It is below the stomach along the posterior abdominal wall and leads to the duodenum.

Pancreatic *endocrine functions* include secreting glucose regulatory hormones (i.e., *glucagon* and *insulin*) into the bloodstream using two types of cells.

One of the two hormones targets the liver depending on blood glucose concentration.

From its *exocrine function*, the *pancreas secretes digestive enzymes* and a fluid rich in bicarbonate ions (HCO_3^-) to *neutralize acid* from the stomach.

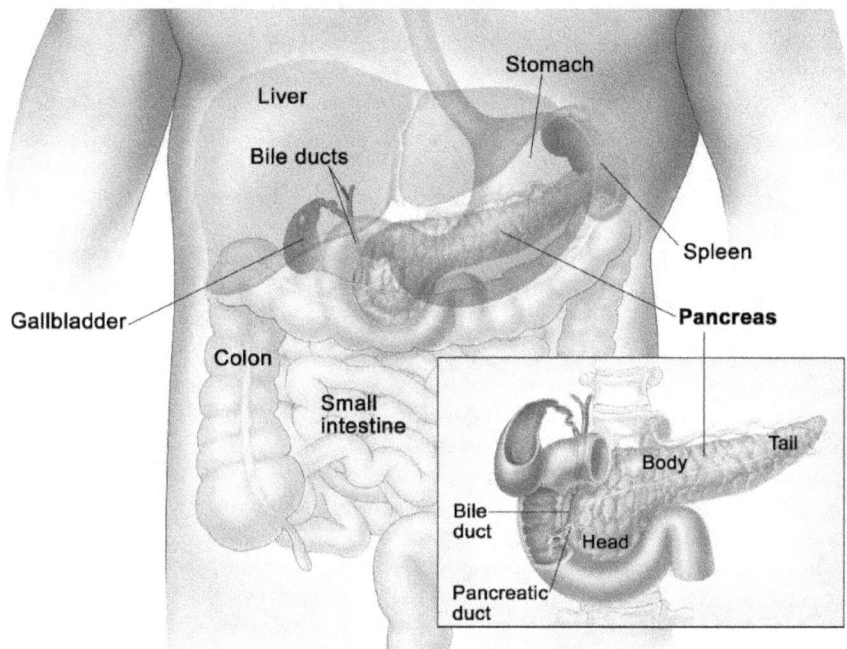

Pancreas as an endocrine and exocrine organ aiding in digestion

Pancreas produces enzymes and bicarbonate

Pancreas secretes pancreatic juice, a mixture of enzymes and ions.

Pancreas releases enzymes from *acinar cells* into the duodenum via the *pancreatic duct*.

Enzymes include *trypsin* and *chymotrypsin* (enzymes that digest proteins), *lipase* (i.e., digests fats), pancreatic amylase (i.e., digests starch), and *deoxyribonucleases* and *ribonucleases* (i.e., digests nucleic acids).

Secretion of pancreatic enzymes is stimulated by *cholecystokinin* (CCK), a GI peptide hormone.

These enzymes exist first as zymogens / proenzymes (inactive forms). Once trypsin becomes activated by intestinal *enterokinase*, it activates digestive enzymes released by the pancreas.

Certain enzymes (e.g., *pancreatic amylase* and *lipase*) are secreted in their active form.

Pancreatic amylase digests starch to *maltose*:

starch + H_2O + *pancreatic amylase* → maltose

Trypsin (and other enzymes) digest protein into peptides:

protein + H_2O + *trypsin* → peptides

Lipase digests fat droplets into *glycerol* and *fatty acids*:

fat droplets + H_2O + *lipase* → glycerol + fatty acids

Cholecystokinin (CCK) hormone, produced in the small intestine, is secreted in response to the presence of nutrients, and it regulates the transport of enzymes into the duodenum.

Acinar cells secrete *pancreatic enzymes*, which organize into *acini* (singular acinus structures), composed of several acinar cells and a duct (which empties into the small intestine).

Bicarbonate ion secretion is stimulated by *secretin*, which is triggered by small intestine *acidity*.

Pancreas secretes *bicarbonate ions* (HCO_3^-) to neutralize HCl from the stomach. Pancreatic enzymes function best in *alkaline* (pH > 7) solutions.

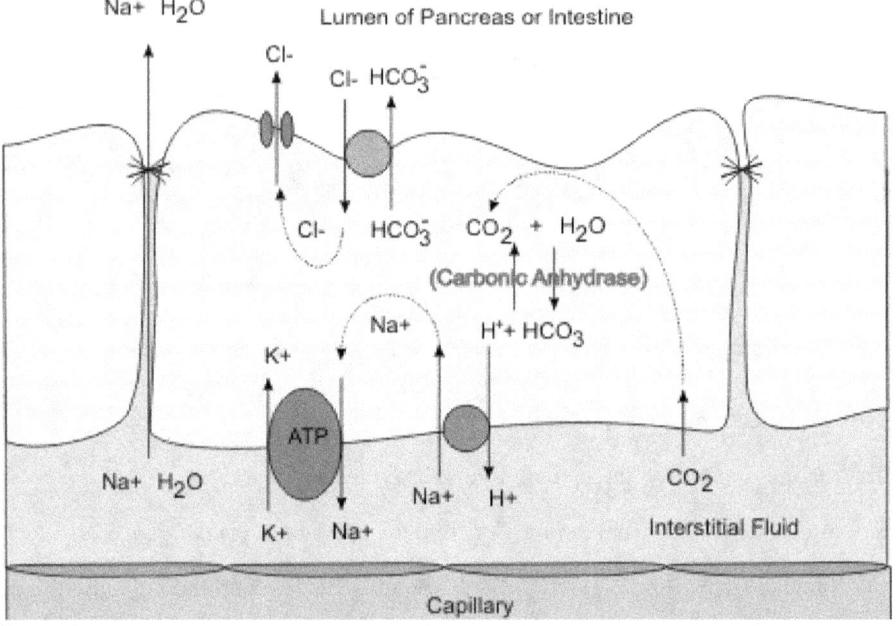

Bicarbonate secretion in the pancreas or intestine aids in digesting lipids

Transport of enzymes to the small intestine

Pancreatic digestive enzymes travel to the small intestine, where the process continues.

Enzymes enter the small intestine through the *pancreatic duct* (or *duct of Wirsung*), which joins the pancreas to the common bile duct so that pancreatic juices can be used in the small intestine.

Secretin is another hormone produced in the small intestine, and it controls the transport of bicarbonate into the small intestine to regulate pH levels.

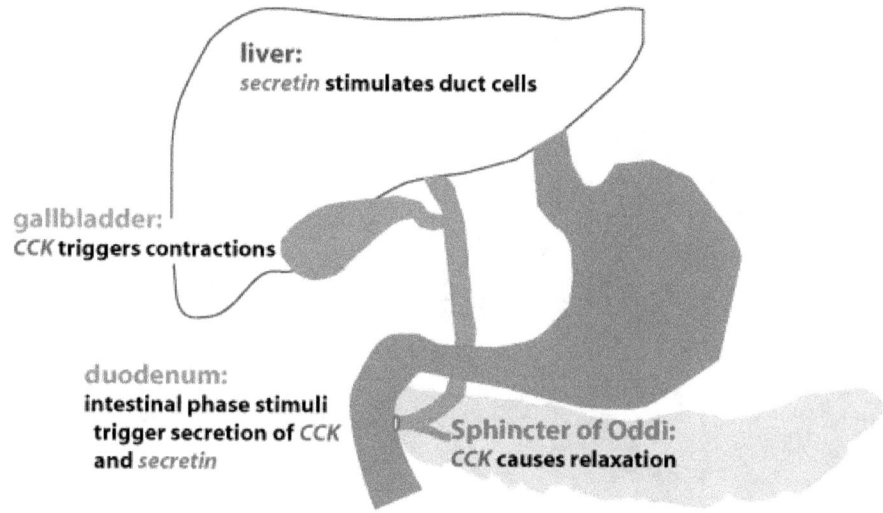

Organs and enzymes associated with digestion

Notes for active learning

Small Intestine

Site of complete digestion and absorption of monomers

Most digestion and absorption of nutrients occur in the small intestine.

Intestinal walls secrete enzymes and receive enzymes from the pancreas.

After chemical digestion, the small intestine's primary function is to complete digestion and absorb food particles' monomers (i.e., individual building blocks comprising polymers).

The small intestine contains many *villi*, structures *increasing the surface area* for absorption.

Absorption of digested food molecules

Most animals must digest food into small molecules to cross plasma membranes.

Complete digestion of complex food molecules is essential for proper absorption.

First, consumed food originates as compounds synthesized by other organisms. Not all the ingested compounds are suitable for use by human tissues. Complex molecules (i.e., polymers) must be broken down into primarily individual subunits (i.e., monomers) and reassembled so the body can use them appropriately.

Second, the food molecules must be small to be absorbed by the villi in the intestine by diffusion, facilitated diffusion, or active transport. Therefore, large food molecules must be broken down for absorption.

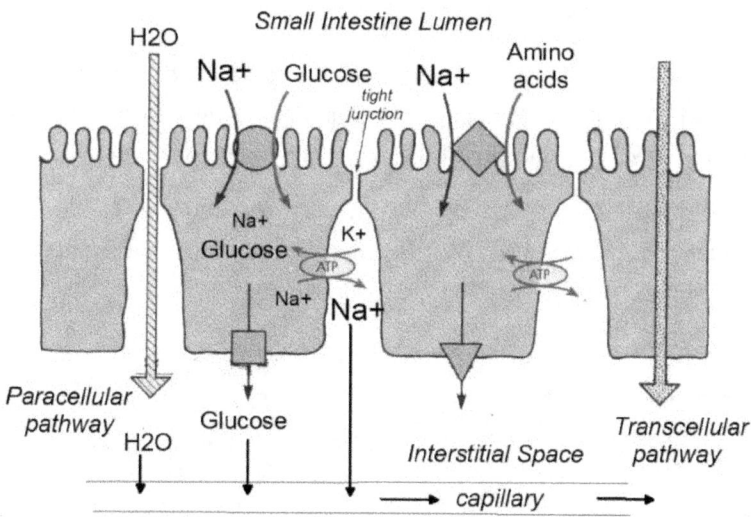

Absorption of glucose in the small intestine

Intestinal folds, villi, and microvilli increase the surface area to absorb digested compounds into circulation.

Absorption uses *lacteals* for fats into lacteals and *capillaries* for *amino acids and sugars*.

Active transport absorbs molecules against the concentration gradient.

The intestinal lumen has less glucose than enterocytes (i.e., intestinal lining); Na^+ / K^+ pump and $Na^+ /$ glucose symport are *secondary active transport*.

Facilitated transport (i.e., passive diffusion) absorbs glucose down its concentration gradient and drives energetically unfavorable reactions.

Enterocytes now have more glucose. It transfers its glucose to the extracellular fluid using *facilitated diffusion*. Glucose then moves from the extracellular fluid to the blood.

Function and structure of villi

Most absorption occurs in the small intestine's duodenum and jejunum (second third).

Intestinal inner surface has circular folds that more than triple the surface area for absorption. Finger-like projections as villi cover the mucous membrane in these ridges and furrows.

Villi increases the surface area for greater digestion and absorption. They are covered with epithelial cells that increase the surface area by another factor of 10.

Epithelial cells are lined with microvilli to increase the surface area; a 6-meter tube has a surface area of 300 square meters. The small intestine is specialized for absorption by the massive number of villi lining the intestinal wall. If the small intestine were a smooth tube, it would have to be 500–600 meters long to have a comparable surface area.

The structure of the villus is specific. Their numbers increase the surface area for absorption in the small intestine. The villi have projections (microvilli).

Microvilli are minute projections (collectively as the brush border) on the intestinal villi's surface of cells. Microvilli have protein channels and pumps in their membranes to allow the rapid absorption of food by facilitated diffusion and active transport.

Villi contains an epithelial layer (one cell layer thick) so that food can pass through easily and be absorbed quickly. Blood capillaries in the villus are associated with the epithelium, so the distance for the diffusion of the food molecules is negligible.

This thin layer of epithelial cells contains mitochondria to provide the ATP needed for the active transport of specific food molecules.

Lacteals branch at the center of the villus carries away fats after absorption.

Lacteals

Sugars and amino acids enter villi cells and are absorbed into the bloodstream.

Glycerol and fatty acids enter villi cells, reassemble fat molecules, and move into lacteals.

Villi have *lacteals*, a lymphatic vessel surrounded by a capillary network in an intestinal villus that aids fat absorption.

Absorption involves diffusion and active transport, requiring the expenditure of cellular energy.

Villi cells produce intestinal enzymes to complete the digestion of peptides and sugars.

Villi have many capillaries that shuttle *amino acids* and *glucose* from digestion to the *hepatic portal vein* and *liver*.

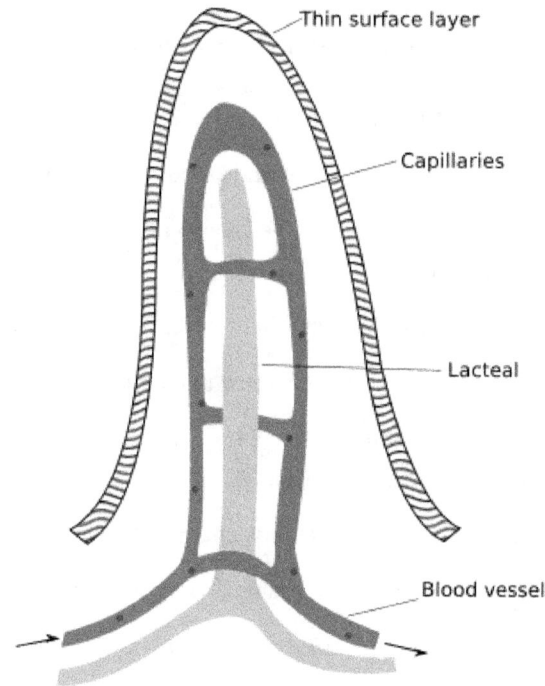

Intestinal villus with lacteals for fat absorption and capillaries for other nutrients

Absorption occurs in the small intestine's specialized villi when food molecules pass through a layer of cells and into the body's tissues.

Absorption is followed *by assimilation* when food molecules become part of the body's tissue.

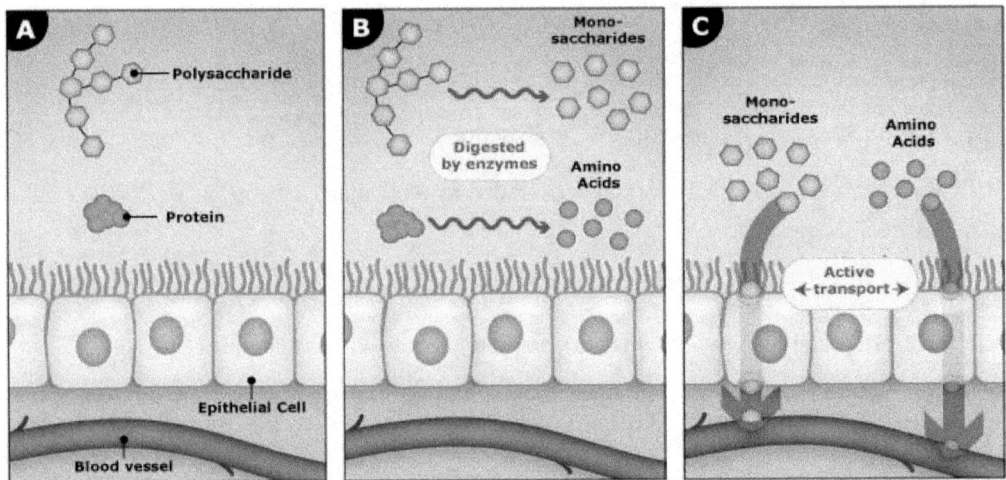

Digestion and absorption of amino acids and monosaccharides in the small intestine

Enzyme production and site of digestion

Chyme enters the duodenum with proteins and carbohydrates partially digested.

Fat has not been digested yet because the liver and pancreas' secretions released into the duodenum are essential for fat digestion.

Digestion of carbohydrates, proteins, and fats continues in the small intestine.

Starch and *glycogen* polymers are broken down into *maltose* (i.e., monomer)

Proteases (enzymes secreted from the pancreas) continue the breakdown of proteins into small peptide fragments and individual amino acids.

The upper part of the small intestine, the duodenum, is the most active during digestion.

Duodenum uses secretions from the liver and pancreas to break down ingested compounds.

Epithelial cells of the duodenum form *Bruner's glands* and secrete watery *mucus.*

Mucus protects duodenal epithelium from the acidic chyme (entered from the stomach), lubricating intestinal walls and providing an alkaline environment for pancreatic enzymes.

Peptidase and maltase

Epithelial cells of villi produce intestinal enzymes attached to microvilli's plasma membrane.

Intestinal secretions complete the digestion of peptides and sugars.

Peptidases digest peptides into amino acids:

$$\text{peptides} + H_2O + \textit{peptidases} \rightarrow \text{amino acids}$$

Maltose (from the first step in starch digestion) is converted by maltase to glucose:

$$\text{maltose} + H_2O + \textit{maltase} \rightarrow \text{glucose} + \text{glucose}$$

Maltose, sucrose, and lactose are the main carbohydrates in the small intestine; the microvilli absorb them. Starch is broken down into two glucose units (i.e., maltose).

Epithelial cell enzymes convert disaccharides (i.e., two sugars) into monosaccharides (i.e., single sugar) that exit the cell and enter the capillaries.

Lactose (i.e., milk sugar) intolerance results from a genetic deficiency of lactase (enzymes with ~*ase*) produced by the intestinal cells. Lack of lactase results in incomplete digestion of *lactose* to *glucose* and *galactose* monomers.

While the pancreas is the primary enzyme source, the small intestine makes enzymes, including *protease, amylase, lipase,* and *nuclease*.

Cellulose is a polysaccharide similar in structure to starch and cannot be digested by humans. Humans lack the cellul*ase* needed to hydrolyze β glycosidic bonds of *cellulose*.

Pancreatic juices neutralize stomach acid

Pancreas secretes *pancreatic juice*, which contains *sodium bicarbonate* [$NaCO_3$], neutralizing the acidity of chyme (due to the HCl from the stomach).

pH of the small intestine is, therefore, slightly basic. This neutralization process facilitates enzymes in the small intestine, which would typically be denatured by stomach pH.

Anatomical subdivisions of the small intestine

Small intestine is divided into three segments:

duodenum, jejunum, and *ileum.*

The small intestine is a coiled tube up to 6 meters long and 2 to 3 cm wide. Coils and folding, along with villi, of 6–meters tube a surface area of a tube 500-600 m.

Food moves from the stomach to the small intestine through the *pyloric sphincter* (into the first 25 cm of the small intestine, the duodenum).

Duodenum has a pH of 6, mainly due to bicarbonate ions secreted by the pancreas.

Breakdown of starches, proteins, and foods (fats, nucleotides) continues in the duodenum.

Ileocecal valve separates the *small intestine* from the large intestine.

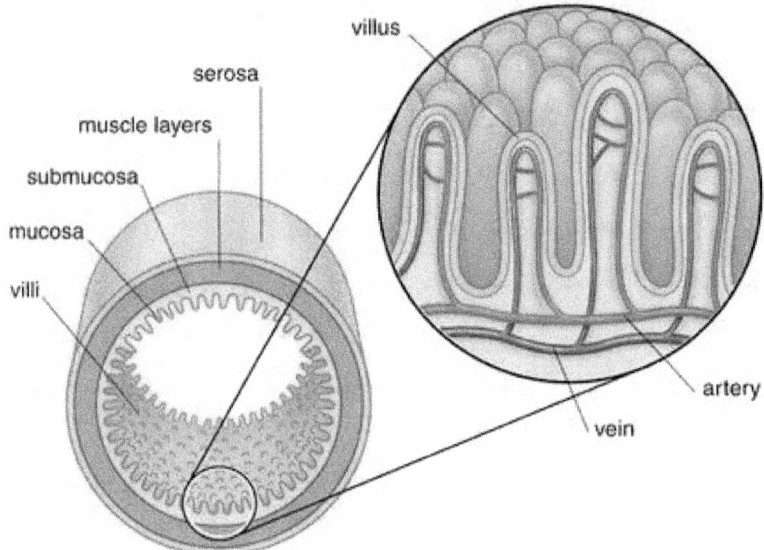

Small intestine

Duodenum is responsible for *digestion*, with the jejunum and ilium mainly responsible for *absorption*. 90% of digestion and absorption occurs within the small intestine.

Goblet cells secrete mucus to lubricate and protect from mechanical or chemical damage.

Tissue stratification of the small intestine

While the entire intestinal tract's length contains lymphoid tissue, only the ileum has abundant *Peyer's patches* (i.e., unencapsulated lymphoid nodules) containing large numbers of lymphocytes and immune cells.

A single epithelium layer containing *exocrine* and *endocrine* cells covers the small intestine's luminal surface.

Epithelia are mucosa with an underlying layer of *lamina propria* (i.e., connective tissue) and *muscularis mucosa* (i.e., muscle).

Below the mucosa is a layer of *inner circular* and an *outer longitudinal smooth muscle* of *muscularis externa*, providing the force for moving and mixing the GI contents.

Serosa is the outermost layer of the tube made of connective tissue.

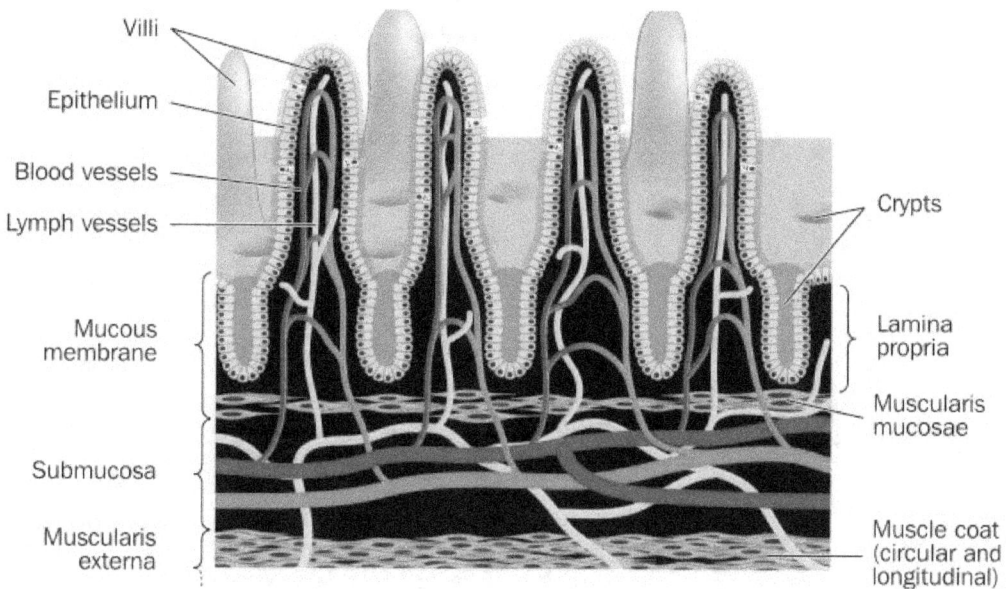

Circulatory and muscular system of the small intestine

Notes for active learning

Large Intestine

Structure of large intestine

Large intestine is the gastrointestinal tract region following the small intestine.

Large intestine has four parts:

>*cecum* (blind pocket; the appendix), colon, rectum, and anal canal.

Chyme enters cecum through ileocecal sphincter, relaxing and opening by gastroileal reflex.

Large intestine terminates at the anus, an external opening.

Large intestine has lobes (pockets) along its length due to muscle tone.

Unlike the small intestine, the large intestine has *no folds or villi* because its primary function is to *store and concentrate fecal material* for elimination.

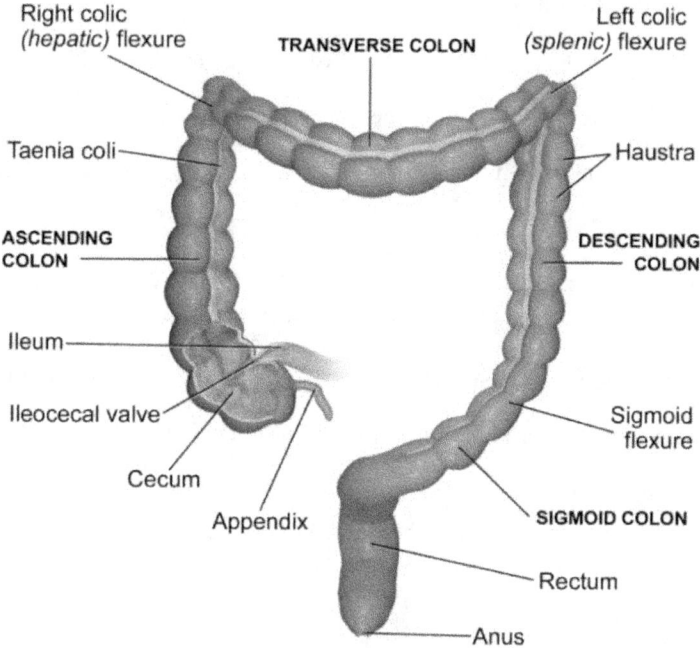

Large intestine with colon, rectum, and anal canal

Appendix is a finger-like projection extending from the cecum, a blind sac at the junction of the small and large intestines. It may play a role in fighting infections.

If an infected appendix bursts, the result is a general abdominal infection, such as peritonitis.

Large intestine secretes an alkaline mucus (HCO_3^- ions) into the lumen, protecting epithelial tissue and neutralizing acids produced by bacterial metabolism.

Water absorption by the large intestine

Material entering the large intestine is mostly indigestible residue and liquid.

Undigested chyme is passed to the large intestine, temporarily stored, and concentrated by reabsorption of salts and water.

About 2,500 milliliters (2.5 liters) of water enters the digestive tract daily by consumption.

Small intestine reabsorbs most of this liquid.

Large intestine (or *large bowel*) absorbs most of the remaining water not absorbed by the small intestine. If water is not reabsorbed, it causes diarrhea, which can cause severe dehydration and ion loss.

However, if too much water is reabsorbed, the result is *constipation* with a blocked passage.

Sodium ions (Na^+) are absorbed whenever water is reabsorbed.

Rectum stores and eliminates waste

Large intestine moves material that is not digested from the small intestine.

Water, salt, and vitamins are absorbed in the large intestine.

Remaining contents in the lumen form feces stored in the rectum and egested through the anus.

Feces consist of about 75% water and 25% solid matter.

One-third of the solid matter is intestinal bacteria. The remainder are undigested waste, fats, organic material, mucus, and dead cells from intestinal linings.

Following a meal, there is a wave of intense contraction (i.e., *mass movement*).

Mass movement of fecal material into the anus initiates the defecation reflex.

Contractions of the rectum expel the feces through the anus. During defecation, the anal sphincter opens, and feces are released through the anus.

Muscular Control

Sphincter muscles

Cardiac sphincter (*gastroesophageal sphincter*) is between the esophagus and the stomach.

It prevents the backflow of food.

Pyloric sphincter is between the stomach and the small intestine.

It releases food into the small intestine, a small amount at a time.

Anal sphincter is at the end of the rectum and ties to the end of the rectum.

Internal anal sphincter is made of smooth muscle and closes the anus, while the *external anal sphincter* is made of skeletal muscle and is under voluntary control.

Both sphincters regulate the anal opening and closing.

The defecation reflex, mediated by mechanoreceptors, causes the *two anal sphincters* to open and expel the feces. If defecation is delayed, rectal contents are driven into the colon *by reverse peristalsis* until the next mass movement.

Peristalsis

Peristalsis is regular circular smooth muscle contractions that produce a slow, rhythmic, bidirectional segmentation movement similar to unidirectional material movement. Undigested material moves back and forth slowly to provide resident bacteria time to grow and multiply.

Large intestine bacteria (e.g., *E. coli*) are symbiotic organisms that ferment undigested nutrients, making gas a byproduct. These bacteria produce vitamins (vitamin K) essential to blood clot formation.

Undigested polysaccharides (i.e., fiber) are metabolized to short-chain fatty acids by residing bacteria and absorbed by diffusion. Bacterial metabolism produces *flatus*, a mixture of gases.

Peristalsis is the involuntary movement of smooth muscles that squeeze food along the digestive tract. Chyme moves through the intestines via peristalsis.

Layers of circular and longitudinal smooth muscle enable the chyme (partly digested food and water) to be pushed along the ileum by waves of muscle contractions as peristalsis.

The remaining chyme is passed to the colon.

Stomach produces *peristaltic waves* in response to the arrival of food. With every wave, the *pyloric sphincter* between the stomach and duodenum opens to release small amounts of chyme into the duodenum.

Waves are generated by pacemaker cells in the longitudinal smooth muscle layer and are spread by gap junctions.

Distension of the stomach with gastrin and other factors stimulates gastric motility, while distension of the duodenum inhibits it.

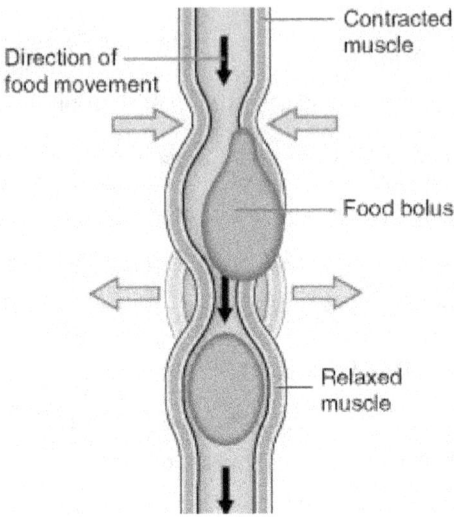

Pacemaker cells in the longitudinal smooth muscle layer produce peristaltic waves

Segmentation by the small intestine mixes chyme

Typical motion of small intestine is stationary contraction and relaxation, called *segmentation*.

Segmentation mixes chyme with digestive juices but results in little net movement.

Chyme is mixed, brought into contact with the intestine wall, and moved slowly toward the large intestine. Movements are initiated by *pacemaker cells* in the smooth muscle layer.

After most materials are absorbed, segmentation is replaced by peristaltic activity as a migrating motility complex, moving undigested material to the large intestine.

Intestinal hormone *motilin* initiates migrating motility.

In the large intestine (due to involuntary contractions), movements shuffle contents back and forth, and propulsive contractions move material through the large intestine.

Gastrointestinal Tract Summary

Anatomy and function of the gastrointestinal (GI) tract

Human digestive tract is a complete tube-within-a-tube system, with each part of the digestive system having a specific function.

In humans, the digestion of food is an extracellular process.

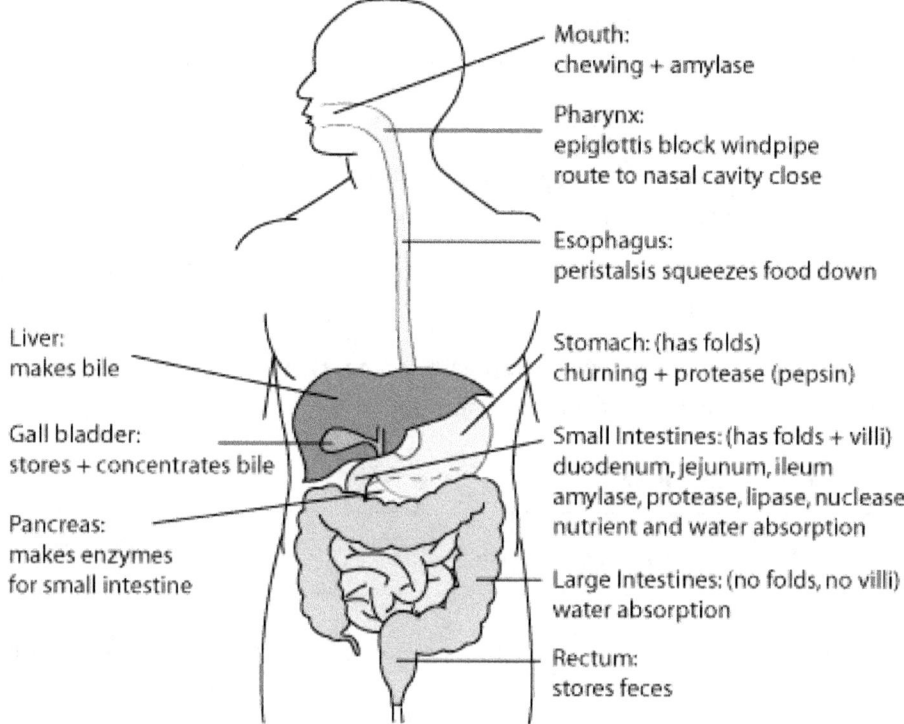

Digestive tract begins at the mouth and continues to the anus, with enzymes assisting

Enzymes are secreted in the digestive tract by nearby glands.

Food is never within the accessory glands, only within the tract.

Digestion is a cooperative effort that produces hormones through actions of the nervous system.

Summary of the digestive system

- *Mouth*: grinds and moistens food by mastication (chewing for mechanical digestion); begins chemical digestion of starch by amylase (~*ase* for enzymes) and lipase in saliva.
- *Esophagus*: moves food to the stomach.

- *Stomach*: churning chyme (i.e., mechanical digestion), acid digestion by HCl, protein digestion by pepsin (chemical digestion), and temporary food storage.

- *Small intestine*: the longest and extensively folded part of the GI tract and is where most of the digestion and absorption of nutrients and water occurs.

  Chyme is subjected to bile (to emulsify fats) from the liver and digestive enzymes (amylase, protease, lipase, nuclease) for chemical digestion.

  Enzymes are predominantly from the pancreas.

- *Large intestine*: remaining water is reabsorbed from chyme to produce a relatively solid indigestible waste (i.e., feces).

Bacteria in the large intestine produce vitamin K.

Enzymes are needed for digestion as biological catalysts, breaking large food molecules into mostly monomers for absorption in the small intestine.

Digestion can occur naturally at body temperature; however, this process takes a long time because it happens slowly.

Enzymes are vital because they speed the digestive process by lowering the activation energy required for the reaction to occur at body temperature.

Amylase, protease and lipase

	Amylase	**Protease**	**Lipase**
Enzyme	Salivary amylase	Pepsin	Pancreatic lipase
Source	Salivary glands	Chief cells in the stomach lining	Pancreas
Substrate	Starch	Proteins	Triglycerides (e.g., fats and oils)
Products	Maltose	Small polypeptides	Fatty acids and glycerol
Optimum pH	pH 7	pH 1.5 – 2	pH 7

Endocrine Control

Digestive glands and associated hormones

Gastric glands produce *gastrin* in the stomach lining by sensing food reaching the stomach.

Gastrin stimulates and increases *gastric motility*.

Gastrin secretion is stimulated by meals rich in protein.

- *Secretin* is produced by cells lining the duodenum when food enters the duodenum. Secretin stimulates the pancreas to secrete fluids rich in $NaCO_3$ into the duodenum. This secretion is stimulated by acidic chyme.

- *Cholecystokinin* (CCK) is produced in the duodenal wall of the small intestine in response to fats. CCK stimulates the pancreas to increase pancreatic juice. It induces the liver to increase bile output and causes the gallbladder to release bile.

- *Gastric Inhibitory Peptide* is produced by the duodenal wall in response to fat and protein as chyme enters the duodenum. It causes a mild decrease in the rate of digestion in the stomach by inhibiting gastric gland secretion and stomach motility.

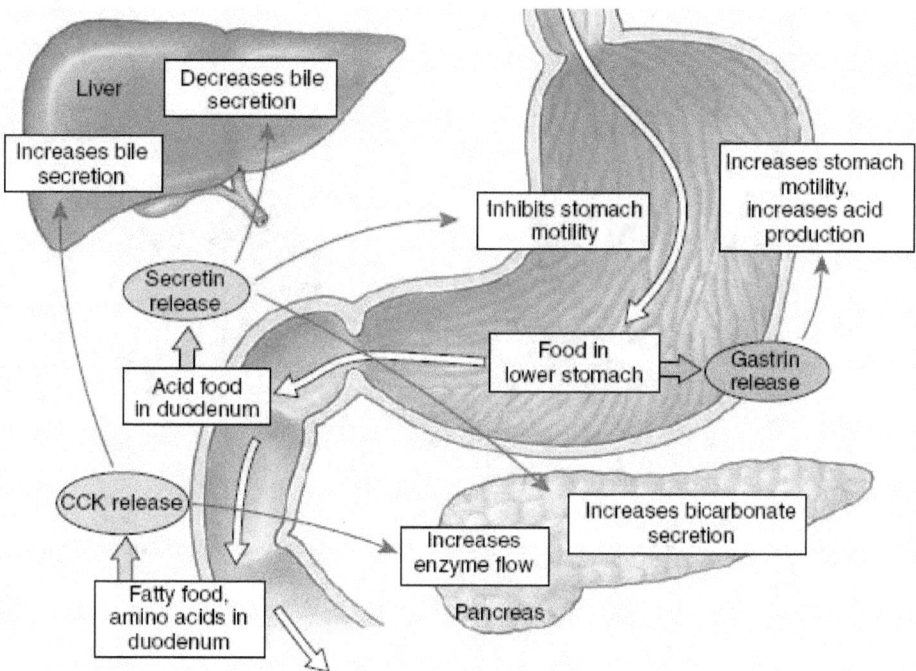

Digestive tract with glands and associated hormones

Endocrine cells are scattered within GI epithelia, and the surface is exposed to the lumen. Chemical substances in the chyme stimulate endocrine cells to release hormones into the blood.

Islets of Langerhans, gastrin, histamine and HCl secretions

Scattered throughout the stomach lining are *enterochromaffin-like* (ECL) cells and other cells that secrete *somatostatin*, an inhibitory protein influencing the release of glucagon and insulin.

ECL cells are neuroendocrine digestive tract cells; gastrin stimulates them to release histamine, stimulating parietal cells to produce gastric acid.

Pyloric antrum, a lower portion of the stomach, secretes gastrin.

Islets of Langerhans of the pancreas are irregularly shaped patches of endocrine tissue secreting insulin and glucagon. Islets have specific cells, including *alpha, beta, delta, F, and C cells*.

Increased meal protein stimulates gastrin and histamine release, stimulating HCl secretion.

Somatostatin inhibits acid secretion by *inhibiting* the release of *gastrin* and *histamine*.

Enterogastrone in the duodenum inhibits gastric acid secretion.

Precursor pepsinogen produced by chief cells is converted to pepsin by excess stomach acid.

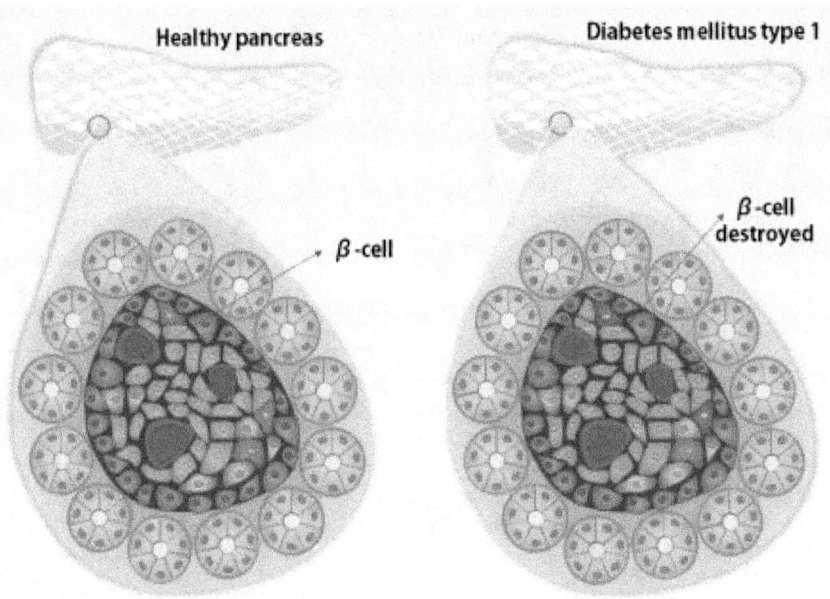

Islets of Langerhans with β-cells producing insulin in nondiabetic patients

Vitamin D and calcium

Vitamin D is a *fat-soluble* nutrient that promotes calcium absorption in the digestive system.

Vitamin D modulates cell growth, supports the immune system, and reduces inflammation.

Cells in the digestive system have vitamin D receptors necessary for protein synthesis.

Vitamin D provides nerve cells with calcium needed to send adequate signals, which is essential because nerves in the digestive tract must communicate to control the digestive process.

Receptor regulation and gastrin

Eighteen types of endocrine cells have been identified within the gastrointestinal tract.

Agonists are peptide ligands that bind a target cell receptor and stimulate target cell response.

Antagonists are peptide ligands (i.e., a molecule that binds a receptor) that bind the receptor but do not cause a reaction within the cell.

An antagonist's (no response) ability to occupy a receptor prevents an agonist's access (i.e., eliciting response). Inhibition is used to treat peptic ulcers with histamine receptor blockers. By occupying the receptors on the parietal cells, antagonists (e.g., medication) inhibit histamine production of hydrochloric acid, a significant cause of peptic ulcers.

The discharge of gastrin granules from G cells occurs when a meal is consumed.

While the concentration of hydrogen ions remains low because of the buffering effect of the food, the release of gastrin continues. As digestion occurs and the stomach starts to empty, acidity increases because of the diminishing neutralizing effect of food.

When the stomach contents contact the mucosa of the antrum to reach a certain acidity level, gastrin release stops. Failure of this process causes inappropriate acid secretion when the stomach is empty and may cause *peptic ulcers* in the duodenum.

Some endocrine cells contain surface microvilli projecting into the lumen of glands, the stomach, or intestine's main channel. These cells continuously sample local luminal contents.

When the production and secretion of a peptide hormone are excessive, it increases the number of target cells and may increase the size of the individual cells. This phenomenon is *trophism* and is similar to the increase in skeletal muscle size in response to appropriate exercise. Such trophism is observed in certain disease states that involve gastrointestinal hormones.

Thus, when gastrin is secreted into the blood by a tumor of G cells (gastrinoma) of the pancreas, it is a continuous process because there is no mechanism at that site to inhibit secretion. This process significantly increases the number of parietal cells in the stomach and the overproduction of acid. Intractable and complicated peptic ulceration occurs because the upper gastrointestinal tract mucosa defenses cannot manage autodigestion.

Notes for active learning

Neural Control by Enteric Nervous System

Neural regulation of the GI tract

Enteric nervous system supplies impulses to the GI muscles and exocrine glands, the local nervous system of the GI tract.

Neural regulation allows local, short reflexes independent of the CNS.

Long reflexes through the CNS are possible via sympathetic and parasympathetic nerves innervating the GI tract.

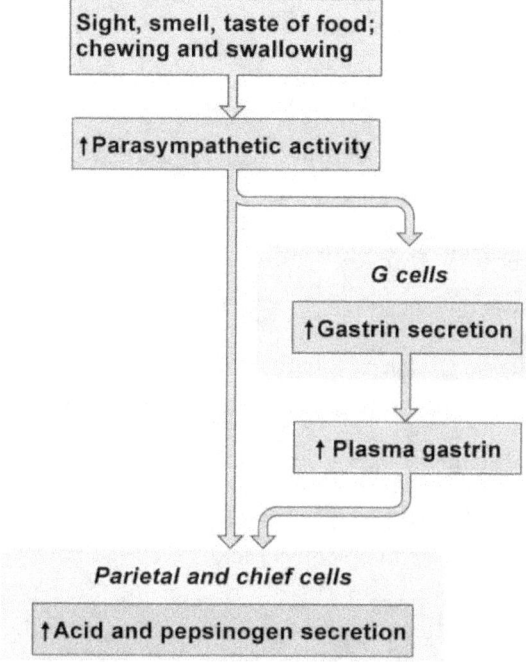

Neural activity stimulates gland secretions

Somatic nerves control chewing by skeletal muscles and the reflex activation of mechanoreceptors on the palate, gums, and tongue.

Autonomic nerves stimulate saliva secretion in response to chemoreceptors and pressure receptors in the mouth.

Swallowing is mediated by pressure receptors on the pharynx walls, sending impulses to the swallowing center in the *medulla oblongata*. The swallowing center activates muscles in the pharynx and esophagus.

Multiple responses occur in a temporal sequence. The palate is elevated to prevent food from entering the nasal cavity, respiration is inhibited, and the epiglottis covers the glottis to prevent food from entering the trachea (windpipe).

Unidirectional movement of food

The upper esophageal sphincter opens, and food enters the esophagus and moves toward the stomach by muscle contractions as peristaltic waves.

Food moves to the stomach when the lower esophageal sphincter opens.

A less efficient (or faulty) lower esophageal sphincter results in the reflux of gastric contents into the esophagus (gastroesophageal reflux); this reversal results in heartburn over time and contributes to ulceration of the esophagus.

Vomit reflex as a survival mechanism

Vomit reflex results in the forceful expulsion of toxic gastric contents and is coordinated by the vomiting center in the medulla oblongata.

Various mechano- and chemoreceptors in the stomach and elsewhere can trigger this reflex.

Increased salivation, sweating, heart rate, and pallor accompany the reflex.

Abdominal muscles contract to raise abdominal pressure while the *lower esophageal sphincter* opens, and gastric contents are forced into the esophagus (retching).

If the upper esophageal sphincter opens, contents are expelled from the mouth (vomiting).

Excessive vomiting leads to water and salt loss, resulting in dehydration and degradation of teeth enamel from the stomach's hydrochloric acid.

Three phases of gastrointestinal control

Location of the receptor names each reflex phase, and they do not occur in a temporal sequence.

1. *Cephalic phase* is initiated when sight, smell, taste, chewing, and emotional states stimulate receptors in the head.
   Reflexes mediated by sympathetic and parasympathetic fibers activate secretory and contractile activity.

2. *Gastric phase* is initiated by distension, acidity, amino acids, and peptides in the stomach. Short and long reflexes mediate and activate gastrin secretion.

3. *Intestinal phase* is initiated by the distension, acidity, and osmolarity of digestive products in the intestine. GI hormones and short and long neural reflexes mediate the phase.

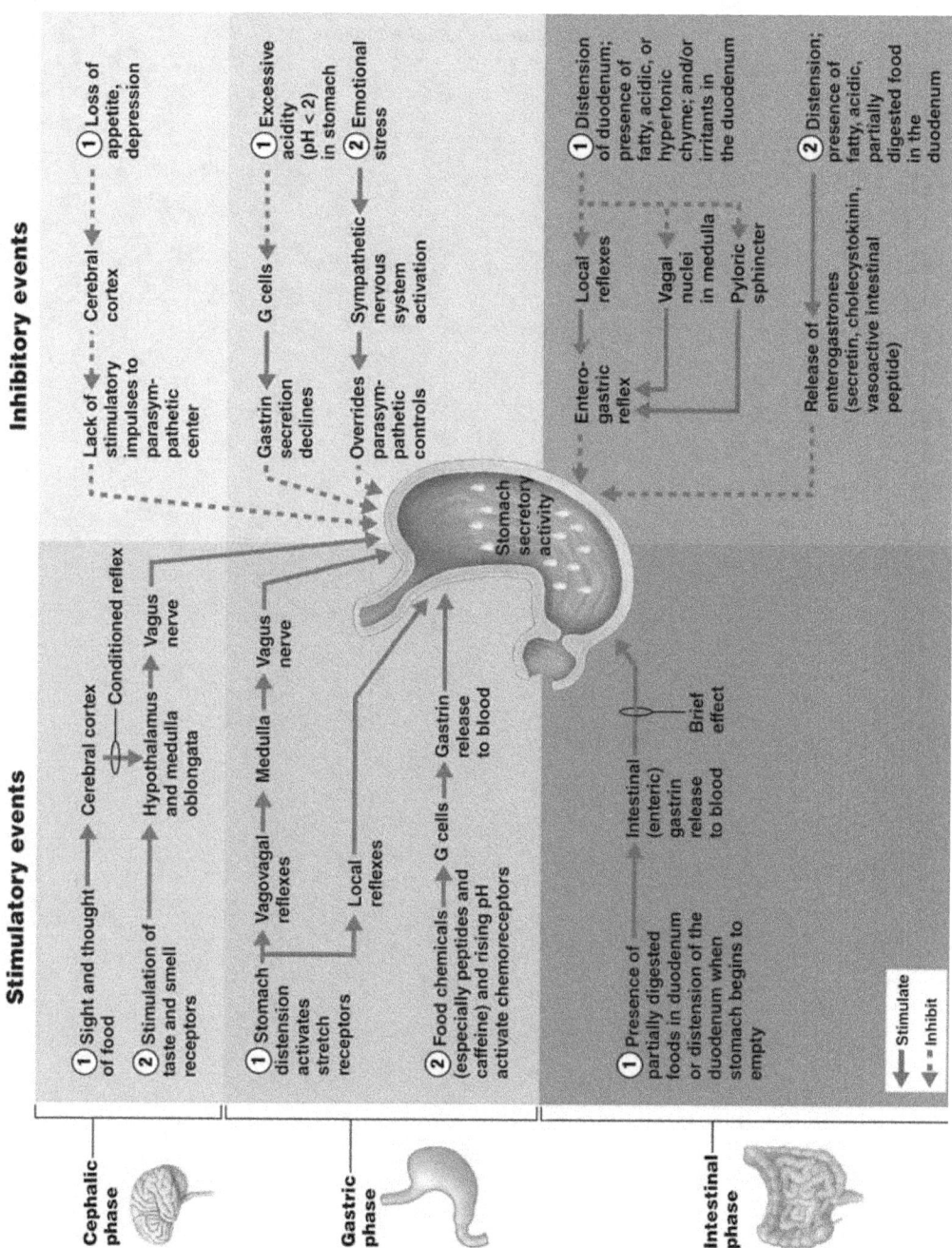

Stimulation and inhibition are sensory with PNS and glandular involvement

Notes for active learning

Human Nutrition

Macronutrients

Nutrition focuses on food composition, energy content, and synthesized organic molecules.

There is a quantitative relationship between nutrients and health. A *balanced diet* for good health includes a correctly proportioned variety of foods. Imbalances can cause disease.

Nutrition is a significant factor in cardiovascular disease, hypertension, and cancer.

Macronutrients are foods required in large quantities each day. These include carbohydrates, lipids, and proteins.

Water is essential because it supports metabolism. Correct water balance is a must for the proper functioning of the body.

Transporter-mediated processes absorb monosaccharides, amino acids, and mineral salts, while fatty acids and water diffuse passively.

Carbohydrates

Digestion begins in the mouth by salivary amylase and is completed in the small intestine by pancreatic amylase.

Monosaccharides (e.g., glucose, galactose, fructose) result from the breakdown of polysaccharides and are transported to the intestinal epithelium by facilitated diffusion or active transport.

Facilitated diffusion moves sugars into blood.

During the absorptive state, glucose is the major energy source, and some of it is converted to glycogen and stored in skeletal muscle and the liver. In adipose tissue, glucose is transformed and stored as fat.

Glucose sparing is the reduction of glucose catabolism and the increase in fat utilization by most tissues. Glucose is spared for the brain, resulting in minimization of protein breakdown.

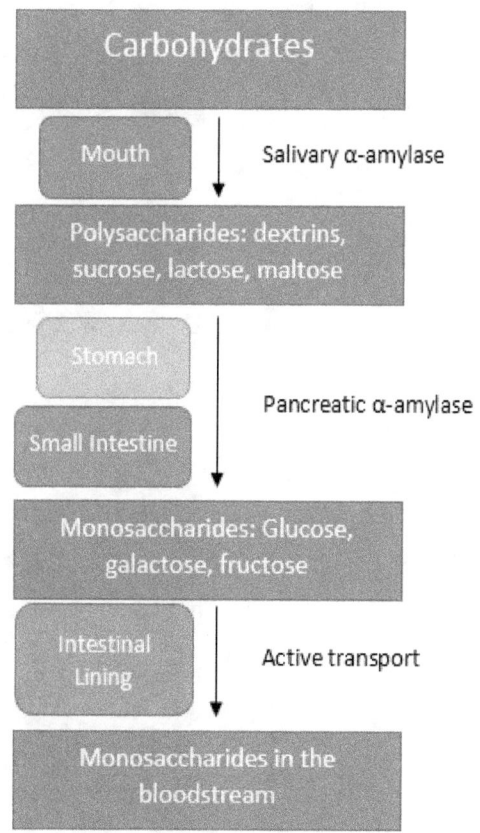

Carbohydrate digestion and absorption

Proteins

Proteins are polymers composed of amino acids. Proteins are in meat, milk, poultry, fish, cereal grains, and beans. They are needed for cellular growth and repair.

Twenty common amino acids are found in proteins, of which humans can naturally synthesize eleven. The remaining nine amino acids are essential (i.e., must be in the diet).

Proteins are generally not used for energy; muscle proteins are broken down for energy during starvation. Excess protein can be used for energy or converted to fats.

Proteins are broken down into peptide fragments by pepsin in the stomach and by pancreatic trypsin and chymotrypsin in the small intestine.

Fragments are digested to free amino acids by *carboxypeptidase* from the pancreas and *aminopeptidase* from the intestinal epithelium.

Free amino acids enter the epithelium by secondary active transport and exit by facilitated diffusion. Small amino acid chains can enter interstitial fluid by endo- and exocytosis. Most amino acids enter cells and are used to synthesize proteins. Excess amino acids are converted to carbohydrates or fat.

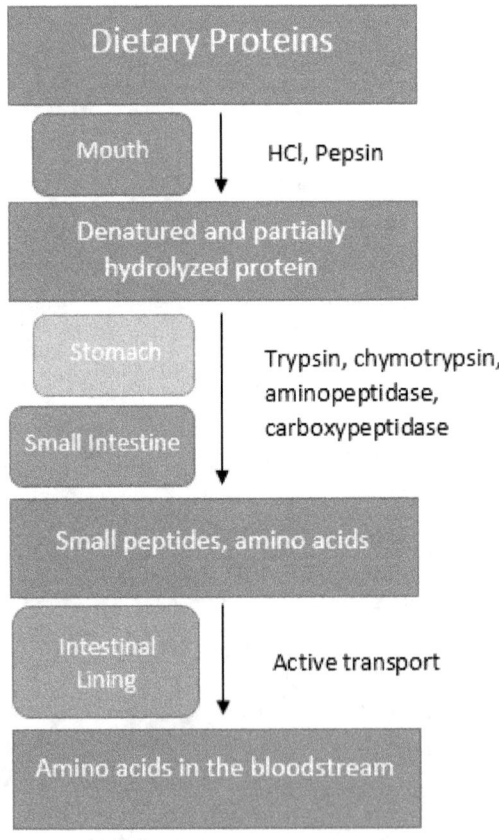

Protein digestion and absorption

Lipids

Lipids generate the greatest energy yield. Therefore, many plants and animals store energy as fats (a type of lipid). Lipids are present in oils, meats, butter, and plants (e.g., avocado and peanuts). Some fatty acids, such as linoleic acid, are essential and must be included in the diet.

When present in the intestine, lipids promote the uptake of fat-soluble vitamins A, D, E and K.

Fatty acids of plasma chylomicrons are released within the adipose tissue capillaries and form triacylglycerols.

Fat digestion occurs by pancreatic lipase in the small intestine, producing a monoglyceride and two fatty acids. Large lipid droplets are first degraded into smaller droplets by *emulsification*.

Emulsification is driven by mechanical disruption (by the contractile activity of the GI tract) and by emulsifying agents (amphipathic bile salts). Pancreatic colipase binds the water-soluble lipase to the lipid substrate.

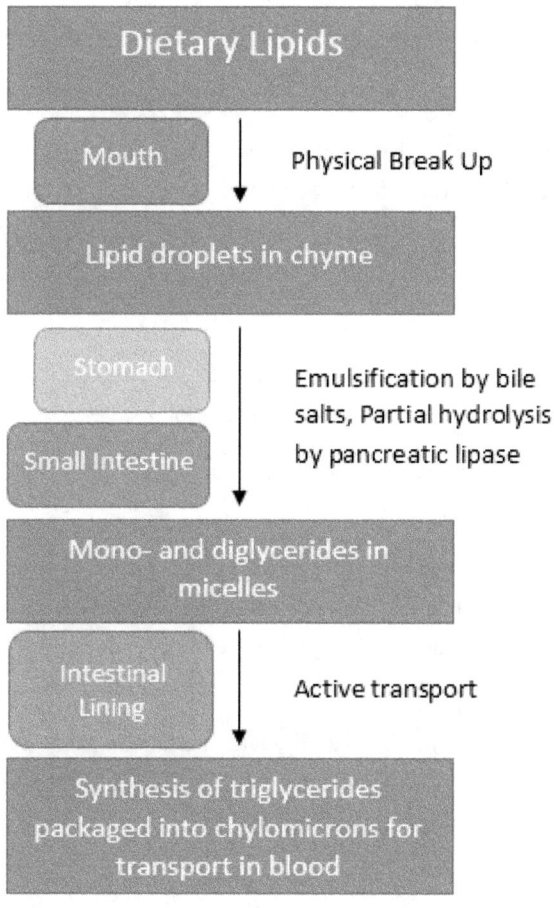

Lipid digestion and absorption

Digested products and bile salts form amphipathic micelles. Micelles keep the insoluble products insoluble aggregates, from which tiny amounts are released and absorbed by epithelial cells via diffusion.

Free fatty acids and *monoglycerides* then recombine into *triacylglycerols* at the smooth ER. They are processed in the Golgi and enter the interstitial fluid as chylomicron droplets, which are then taken up by the lacteals in the intestine.

Absorptive and post-absorptive states

Absorptive state is when ingested nutrients enter the blood. Some nutrients supply the body's energy needs while the remainder is stored.

Carbohydrates and proteins are absorbed into the blood primarily as monosaccharides and amino acids, respectively, while fat is absorbed into the lymph as triacylglycerols.

Post-absorptive state is when the GI tract depletes nutrients, and the body must supply the required energy. In this state, the net synthesis of glycogen, fat, and protein ceases, and net catabolism of these substances begins. Plasma glucose level is maintained by:

>*Glycogenolysis*, hydrolysis of glycogen in the liver and skeletal muscles.

>*Lipolysis*, catabolism of triacylglycerols into glycerol and fatty acids in adipose tissues. Glycerol, when reaching the liver, is converted to glucose.

>*Gluconeogenesis*, catabolism of non-carbohydrate substances to glucose.

Vitamins

Vitamins are *necessary organic compounds* required for metabolic reactions. They usually cannot be made by the body and are needed in trace amounts.

Vitamins may act as enzyme cofactors, known as *coenzymes*. Some vitamins are soluble in fats, while others are soluble in water.

Fat-soluble vitamins are absorbed and stored along with fats. Most water-soluble vitamins are absorbed by diffusion or mediated transport. Fat-soluble vitamins necessitate more complex mechanisms to cross the phospholipid bilayer. For example, due to its large size and charged nature, Vitamin B-12 must bind to the intrinsic factor protein to be absorbed via endocytosis.

The body cannot make some vitamins required for metabolic activities—a lack of vitamins results in vitamin deficiencies. The 13 vitamins are divided into fat-soluble (A, D, E, K) and water-soluble vitamins (8 B vitamins and vitamin C).

Many vitamins are portions of coenzymes; for example, niacin is part of NAD^+ and riboflavin is part of FAD. Coenzymes are needed in small amounts because they are used repeatedly. Vitamin A is not a coenzyme but a precursor for visual pigments that prevent night blindness.

Vitamin A is part of a group of hydrophobic unsaturated nutritional organic compounds, including retinol, retinal, retinoic acid, and several carotenoids (e.g., beta-carotene). Vitamin A has multiple functions. It is vital for growth and development, the maintenance of the immune system, and good vision.

For example, the eye's retina needs vitamin A in the form of *retinal*, which combines with protein *opsin* to form *rhodopsin* (i.e., light-absorbing molecule). Rhodopsin is necessary for low-light (night vision) and color vision.

Skin cells contain a precursor cholesterol molecule converted to vitamin D by UV light. Only a tiny amount of UV is needed to cause this change. Vitamin D leaves the skin and is modified in the kidneys and liver to become calcitriol.

Calcitriol circulates throughout the body, regulating calcium uptake and metabolism. It promotes the absorption of calcium by the intestines.

Vitamin D deficiency causes *rickets* in children, a condition in which poor mineralization of the skeleton causes the legs to bow. Most milk is *fortified* (i.e., added during processing) with vitamin D to prevent *rickets*.

Cell metabolism generates *free radicals*, unstable molecules with an extra electron. O_3^- is a common free radical. Free radicals are stabilized by donating electrons to another molecule; however, doing so damages cellular molecules, such as DNA and proteins. This damage may cause plaque in arteries or cancer.

Vitamins C, E, and A—abundant in fruits and vegetables—are antioxidants for free radicals.

While vitamin supplements can assist in fighting vitamin deficiencies, they do not replace fruits and vegetables which contain *phytochemicals* and other beneficial compounds.

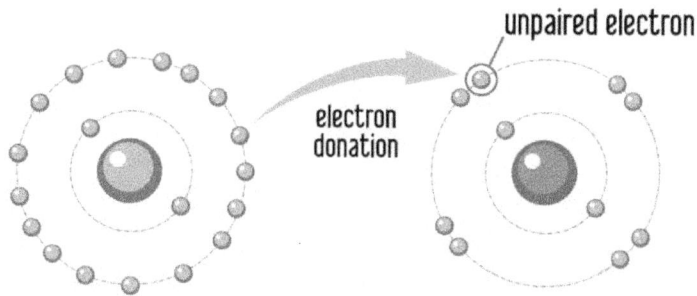

Antioxidants reduce free radicals

Minerals

Minerals are trace elements required for normal metabolism, cell and tissue structure, nerve conduction, and muscle contraction. They are essential and can only be obtained from the diet. Iron, iodine, calcium, and sodium are examples of minerals.

Humans require *macrominerals* (e.g., calcium, phosphorus) in amounts of over 100 mg per day. They are constituents of cells and body fluids and are structural components of tissues.

Calcium (Ca^{2+}) is needed for bones and tooth enamel, generate nerve conduction, and muscle contraction.

Sodium (Na^+) is a crucial macromineral used to control blood pressure and volume and keep nerves and muscles functioning correctly.

Microminerals are elements (e.g., zinc, iron) recommended in amounts less than 20 mg daily.

Microminerals often have specific functions. For example, iron is needed to produce hemoglobin, which adult females need more due to menstrual blood loss.

Iodine is used to produce *thyroxin*, a hormone of thyroid glands.

Minute amounts of molybdenum, selenium, chromium, nickel, vanadium, silicon, and arsenic (among others) are also essential to keep the body functioning properly.

Notes for active learning

Notes for active learning

CHAPTER 10

Excretory System

General Anatomy of Excretory System

Nephron Structure and Function

Kidneys and Homeostasis

Urine Formation

Urine Storage and Elimination

Page intentionally left blank

General Anatomy of Excretory System

Excretory system and kidneys

Human excretory system is an organ system that removes excess fluids and materials to prevent damage to the body. It consists of several parts.

Kidneys are two bean-shaped, reddish-brown organs about the size of a fist. They are on each side of the vertebral column (below diaphragm) and partially protected by the lower rib cage.

Kidneys are urine formation sites, and each is connected to a *ureter*, which moves urine from the kidney to the *urinary bladder*.

Urinary bladder stores urine from the kidneys until it is voided through the *urethra*.

Urinary bladder and urethra

In males, the urethra runs through the penis and conducts semen.

In females, the urethra opens the ventral to the vaginal opening.

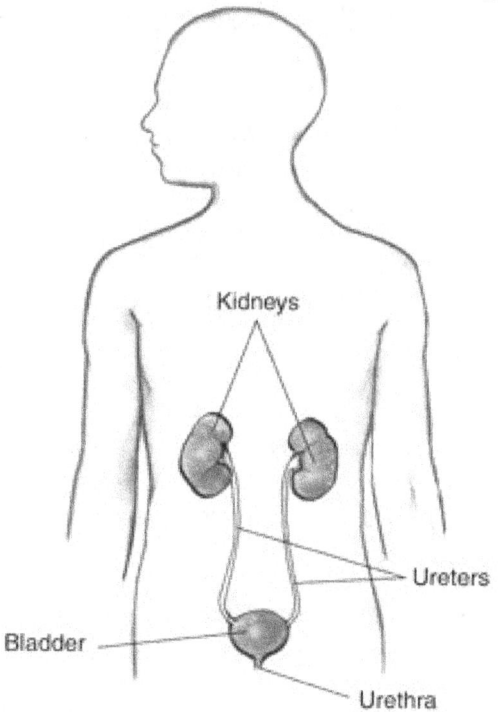

Two kidneys connect by ureters to the urinary bladder.

Kidneys regulate fluid volume

Kidneys remove and add substances to and from the plasma. They regulate water concentration, inorganic ion concentrations, and aqueous volume of the internal environment by controlling excretion.

In urine, the kidneys excrete metabolic wastes (e.g., urea, creatinine, foreign chemicals). They synthesize glucose from amino acids and other precursors through gluconeogenesis.

Kidneys secrete hormones, erythroproteins, renin, and 1,25-dihydroxy vitamin D_3.

Anatomy of the kidney

Kidney has three regions:

renal cortex (outer), *medulla* (inner), and *renal pelvis* (innermost, hollow structure).

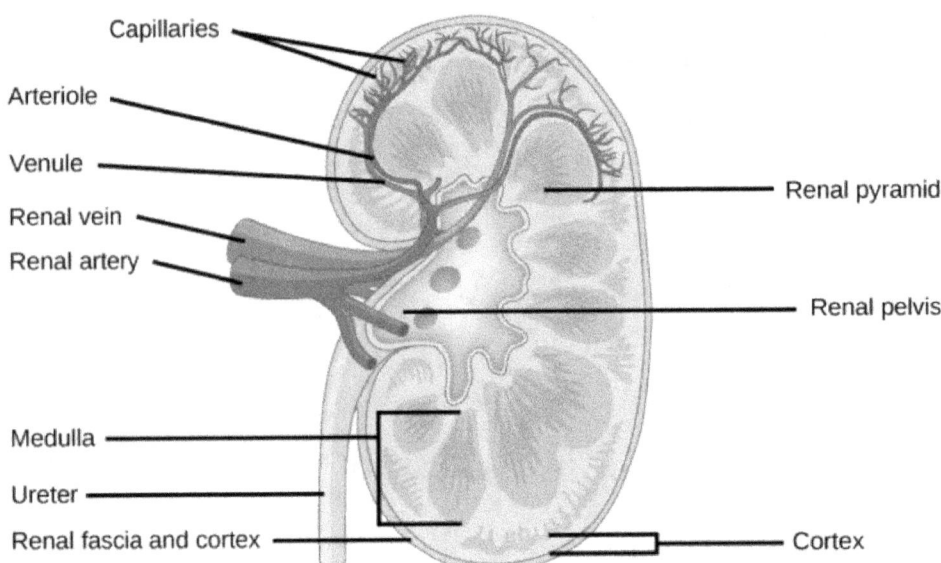

Anatomy of the kidney with renal cortex, medulla, and renal pelvis

Renal cortex is the kidney's thin outer region (or shell), composed of many convoluted tubules that give it a granular appearance.

Renal medulla is the kidney's inner region consisting of the striped, pyramid regions that lie on the cortex's inner side and the loop of Henle.

Renal pelvis is a hollow, funnel-shaped structure in the kidney's innermost part that collects urine. It receives urine from *collecting ducts* and *papillary ducts*, releasing urine into the *ureter*, which leads to the *bladder*.

Nephron Structure and Function

Nephron as the functional unit of the kidney

Each kidney has approximately one million subunits called *nephrons*.

Nephrons are the kidney's functional units because they reabsorb nutrients, salts, and water.

Nephrons are composed of the *renal corpuscle* and *renal tubule*.

Glomerulus as a capillary bed for blood filtration

The *glomerulus* is a ball of fenestrated capillaries that acts like a sieve (or colander).

Small molecules dissolved in the fluid pass through the glomerulus (e.g., glucose, which is later reabsorbed), while large molecules, such as plasma proteins and blood cells, do not.

If blood cells or proteins are in the urine, this indicates a problem with the glomerulus.

Juxtaglomerular apparatus (JGA), named for its proximity to the glomerulus, consists of macula densa and juxtaglomerular (JG) cells.

Macula densa cells are essential in blood flow regulation and affect glomerulus filtration rate. They are in the ascending limb, passing between the afferent and the efferent arterioles.

Walls of afferent arterioles near the Bowman's capsule have juxtaglomerular cells, which secrete the hormone renin.

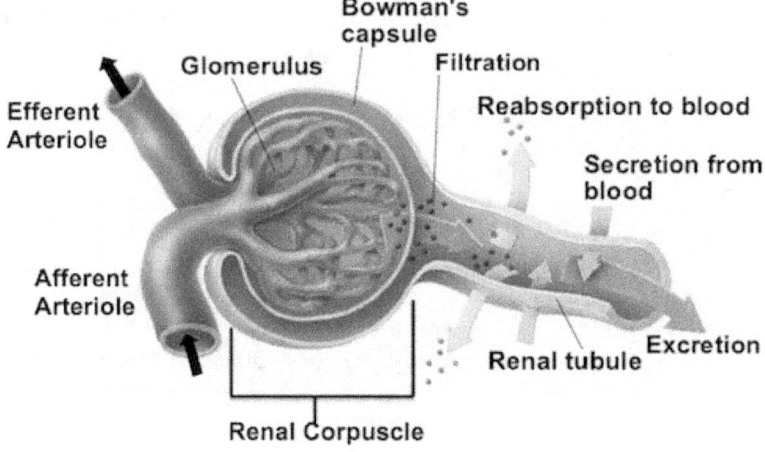

Nephron as the functional unit of the kidney.
Blood enters via the afferent arteriole and exits via the efferent arteriole.

Bowman's capsule

Bowman's capsule is a structure surrounding the glomerulus. It performed the first step in blood filtration to form urine.

Bowman's capsule encloses the glomerulus that filters liquids and microscopic components from blood.

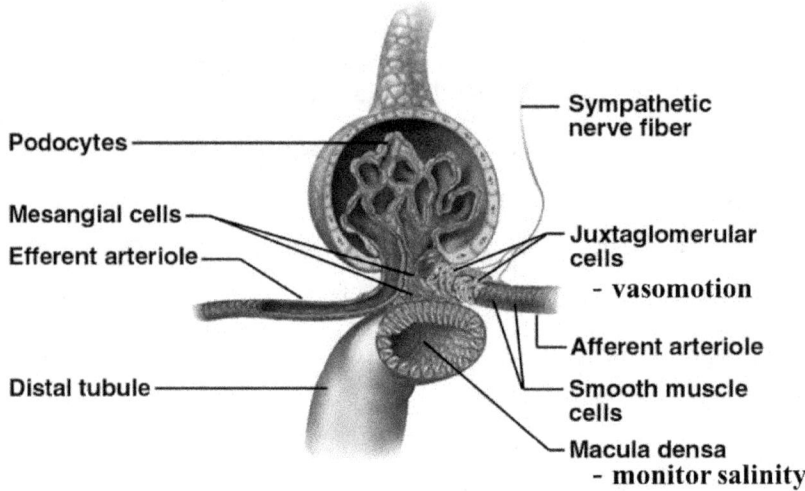

Juxtaglomerular apparatus of the kidney

Proximal tubule

Proximal tubule is a convoluted tubule on the side of Bowman's capsule and is the primary site of active reabsorption of glucose, ions, and amino acids.

Additionally, it is responsible for the secretion of ions, except potassium.

Proximal tube divides into initial *convoluted* and *straight* (descending) portions.

Fitrate fluid entering the proximal convoluted tubule is reabsorbed into peritubular capillaries. Reabsorption includes approximately two-thirds of salt and water filtered by the glomerulus.

Proximal convoluted tubule secretes chemicals, such as ammonium, formed by the deamination processes that convert glutamine to alpha-ketoglutarate. It drains into the loop of Henle.

Loop of Henle structure

Most of the nephron is the *loop of Henle*, a U-shaped tube that extends from the proximal tubule and consists of descending and ascending limbs.

Loop begins in the *cortex*, receiving filtrate from the *proximal convoluted tubule*.

Loop of Henle extends into the *medulla* as the *descending limb* and returns to the *cortex* as the *ascending limb* continues into the *distal convoluted tubule*.

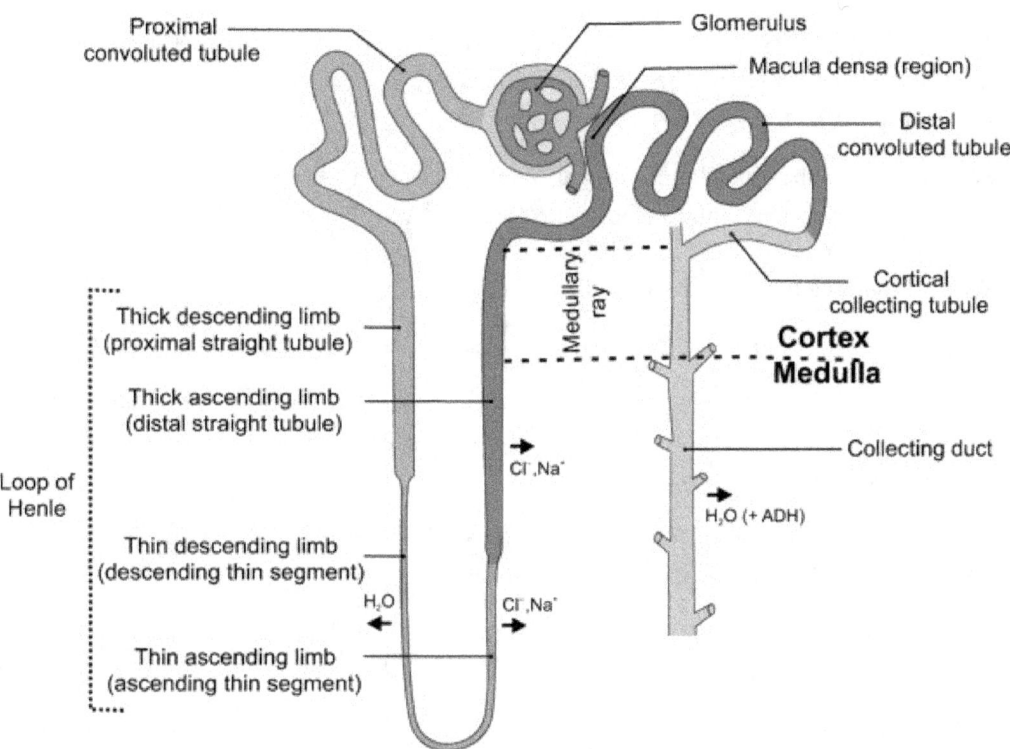

Cross-section of a nephron including glomerulus and loop of Henle

Loop of Henle reabsorbs salt and water

Pimary role of the loop of Henle is to concentrate salt in the surrounding tissues (interstitium). This is accomplished using a countercurrent multiplier mechanism.

> *Descending limb* of the loop of Henle is the site of *water reabsorption*.

> *Ascending limb* of Henle is the site of *salt absorption*.

Considerable differences distinguish the ascending and descending limbs of the loop of Henle.

Thin descending limb is permeable to H_2O and noticeably less permeable to salt. This part of the loop of Henle indirectly contributes to the concentration of the interstitium.

Excess water is picked up by the *vasa recta* and returned to the blood.

As the filtrate descends deeper into the renal medulla's hypertonic interstitium, H_2O flows freely out of the descending limb by osmosis until tonicity of the filtrate and interstitium equilibrate.

Longer descending limbs allow time for H_2O to flow out of the filtrate; thus, longer limbs make the filtrate more hypertonic than shorter limbs.

The *thick ascending limb* of the loop of Henle is *impermeable to H_2O*, a critical feature of the *countercurrent exchange* mechanism.

Ascending limb actively pumps Na^+ out of the filtrate, generating the hypertonic interstitium that drives countercurrent exchange. This is done through secondary active transport via Na-K-Cl cotransporters.

Passing through the ascending limb, the filtrate becomes hypotonic since it has lost a lot of sodium. The hypotonic filtrate is passed to the distal convoluted tubule in the renal cortex.

Distal tubule regulates calcium levels

Loop of Henle leads to the *distal convoluted tubule* on the side of the collecting ducts.

Distal convoluted tubule is hormone-controlled, fine-tunes the proximal tubule's effects, continues the reabsorption of *salts* and *water,* and is partially responsible for glucose, ions, and water reabsorption.

Distal convoluted tubule cells contain numerous mitochondria, producing energy (ATP) for active transport. Endocrine system regulates much ion transport in the distal convoluted tubule.

Additionally, the distal convoluted tubule regulates the pH by secreting *protons*, absorbing protons, and secreting *bicarbonate ions*.

Calcium reabsorption occurs in the *distal convoluted tubule* in response to low blood calcium.

When blood calcium levels are low, parathyroid hormone is released. In the presence of parathyroid hormone, the distal convoluted tubule reabsorbs Ca^{2+}, osteoclast activity is stimulated (Ca^{2+} released from bone), and additional phosphate is secreted.

Aldosterone controls sodium levels (absorption) and potassium levels (through secretion). When aldosterone is present, more Na^+ is reabsorbed (along with H_2O), and K^+ is secreted.

Atrial natriuretic peptide causes the *distal convoluted tubule* to *secrete Na^+*.

Collecting ducts and the antidiuretic hormone (ADH)

Many distal convoluted tubules drain into *collecting ducts*, comprised of the connecting tubules, the cortical collecting ducts, and the medullary collecting ducts.

Medullary collecting ducts from numerous nephrons merge and drain into the renal pelvis, which is connected to the ureter. Tubules are connected to another set of blood vessels, the *peritubular capillaries*.

Nephrons share each collecting duct, where the antidiuretic hormone (ADH)-controlled reabsorption of water and hormone-controlled reabsorption / secretion of sodium occur.

Collecting ducts are generally impermeable to water. However, if the hormone ADH is present, collecting ducts become permeable to water, and water reabsorption occurs.

ADH causes blood pressure to rise and is vital in homeostasis by regulating glucose, sodium, and water levels.

Kidneys and Homeostasis

Kidneys' role in blood pressure regulation

Kidneys function to excrete waste, control plasma pH, and maintain homeostasis of fluid volume and solute composition.

Since sodium is the major extracellular solute, changes in sodium levels result in changes in extracellular fluid volume. These changes lead to changes in plasma volume and blood pressure, which *baroreceptors* detect.

Usually, more than 99% of the Na^+ filtered at the glomerulus is returned to the blood. Most are reabsorbed at the proximal tubule, the ascending limb extrudes 25%, and the remaining Na^+ is reabsorbed from the distal convoluted tubule and collecting duct.

Juxtaglomerular cells

Blood pressure is continuously monitored within the *juxtaglomerular apparatus*. If the blood pressure is insufficient to promote glomerular filtration, the afferent arteriole cells secrete *renin*.

Renin catalyzes the conversion of *angiotensinogen* (i.e., liver protein) into *angiotensin I*.

Angiotensin I is converted to *angiotensin II* by *angiotensin-converting enzyme* (ACE); the rate-limiting step of this reaction is controlled by renin from juxtaglomerular (JG) cells.

JG cells are internal baroreceptors and receive sympathetic inputs from external baroreceptors.

Aldosterone regulates sodium ion reabsorption

Angiotensin II increases blood pressure as a *vasoconstrictor* by promoting sodium ion retention. This hormone stimulates cells in the adrenal cortex to produce aldosterone, stimulating sodium reabsorption by *cortical collecting ducts* (and large intestine, sweat, and salivary glands).

Aldosterone acts on *distal convoluted tubules* to increase *reabsorption* of Na^+ and *excretion* of K^+. Increased Na^+ causes water to be reabsorbed, increasing blood volume and pressure.

Renin-angiotensin-aldosterone system triggers aldosterone production.

Thirst is stimulated by lower extracellular volume, higher plasma osmolarity, or angiotensin II. The brain centers for thirst are in the hypothalamus.

Atrial natriuretic hormone (ANH) is produced by atria of the heart when cardiac cells stretch. When blood pressure rises, the heart produces ANH to inhibit renin's secretion and the release of ADH, which decreases blood volume and pressure.

Additionally, the heart can release atrial natriuretic peptide (ANP), the antagonist for aldosterone, which causes kidneys to excrete more sodium ions and water, causing vasodilation.

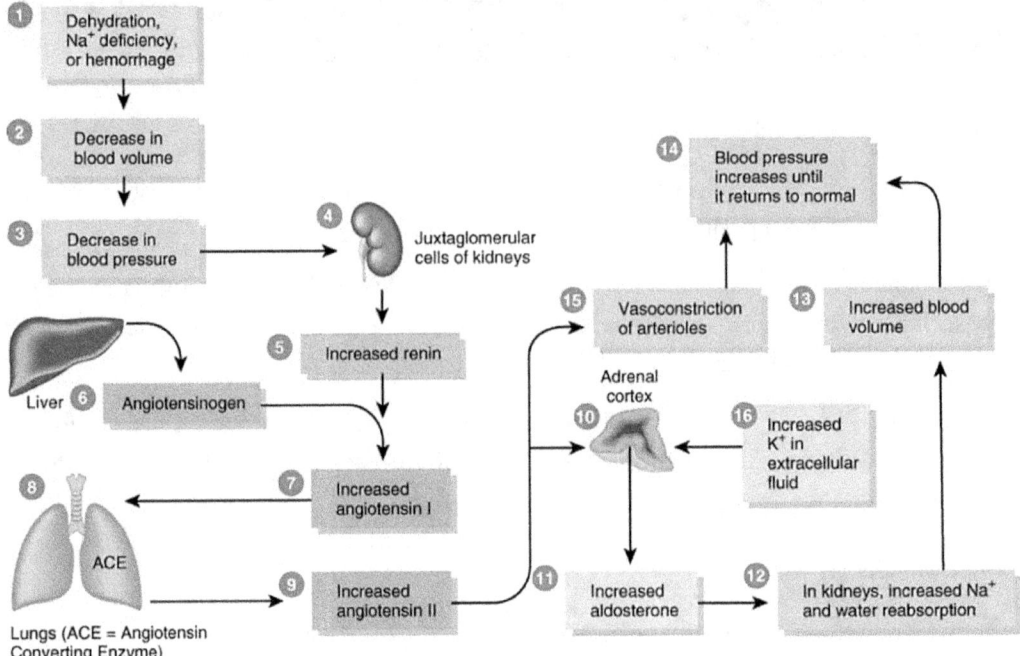

Renin-angiotensin-aldosterone (RAA) pathway

Kidneys' role in osmoregulation

If osmolarity differs between two regions, water moves toward higher solute concentrations.

Marine environments are high in salt and promote the loss of water and the gain of ions when drinking saltwater. Freshwater promotes water gain by osmosis and a loss of ions as this excess water is excreted.

For example, the body of a marine fish living in saltwater is hypotonic relative to its environment, resulting in water being constantly lost by osmosis. To account for this, marine fish constantly consume water, rarely urinate, and secrete accumulated salts through their gills.

Conversely, freshwater fish live in an environment where their bodies are hypertonic relative to the environment. Water, therefore, is being constantly gained. This characteristic makes freshwater fish rarely consume water, constantly urinate, and readily absorb salts through gills.

The excretory system regulates ions and water in body fluids. Regulation depends on the concentration of mineral ions (i.e., Na^+, Cl^-, K^+ and HCO_3^-).

Body fluids gain ions when food and fluids are consumed and lose them by excretion.

Water enters the body through food or drink and is metabolized by cellular respiration, which produces water. Water is lost by evaporation from the skin and lungs and excretion (i.e., in urine or feces).

For balance, the water volume entering the body must equal the water lost.

The kidneys function to eliminate wastes (urea, H^+) generated by metabolic activity while reabsorbing important substances (glucose, amino acids, sodium) for reuse by the body.

Generating a solute concentration gradient from the kidney's cortex to its medulla allows a considerable amount of water to be reabsorbed.

Concentrated urine excretion limits body water loss and preserves blood volume.

Nephron's long loop comprises a:

descending limb (cortex → medulla)

ascending limb (medulla → cortex).

Salt (NaCl) passively diffuses out of the lower portion of the ascending limb, but the upper, thick portion of the limb actively transports salt out into the tissue of the renal medulla.

Less salt is available for transport from the tubule as the fluid moves up the thick portion of the ascending limb. Urea leaks from the lower portion of the collecting ducts, causing the concentrations in the lower medulla to be highest.

Because of the solute concentration gradient within the renal medulla, water leaves the descending limb of the loop of Henle along its length.

The decreasing water concentration in the descending limb encounters an increasing solute concentration; this is a countercurrent mechanism.

Fluid received by a collecting duct from the distal convoluted tubule is isotonic to cortex cells.

Water diffuses from the collected duct into the renal medulla as this fluid passes through the renal medulla. The urine delivered to the renal pelvis is usually hypertonic to the blood plasma.

Some terrestrial animals near oceans drink seawater despite its high osmolarity. Such birds and reptiles have a nasal salt gland that excretes concentrated salt solution. In general, terrestrial animals lose water and ions to the environment.

Humans gain water and sodium from ingesting and oxidizing organic nutrients. Water is then lost via sweat glands, respiratory passageways, and the gastrointestinal and urinary tracts.

Aldosterone regulates blood osmolarity

Blood plasma mainly contains sodium and chloride ions, whereas cells mainly contain potassium and hydrogen ions.

Blood osmolarity is determined predominantly by the concentrations of sodium and potassium ions. If the osmolarity is too low, aldosterone is released so that reabsorption can occur.

Aldosterone controls potassium concentrations by allowing the renal system to reabsorb sodium ions and excrete potassium ions in urine.

Secretions and reabsorptions of the kidney tubules regulate osmolarity.

ADH increases the permeability of collecting ducts

Antidiuretic hormone (ADH) is released from the posterior lobe of the pituitary gland. It acts on collecting ducts by increasing permeability to H_2O, thereby increasing H_2O retention.

When ADH is released, water is reabsorbed, and there is less urine.

When ADH is not released, water is excreted, and more urine forms. Thus, if an individual does not drink, the pituitary releases ADH; if hydrated, ADH is not released.

Diuresis is increased urine production, while *antidiuresis* is decreased urine.

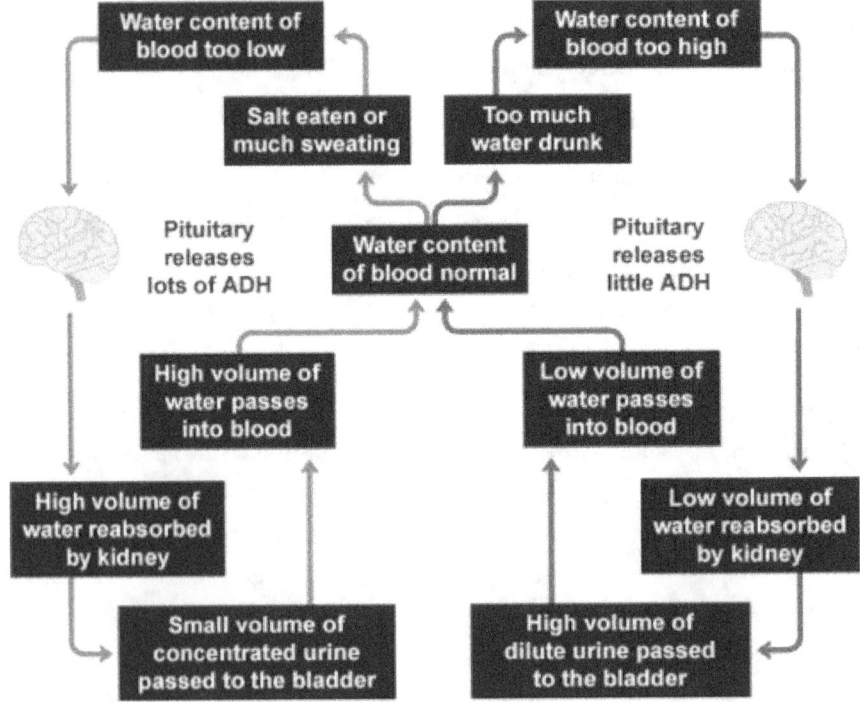

Feedback loops used by ADH for homeostasis of blood volume

While aldosterone and ADH ultimately do the same thing (i.e., increase water reabsorption in the kidneys), they have different mechanisms of action.

ADH increases water reabsorption from the nephron's collecting duct, while aldosterone indirectly increases H_2O reabsorption by increasing Na^+ reabsorption from the collecting duct.

Acid-base balance

The balance between acids and bases within the blood keeps the blood pH steady. This balance is primarily regulated through the bicarbonate HCO_3^- buffer system in blood and extracellular fluid and the phosphate buffer system inside the cells.

During bicarbonate regulation, HCO_3^- is filtered at the renal corpuscle. It then undergoes reabsorption in the proximal tubule and can be secreted in the collecting ducts.

$$HCO_3^- \text{ excreted} = HCO_3^- \text{ filtered} + HCO_3^- \text{ secreted} - HCO_3^- \text{ reabsorbed}$$

CO_2 and H_2O combine inside red blood cells to form H_2CO_3, dissociating into H^+ and HCO_3^- ions. HCO_3^- moves to the interstitial fluid by diffusion, while H^+ ion is secreted into the lumen by an active process involving H-ATPase pumps.

Secreted H^+ ion combines with filtered HCO_3^- in the lumen, generating CO_2 and H_2O. These two compounds diffuse into the cell, and the process is repeated.

If excess H^+ ions are secreted, they combine with a nonbicarbonate buffer, usually HPO_4^{2-}, in the lumen and are excreted.

HCO_3^- generated within the cell and entering the plasma produces a net gain of HCO_3^-.

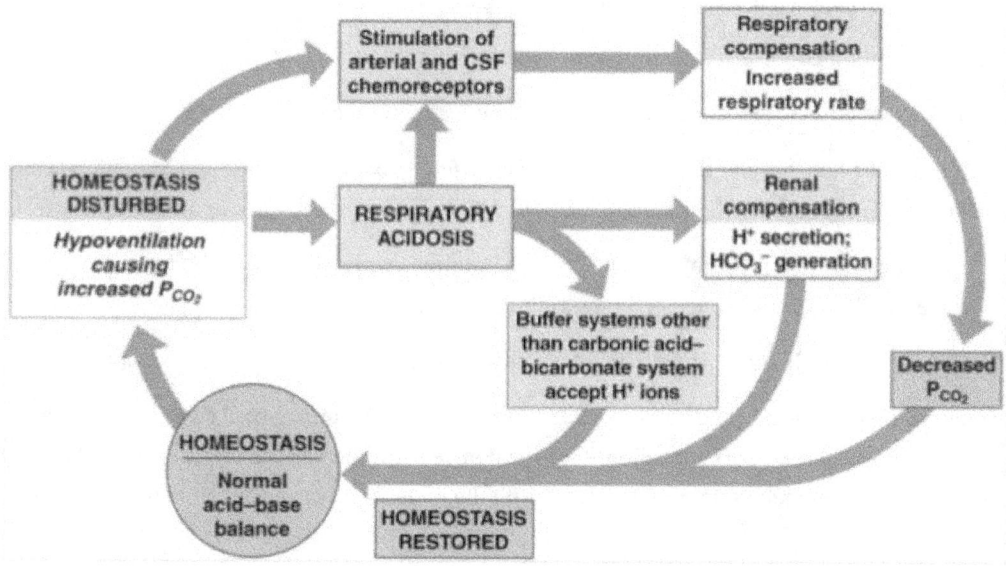

Respiratory and excretory systems function to maintain homeostasis

Bicarbonate buffer system and the respiratory system maintain blood pH.

Exhaling CO_2 decreases blood acidity. Bicarbonate ions lower blood pH. Then, the excretion of H^+ ions and NH_3 and the reabsorption of bicarbonate ions (HCO_3^-) is adjusted.

If blood is basic (pH is high), fewer H^+ ions are excreted, and fewer (HCO_3^-) ions are reabsorbed to lower the pH.

$$H^+ + HCO_3^- \rightleftarrows H_2CO_3 \rightleftarrows H_2O + CO_2$$

Ammonia is produced by the *deamination of amino acids* in the tubule cells.

Reabsorption or excretion of ions by kidneys regulates blood pH and osmolarity.

Kidneys' role in removing soluble nitrogenous waste

The breakdown of nucleic acids and amino acids produces nitrogenous wastes.

Amino acids derived from protein are used to synthesize bodily proteins or nitrogen-containing molecules. Unused amino acids are oxidized to generate energy or stored as fats or carbohydrates. The resulting *amino groups* ($-NH_2$) must be removed.

Depending on the organism, nitrogenous wastes are excreted as *ammonia, urea,* or *uric acid.*

Amino groups removed from amino acids form *ammonia* (NH_3) by adding a third H^+, which requires little or no energy.

Ammonia, while quite toxic, is water soluble and requires a significant amount of water to wash away from the body (e.g., aquatic animals).

Urea ($CO(NH_2)_2$) is a harmless form of ammonia.

Amino acids are converted into ammonia, which is converted to urea.

Urea is excreted as urine, concentrated urea in ionized water (e.g., humans).

Mammals like humans and terrestrial amphibians usually excrete urea as their main nitrogenous waste because urea is much less toxic than ammonia.

Urea is excreted in a moderately concentrated solution, which conserves body water. Urea is produced in the liver by the energy-requiring *urea cycle.*

Urea cycle molecules take up carbon dioxide and two ammonia molecules, releasing urea.

Some animals have adapted to survival in dry, arid environments and can altogether avoid drinking water. They form concentrated urine and fecal matter that is almost completely dry, and they can meet their water requirements with the metabolic water generated through aerobic respiration.

Insects, reptiles, and birds excrete *uric acid* as their main nitrogenous waste. Uric acid is not toxic and is poorly soluble in water, but is concentrated for water conservation. Uric acid is synthesized through enzymatic reactions using even more ATP than urea synthesis, demonstrating the tradeoff between water conservation and energy expenditure.

Osmoregulation: reabsorption of H_2O, glucose, ions

Kidneys remove and add substances to and from blood plasma. Kidneys regulate water concentration, inorganic ion concentrations, and the aqueous volume of the internal environment by controlling excretion.

In urine, the kidneys excrete metabolic waste (e.g., urea, uric acid, creatinine, and chemicals). They synthesize glucose from amino acids and other precursors through gluconeogenesis.

Kidneys secrete hormones, erythroproteins, renin, and 1,25-dihydroxyvitamin D_3.

Tubule cells synthesize glucose, ammonia, and other products and release them into the blood.

Sodium and water filter freely from glomerular capillaries to Bowman's space. They undergo reabsorption in the proximal tubule, but the major hormonal controls on reabsorption in the collecting ducts.

Hormones and neurotransmitters regulate channels and transporters.

Glomerular filtration rate (GFR) must be high to excrete waste products, resulting in more filtered substances. The primary role of the *proximal tubule* and the *loop of Henle* is to reabsorb enormous quantities of substances. Such extensive reabsorption ensures that distal segments receive tiny amounts of substances and that their quantities in urine can be further regulated.

Most homeostatic controls are therefore exerted on distal segments. Lower total body sodium can decrease GFR by vasoconstriction, resulting in lower pressure in renal arteries.

Amount of water excreted equals the amount of filtered water, subtracted by the amount of reabsorbed water. Water excretion is regulated mainly at the level of reabsorption by ADH (vasopressin). Changes in total body water are regulated by reflexes that alter water excretion without altering sodium excretion.

Receptors for vasopressin secretion due to water gain or loss are the osmoreceptors in the hypothalamus. Vasopressin secretions can be triggered by decreased extracellular volume. This baroreceptor reflex plays a lesser role because it has a higher threshold.

Potassium is filtered in the renal corpuscle, most of which is absorbed in the tubules. Changes in potassium excretion are mainly due to changes in potassium secretion by cortical collecting ducts. This secretion is associated with the reabsorption of sodium by Na/K−ATPase.

Aldosterone-secreting cells are sensitive to extracellular fluid potassium (K^+) concentrations, and an increased K^+ concentration stimulates aldosterone production, thereby increasing potassium secretion and its excretion from the body.

Calcium is filtered in the renal corpuscle, and most of it is reabsorbed. There is no tubular secretion of calcium:

>Calcium excreted = calcium filtered − calcium absorbed

Calcium reabsorption in the GI tract is under hormonal control and is a significant means of controlling calcium balance.

Urine Formation

Afferent and efferent arterioles at the glomerulus

Urine formation follows the sequence of *filtration*, *secretion*, and *reabsorption*.

Filtration of plasma from glomerular capillaries into Bowman's capsule is *glomerular filtration*.

Glomerular filtrate passes the glomerulus (afferent arteriole → glomerulus → efferent arterioles) to the rest of the nephron.

It is bulk flow because water and solutes are moved together due to a pressure gradient. Glomerular filtrate contains plasma substances in the same concentrations as plasma, except plasma proteins and the molecules bound to these proteins.

Afferent arterioles carry blood into the glomerulus, while *efferent arterioles* carry blood away from the glomerulus.

Efferent arterioles exit the glomerulus and web around the nephron as *peritubular capillaries*.

Peritubular capillaries surround the *proximal convoluted tubule* (PCT) and *distal convoluted tubule* (DCT). Peritubular capillaries reabsorb nutrients and ions filtered by the glomerulus.

Tubular reabsorption

Efferent arterioles continue to form the *vasa recta*, surrounding the loop of Henle (maintaining the concentration gradient) before merging with the renal branch of the renal vein.

Peritubular capillaries drain into a venule. The venules from many nephrons drain into a small vein. Many small veins join to form the *renal vein*, which enters the *inferior vena cava*.

During passage through tubules, substances move from tubules to peritubular capillaries as *tubular reabsorption*.

Tubular secretion, substances move from peritubular capillaries to tubules. Waste (e.g., urea, creatine, uric acid) and small useable ions and nutrients are filtered out.

Nutrients and usable ions are reabsorbed while the waste is excreted.

Particles too large to filter through (e.g., blood, albumin) remain in the circulatory system. This is a passive process driven by the hydrostatic pressure of blood. The filtrate is pushed (i.e., *hydrostatic pressure*) from the glomerulus into Bowman's capsule during filtration.

Juxtaglomerular apparatus monitors filtrate pressure in the distal tubule via granular cells. It is responsible for renin secretion, initiating a signal transduction cascade involving angiotensin. The adrenal cortex is stimulated to create *aldosterone*, which stimulates *sodium retention*.

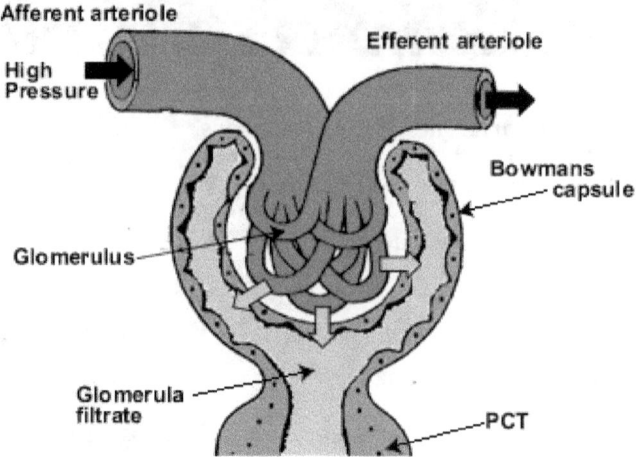

Glomerulus and Bowman's capsule with afferent and efferent arterioles

Nephron regions and the passage of substances

When blood enters the glomerulus (i.e., a cluster of capillaries), hydrostatic pressure (i.e., blood pressure) forces small molecules from the glomerulus across the glomerular capsule's inner membrane into the lumen of the glomerular capsule, a process of *pressure filtration*.

Glomerular walls are a hundred times more permeable than capillary walls.

Glomerular filtrate is molecules leaving the blood and entering the glomerular capsules.

Plasma proteins and blood cells are too large for glomerular filtration.

Failure to restore fluids causes death due to loss of water and nutrients and lower blood pressure.

$$A_E = A_F + A_S - A_{RA}$$

where A is the amount: A_E = excreted, A_F = filtered, A_S = secreted, A_{RA} = reabsorbed

For a given substance:

Net glomerular filtration pressure = $P_{GC} - P_{BS} - \pi_{GC}$

where P_{GC} = glomerular capillary hydrostatic pressure favors filtration from capillaries to Bowman's capsule, P_{BS} = the Bowman's capsule hydrostatic pressure favoring movement from Bowman's capsule to capillaries, and π_{GC} = osmotic pressure resulting from the presence of protein in glomerular capillary plasma and the absence of protein in Bowman's capsule.

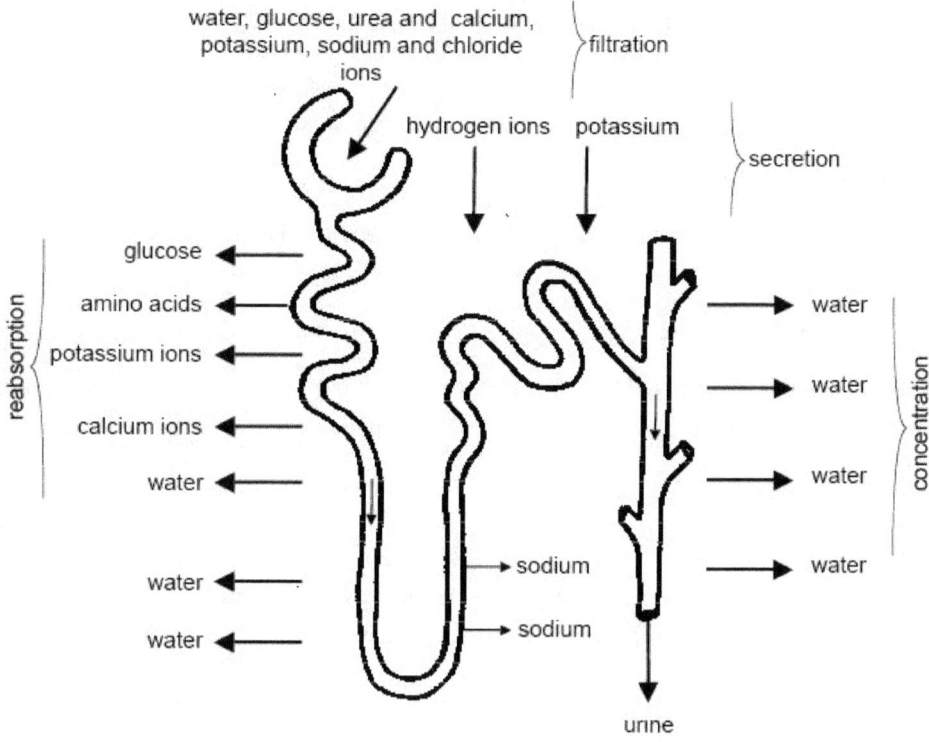

Filtration begins at Bowman's capsule with filtrate exiting through the collecting ducts

Net glomerular filtration pressure is usually positive (fluid moves into Bowman's capsule).

Glomerular filtration rate (GFR) is the volume of liquid filtered from glomeruli into the Bowman's capsule per unit time.

GFR is determined by net filtration pressure, the permeability of the corpuscular membranes, and the surface area available for filtration.

GFR is subject to physiological regulation by neural and hormonal inputs to afferent and efferent arterioles. *Afferent arterioles constriction* decreases P_{GC}, while *efferent arterioles constriction* increases P_{GC}.

Mesangial cells, modified smooth muscle cells, participate in this constriction process.

Filtered load is the total amount of non-protein substances filtered into Bowman's space. It is given by multiplying GFR with the plasma concentration of the substance.

$$\text{Filtered load} = \text{GFR} \times \text{plasma concentration}.$$

If the quantity of a substance excreted in urine is less than the filtered load, tubular reabsorption has occurred; if it is more, tubular secretion has occurred.

Location and mechanism for secretion and reabsorption of solutes

During *secretion*, substances such as acids, bases, and ions (e.g., K^+) may be secreted by passive and active transport in *peritubular capillaries* formed from glomerular efferent arterioles.

Proximal convoluted tubules reabsorb the nutrients and most ions.

Soluble waste (e.g., urea) remains in the filtrate, and NH_4^+, creatinine, and organic acids are excreted.

Loop of Henle reabsorbs water and salt using the countercurrent mechanism.

Distal convoluted tubules selectively reabsorb or secrete ions and compounds based on hormonal control. Collecting ducts reabsorbs water to concentrate urine if ADH is present.

Collecting duct can secrete and reabsorb substances based on *hormonal control*.

Regulation of blood:

> H^+ is secreted from blood when the blood pH is too acidic, whereas HCO_3^- is secreted when the blood pH is too basic.

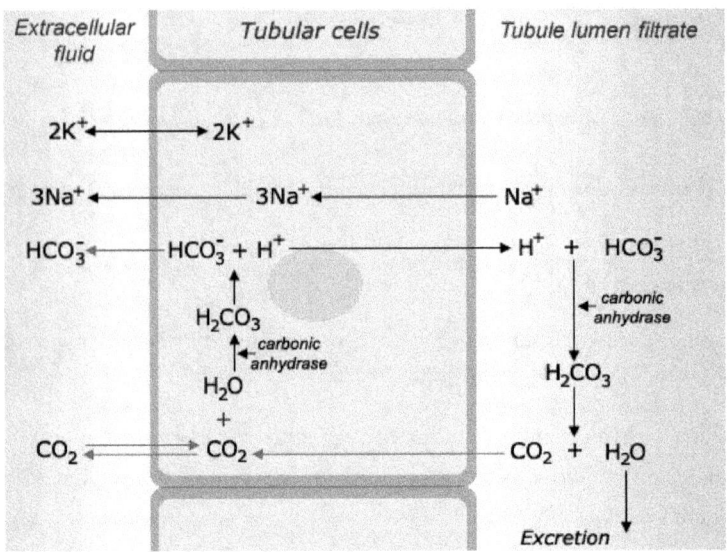

Ion exchange in the tubular cells of the kidney

Tubular secretions and reabsorption

Tubular secretion moves substances (e.g., H^+ and K^+ ions) from *peritubular capillaries* into the *tubular lumen* by diffusion or transcellular mediated transport.

Some movements are coupled with the reabsorption of Na^+ ions.

Secretion back into the filtrate is primarily associated with the distal convoluted tubule. This removes potentially harmful compounds not filtered into the glomerular capsule (e.g., uric acid, hydrogen ions, ammonia, and penicillin).

Tubular reabsorption of substances and fluids (e.g., glucose, salts, amino acids, and water) from the nephron into the blood occurs through the *proximal convoluted tubule walls* and returns to the blood. Reabsorption recovers much of the glomerular filtrate.

Osmolarity (i.e., solute concentration) of blood and filtrate are equal, so water osmosis does not occur. Sodium ions are actively reabsorbed, pulling along chlorine, changing the blood's osmolarity as water moves passively from the tubule to the blood.

Proximal convoluted tubules reabsorb salts

About 60–70% of salt and water is reabsorbed at the *proximal convoluted tubule*. Cells of the proximal convoluted tubule have numerous *microvilli*, which increases the surface area available for absorption. They have *numerous mitochondria*, which supply the energy needed for active transport. Only molecules with carrier proteins are reabsorbed. For example, excess glucose appears in the urine if glucose levels exceed available receptors.

In diabetes mellitus, there is high plasma glucose due to a lack of insulin or insulin-resistant receptor cells. When diabetic, the liver does not correctly convert glucose to glycogen.

Waste products are excreted in the urine. Useful products are reabsorbed and are predominantly not excreted. Mediated transport is the reabsorption mechanism of many substances (e.g., glucose molecules are coupled to sodium reabsorption).

Transport maximum (T_m) is the limit to which mediated transport moves materials per unit time. This limit results from the *saturation of binding sites* on membrane transport proteins.

Sodium moves out of the lumen into epithelium by diffusion (via ion channels) by cotransport with glucose (which is also being reabsorbed) or by countertransport with H^+ ions (which are being secreted).

Sodium-potassium pump (Na^+/K^+–ATPase) transports Na^+ from epithelium into the interstitial.

Removing Na^+ lowers the osmolarity of the lumen and raises that of the interstitial fluid. This causes a net diffusion of water from the lumen into the interstitial fluid through the epithelium.

Water permeability of the *proximal tubule* is high, but only that of collecting ducts is controlled by vasopressin (ADH). ADH stimulates the insertion of aquaporin channels, increasing water permeability.

Low ADH leads to water diuresis or *diabetes insipidus*, a condition caused by the inability to produce ADH and promote water retention. As a result, the person excretes more urine than necessary. Increased urine flow due to increased solute excretion is *osmotic diuresis*.

Concentration of urine

Urine concentration occurs when there is a low fluid volume in the bloodstream. The body produces less amounts of concentrated urine to counter this.

Concentrated urine production is achieved through hormone ADH, which reduces water loss by making the *distal convoluted tubule* (DCT) and *collecting ducts* permeable to water.

When blood pressure is low, aldosterone also increases the reabsorption of Na^+ by DCT, which increases water retention (serum [Na^+] increases blood pressure).

Distal convoluted tubule contains a dilute solution of urea. The collecting duct concentrates this dilute solution by water reabsorption (via facilitated diffusion) using ADH-controlled action. Water reabsorption in the collecting duct is possible because the loop of Henle has high osmolarity (i.e., very concentrated) at the bottom.

Distal convoluted tubules join the collecting duct, and filtrate becomes more concentrated as it descends the collecting duct because the surrounding medulla is salty and water leaves.

Collecting duct leads to the *renal calyx*, emptying into the *renal pelvis* and drains into the *ureter*.

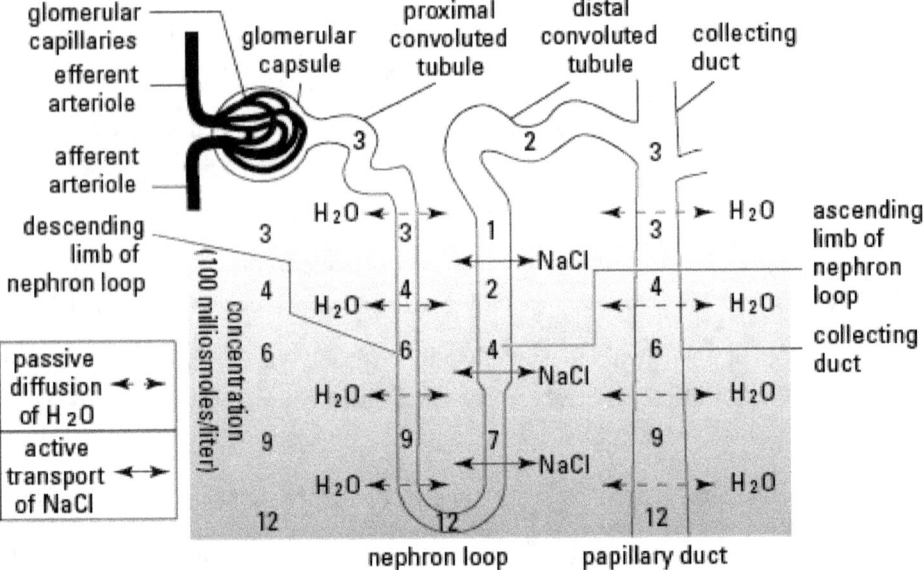

Urine concentration with passive and active transport of substances in the nephron

Countercurrent multiplier mechanism

Countercurrent multiplier creates an osmotic gradient down the loop of Henle, which the collecting duct uses to concentrate urine. Sodium-potassium pump on the ascending limb drives this gradient.

Countercurrent is water flowing out of the filtrate on the descending limb, and salt flows out on the ascending limb.

Descending limb is impermeable to *salt*, and the ascending limb is impermeable to *water*.

The multiplier is the product of the gradient-producing power of each sodium-potassium pump. This gradient-producing power multiplies down the length of the loop of Henle. Therefore, the longer the loop of Henle, the greater the osmotic gradient. Also, the greater the osmotic gradient, the more concentrated the urine.

Urea recycling contributes to the high osmolarity at the bottom of the loop of Henle. It occurs when urea at the bottom of collecting ducts leaks into interstitial fluid and returns to the filtrate.

Fluid from the proximal tubule has the same osmolarity as plasma since it absorbs sodium and water equally. In the ascending limb, sodium, but not water, is actively reabsorbed from the lumen, making the interstitial fluid of the medulla hyperosmotic.

Due to hyperosmolarity, water diffusion from the lumen into interstitial fluid in the descending limb is *passive diffusion*. Fluid in the distal tubule becomes progressively dilute as sodium is transported out. Then, in the cortical and medullary ducts, water diffuses from the tubule into the hyperosmotic interstitial fluid, and urine is concentrated.

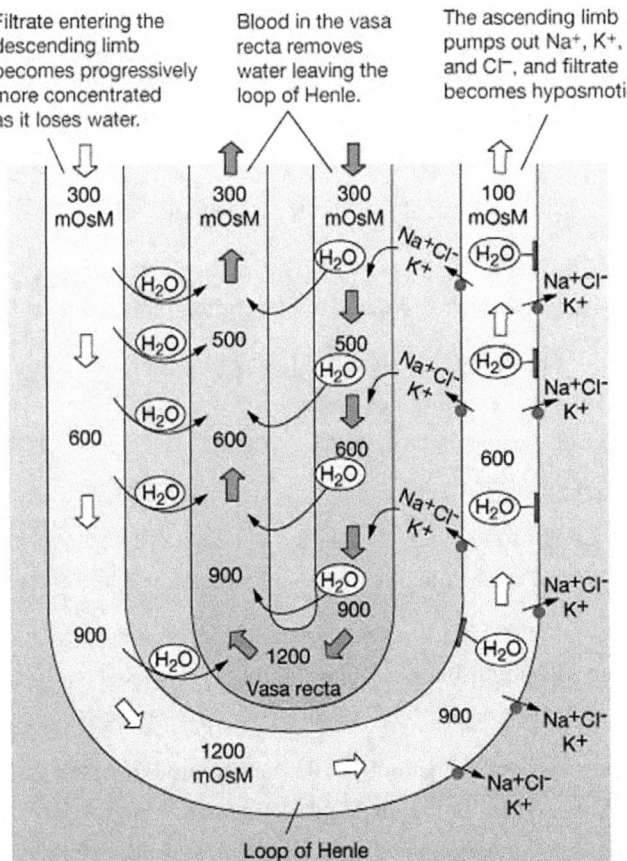

Counter-current multiplier mechanism in the loop of Henle that creates high interstitial osmolarity. Thin descending loop is on the left, and the thick ascending loop is on the right. Note the molecules and ions that pass each section.

Urine Storage and Elimination

Urinary bladder structure and function

Collecting ducts empty into the ureter, draining into the bladder, and storing the urine. Its special epithelium (transitional epithelium) distends to accommodate the storage of large amounts of urine.

Urine is excreted from the bladder through the *urethra*.

Smooth-muscle contractions of the ureter wall allow urine to flow.

Urine is stored in the bladder and ejected during urination (i.e., *micturition*).

The bladder is a chamber with smooth muscle walls (i.e., *detrusor muscle*). Contractions of detrusor muscles produce urination.

Part of the muscle at the base of the bladder, where the urethra begins, functions as the internal urethral sphincter.

Below this sphincter is a ring of skeletal muscle of the external urethral sphincter, which surrounds the urethra.

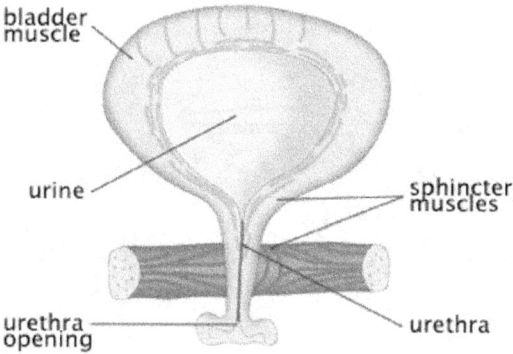

Urinary bladder and sphincter muscles as urine passes into the urethra

Renal clearance rate

Renal clearance is the volume of plasma from which kidneys remove a substance per unit time:

$$\text{Clearance of substance S} = \frac{\text{Mass of S excreted per unit time}}{\text{Plasma concentration of S}}$$

$$C_S = \frac{U_S V}{P_S}$$

where C_S = clearance of S, U_S = urine concentration of S, V = urine volume per unit time, P_S = plasma concentration of S. C_S of a substance equals glomerular filtration rate (GFR) if the substance is filtered but not reabsorbed, secreted, or metabolized.

Neural control of the bladder

Sympathetic neurons innervate the bladder's *detrusor* (i.e., smooth) muscle from the lumbar spinal cord and *parasympathetic fibers* from the sacral spinal cord.

While filling, the detrusor muscle is relaxed, and the sphincters are closed.

When full, stretch receptors stimulate parasympathetic fibers, resulting in detrusor muscle contraction. However, there is strong sympathetic and motor input to sphincters. Consequently, sympathetic and motor input to the sphincters are inhibited, and sphincters open for urination.

There is voluntary control over the external sphincter.

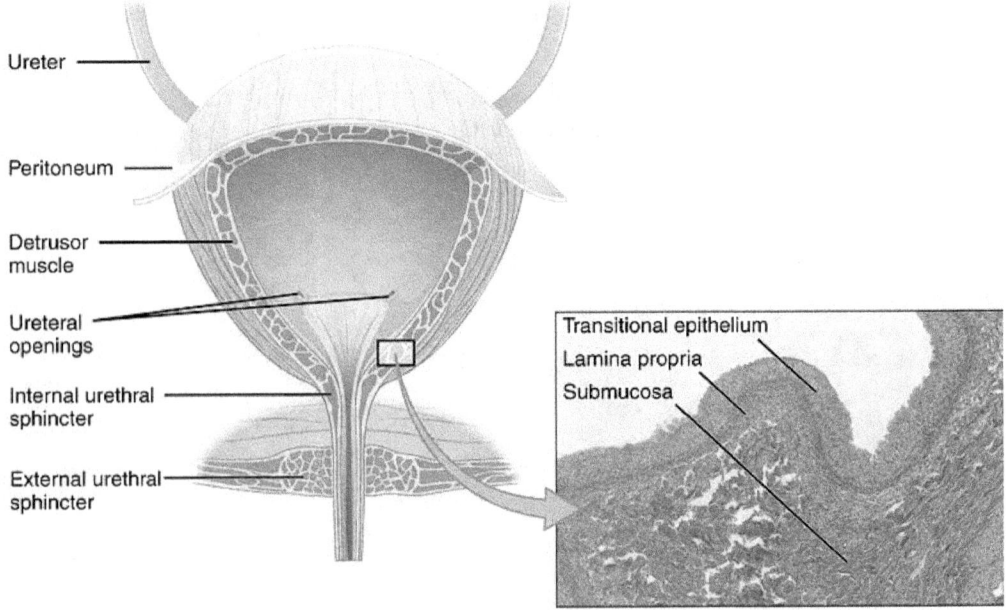

Bladder anatomy and histology (inset)

Notes for active learning

Notes for active learning

CHAPTER 11

Muscular System

Muscular System Functions

Structural Characteristics of Muscles

Muscle Contraction Mechanism

Muscle Regulation

Neural Control of Muscular System

Muscle Cell

Page intentionally left blank

Muscular System Functions

Support and mobility

Muscular system consists of contractile fibers held by connective tissue. Muscle contractions result in movement, position stabilization, movement of substances throughout the body, and generation of body heat.

Muscles provide *support* for stabilizing joints and maintaining posture while sitting or standing.

Muscles provide *mobility*. For example, skeletal muscles facilitate body movement, and smooth muscles move substances through the gut.

Assisting peripheral circulation

Heart is a muscle that pumps blood. Pumping cardiac muscle in the heart causes blood to flow through blood vessels. Other body muscles provide peripheral assistance outside of the heart to help keep the circulatory system flowing.

For example, the contraction of the skeletal muscles of the diaphragm not only draws air into the lungs but also squeezes on the abdominal veins to draw blood back to the heart.

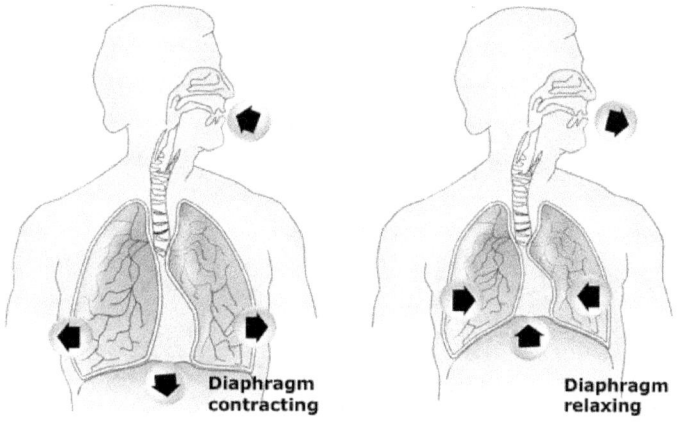

Contraction of the diaphragm: inhaling (left) and exhaling (right).
During inhalation, the diaphragm contracts as the lungs expand.
During expiration, the diaphragm relaxes as air is expelled from the lungs.

Thermoregulation

Thermoregulation allows an organism to keep its body temperature within a specific range. One thermoregulation method is the "*shivering reflex*," generating heat due to rapid skeletal muscle contractions (i.e., hydrolysis of ATP generates heat). Contractions are essential for homeostasis to maintain body temperature in cooler environments.

Notes for active learning

Structural Characteristics of Muscles

Skeletal, cardiac and smooth muscle comparison

Muscles are contractile fibers. Three major types have distinctive properties: skeletal muscle, cardiac muscle, and smooth muscle.

	Skeletal:
	• voluntary
	• striated
	• multinucleated
	• non-branched
	Cardiac:
	• involuntary
	• striated
	• single nucleus
	• branched
	Smooth:
	• involuntary
	• non-striated
	• single nucleus
	• tapered

Voluntary control of skeletal muscle

Skeletal muscle cells are *multinucleated*. Under a microscope, skeletal muscle cells appear as long, non-branched fibers with *striations* (or vertical stripes) due to the presence of *sarcomeres*.

The basic functional unit of myofibrils is the sarcomere, an individualized, organized structure that allows for muscle contraction.

Myofibrils are contractile portions of fibers that lie parallel and run the length of the fiber.

Sarcomeres communicate using *transverse tubules* (T-tubules), which penetrate and contact muscle cells but do not fuse to the *sarcoplasmic reticulum*.

Ions are exchanged through myofibrils using this transverse system.

Skeletal muscles are attached to the skeleton by *fibrous connective tissue tendons*, allowing skeletal muscle contractions to move the skeleton.

Skeletal muscles, under voluntary control, perform everyday movements of the skeleton.

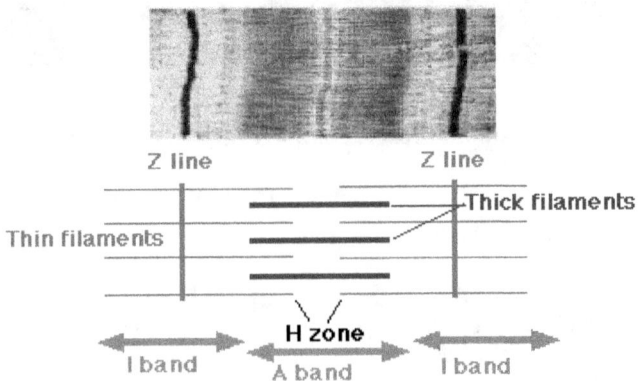

Sarcomere with electron micrograph showing striated pattern and illustration of thin (actin) and thick (myosin) filaments with associated A and I band and H zone

In a healthy state, the skeletal muscle never fully relaxes to its entire length because there is always *muscle tone* (some degree of tension) in the muscle, which provides essential protection to the fibers.

Muscle tone gives the muscle fibers a passive resistance to stretching. This is driven by the viscoelastic properties of muscle fibers and a degree of alpha motor neuron activation (lower motor neurons of the brainstem and spinal cord).

Hypertonia is high muscle tone resulting in brief spasms, prolonged cramps, or rigidity.

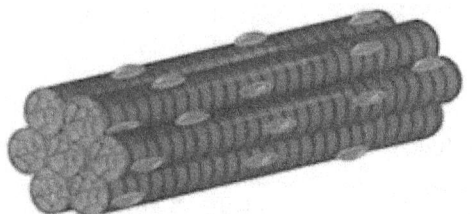

A skeletal muscle with multinucleated myofibrils

Cardiac muscle comprises the heart

Cardiac muscle has a striated appearance due to sarcomeres, and cardiac muscle cells contain one or two central nuclei.

Unlike skeletal muscle, cardiac muscle is branched.

Cardiac muscle is under *involuntary control* and is exclusively in the heart.

Myocardial (i.e., cardiac muscle) cells are separated by intercalated discs with gap junctions, allowing action potentials to flow through electrical synapses.

Cardiac muscle has many mitochondria and is stimulated by *autonomic innervation*.

Cardiac and smooth muscle are *myogenic* and can contract without stimuli from nerve cells.

Some myocardial cells do not function in contraction; instead, they form the conducting system, which initiates the heartbeat and spreads it throughout the heart.

Blood is supplied to cardiac muscle cells by *coronary arteries* and drained by *coronary veins*.

Blood pumped through the chambers *does not exchange* substances with the heart muscle cells.

Vital cardiac muscle cells are innervated with a rich supply of sympathetic fibers, which release norepinephrine, and parasympathetic fibers, which release acetylcholine.

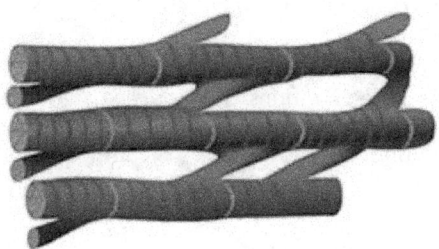

Cardiac muscle with branching between myocardial cells

Involuntary control of smooth muscle

Smooth muscle fibers are composed of *spindle-shaped cells* with a *single nucleus*.

Smooth muscle fibers are *nonstriated* because they do not have the highly organized sarcomeres that form the basic skeletal and cardiac muscle units.

Sliding filament mechanism for the contraction of intermediate filaments uses *myosin* and *actin*.

Thick (i.e., *myosin*) and thin (i.e., *actin*) filaments run diagonally to the cell's long axis, and they are attached to the plasma membrane or *dense bodies* as cytoplasmic structures.

Like skeletal muscle, smooth muscle requires Ca^{2+} ions for contraction, which (like skeletal muscle) is *released from the sarcoplasmic reticulum* inside the cell.

While cardiac and muscle cells do not generally divide in adult humans, smooth muscle cells maintain the ability to divide throughout life.

The autonomic nervous system controls them under involuntary control.

For example, smooth muscle is in the lining of the bladder, the uterus, the digestive tract, and blood vessel walls.

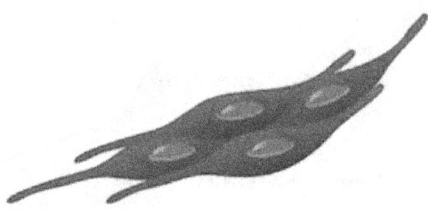

Smooth muscle with spindle-shaped cells and a single nucleus

Plasma membrane of smooth muscles receives excitatory and inhibitory inputs, and the contractile state of the muscle depends on the relative intensity.

However, some smooth muscle fibers generate action potential spontaneously. The potential change during spontaneous depolarizations is the *pacemaker potential*.

Unlike skeletal muscles, smooth muscles do not have motor endplates.

Postganglionic autonomic neurons divide into smooth muscle fibers branches, each containing a series of *varicosities* (i.e., swollen regions).

Varicosities contain vesicles filled with a neurotransmitter released from an action potential. The same neurotransmitter can produce excitation in one fiber and inhibition in another.

Varicosities from a single axon may innervate several fibers, and a single fiber may receive signals from varicosities of sympathetic and parasympathetic neurons.

Smooth muscle plasma membranes bind and respond to hormones. Paracrine agents, acidity, oxygen concentration, osmolarity, and ion composition can influence smooth muscle tension, providing a response mechanism to local factors.

Single-unit and multiunit smooth muscle

Single-unit smooth muscle (or *visceral muscle*) cells are connected by gap junctions, intracellular channels allowing the passage of molecules between cells. Therefore, an action potential can influence many single-unit smooth muscle cells, causing a unified contraction.

In a single-unit smooth muscle, the fibers undergo synchronous activity due to adjacent fibers being linked by gap junctions; an action potential occurring on any of the fibers propagates to the other cells. This allows the whole muscle to respond to stimulation as a single unit.

Some of the fibers may consist of pacemaker cells, which can control the contraction of the entire muscle. However, most of the smooth muscle fibers consist of non-pacemaker cells.

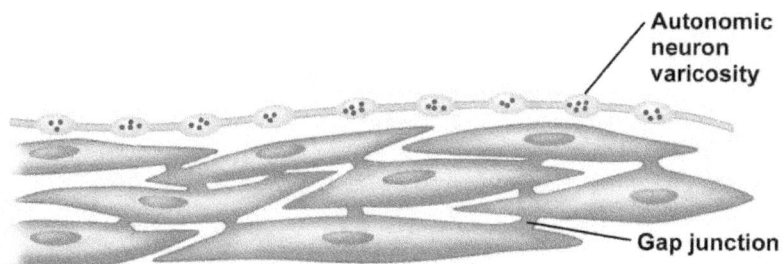

Single-unit smooth muscle with autonomic neural innervation and gap junction

Multiunit smooth muscle is made of cells that contract independently from one another.

Each multiunit smooth muscle cell is directly attached to a neuron. In addition to the neuronal response, smooth muscle cells respond to hormones, changes in pH, O_2 and CO_2 concentration, temperature, and ion concentration.

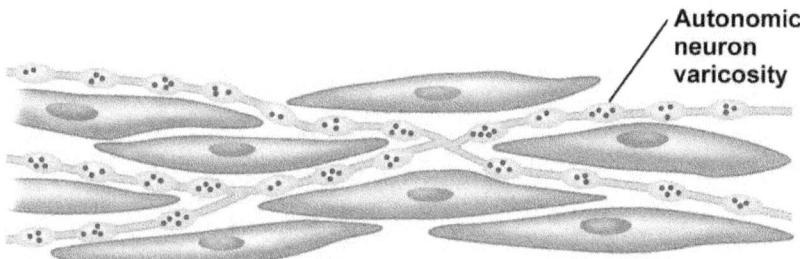

Multiunit smooth muscle contracts independently

Notes for active learning

Muscle Contraction Mechanism

Actin and myosin filaments

Skeletal and cardiac muscle cells show dark and light bands under a microscope.

Electron microscopy shows that the placement of protein filaments within sarcomeres forms the striations of myofibrils.

The light and dark bands correspond to two types of proteins: *actin* and *myosin*.

Actin filaments (i.e., thin filaments) are long actin protein chains in a spherical conformation that include *troponin* and *tropomyosin*, which wrap the actin protein.

Thin myofilaments have two chains that coil around each other. Actin molecules have a unique combination of strength and sensitivity.

These molecules are constantly destroyed and renewed to contribute to the muscle tissue's function. This is controlled by the ATP attached to each actin monomer.

The state of ATP determines the stability of the actin molecules.

Myosin filaments (i.e., thick filaments) are protein molecules arranged in a bipolar structure. They are made of protruding club-like heads that lie towards the thick filaments' ends while their shafts lie towards the middle.

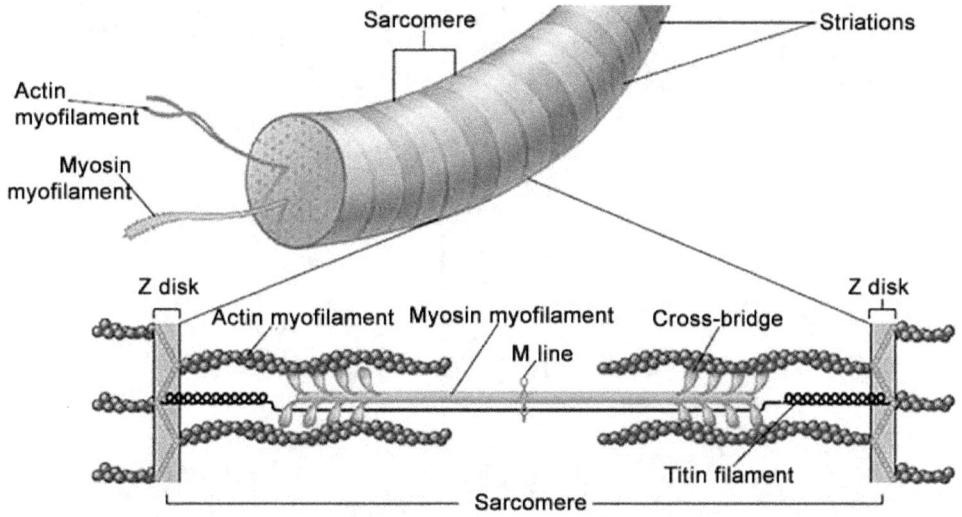

Skeletal and cardiac muscles have a striated appearance from sarcomeres

Each myosin protein thick filament has a central bare zone and an array of protruding heads of opposite polarity at the ends. Myosin molecules possess a tail forming the core of the thick myofilament, while the head projects from the core filament. Myosin heads are cross bridges.

Myosin heads have ATP-binding sites and actin-binding sites. The myosin head contains a hinge at the point where it leaves the core of the thick myofilament to allow the head to swivel, and this swiveling action is the cause of any muscle contraction.

Swiveling action occurs when actin combines with the myosin head, leading to the ATP associated with the head hydrolyzing ATP → ADP + energy. Actin molecules contain a binding site for myosin; myosin molecules contain a binding site for actin and ATP.

Troponin and tropomyosin in muscle contraction

In a resting muscle fiber, tropomyosin, a long protein that spirals along actin, blocks the myosin head or the binding sites on actin, preventing cross-bridge formation with actin. An action potential releases Ca^{2+} from the sarcoplasmic reticulum of the muscle cell and increases the cytosolic concentration of Ca^{2+}.

When Ca^{2+} binds to troponin, it shifts tropomyosin from the myosin-binding site, making it possible for myosin cross bridges to attach with actin. Tropomyosin can be thought of as protecting actin's binding sites from the advances of the myosin head.

In the presence of Ca^{2+}, troponin changes its conformation and moves tropomyosin away from its guard position, allowing myosin heads to bind to actin and muscle contraction to ensue.

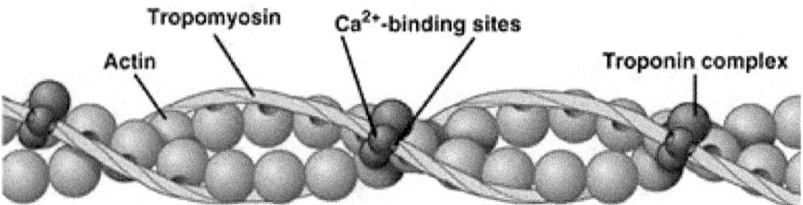

Myosin-binding sites blocked by tropomyosin on actin filament

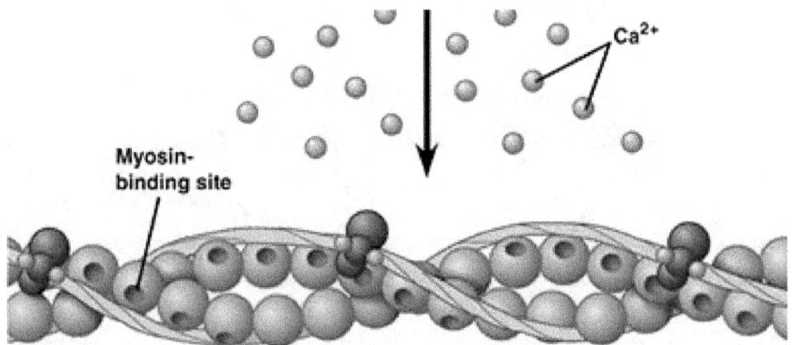

Myosin-binding sites exposed when Ca^{2+} binds to troponin; a conformation change in tropomyosin exposes the myosin-binding sites on actin.

Cross bridges

Overlapping thick and thin filaments form *cross bridges* from the thick myosin filaments.

In a cross bridge, each thick filament is surrounded by a hexagonal array of six thin filaments, and each thin filament is surrounded by a triangular array of three thick filaments.

Thick filaments contain contractile protein *myosin*. Thin filaments contain contractile protein *actin, troponin* and *tropomyosin proteins*.

Power stroke of muscle contraction

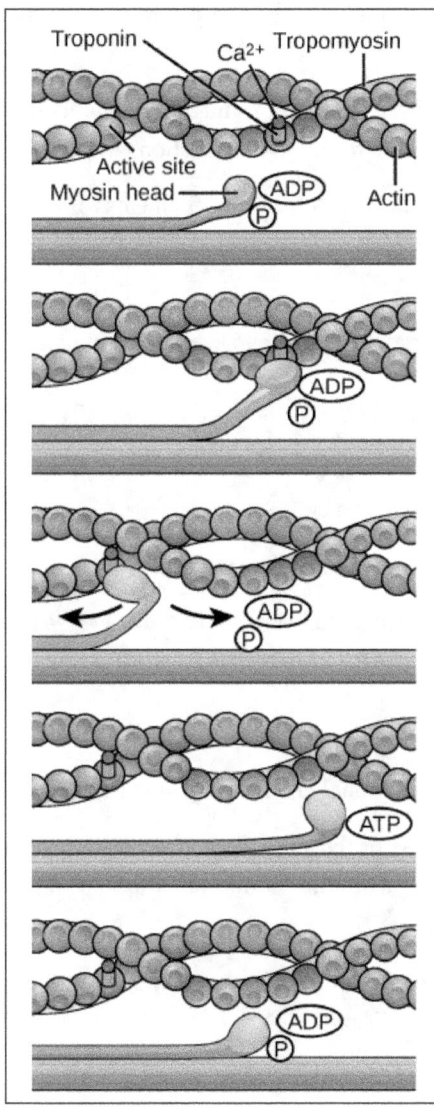

1 - Active site on actin is exposed as Ca^{2+} binds *troponin* and causes a conformational change in *tropomyosin* on actin.

2 – Movement of tropomyosin allows the myosin head forms a cross-bridge with actin.

3 – During the power stroke, myosin head bends, the muscle shortens, and ADP and phosphate are released.

4 – A new molecule of ATP attaches to the myosin head, causing cross-bridges from the myosin head to actin to detach.

5 – ATP hydrolyzes to ADP and phosphate, returning the myosin head to the "cocked" position in preparation for contraction.

Without ATP, cross-bridges between the myosin head and the actin filament remain attached. Cross bridges break due to enzymatic activity in a deceased individual, which gives rise to cadaver movement. This explains why corpses are stiff; non-living bodies do not produce ATP.

Contraction strength of a single muscle fiber cannot be increased, but the strength of the overall contraction can be increased by *recruiting more muscle fibers*.

Sliding filament theory for muscle contractions

Sliding filament model proposes that muscle fiber contracts, causing the sarcomeres within the myofibrils to shorten. As a sarcomere shortens, actin filaments slide past myosin; the I band shortens, and the H zone disappears.

The swivel movement of the cross-bridges makes the overlapping thick and thin filaments slide past each other. Actin and myosin fibers *do not change length* during contraction.

Z line is the boundary of a single sarcomere and anchors thin actin filaments. Electron microscopy shows a zigzag line on the sides of the sarcomere that connects the filaments of adjacent sarcomeres.

M line is a line of myosin in the middle of the sarcomere linked by accessory proteins.

I band is the region containing thin filaments (actin) only.

H zone is the region containing thick filaments (myosin) only.

A band is made of an actin end overlapping with a myosin end.

H zone and I band reduce during contraction, while the A band remains constant.

In the sliding filament model, cross-bridge forms, and the myosin head bends, the *power stroke*.

Power stroke causes actin to slide toward the *M line*, allowing the muscle fiber to contract.

ATP binds to myosin head and is converted to ADP + Pi, which remains attached to the head.

Release of myosin Ca^{2+} binds to troponin with a conformational change in *tropomyosin*.

Tropomyosin exposes myosin attachment sites, and cross bridges are formed between myosin heads and actin filaments. ADP + Pi is released, causing a sliding motion of actin to bring the sarcomere's Z lines together (contraction, power stroke).

A new ATP molecule attaches to the myosin head, and the cross-bridges unbind, resulting in sarcomere relaxation as phosphorylation breaks the cross-bridge.

Though counterintuitive, ATP is not directly needed for the power stroke.

ATP binding is needed to detach the myosin head from actin and reset the power stroke by cocking the myosin head (in preparation for the next power stroke).

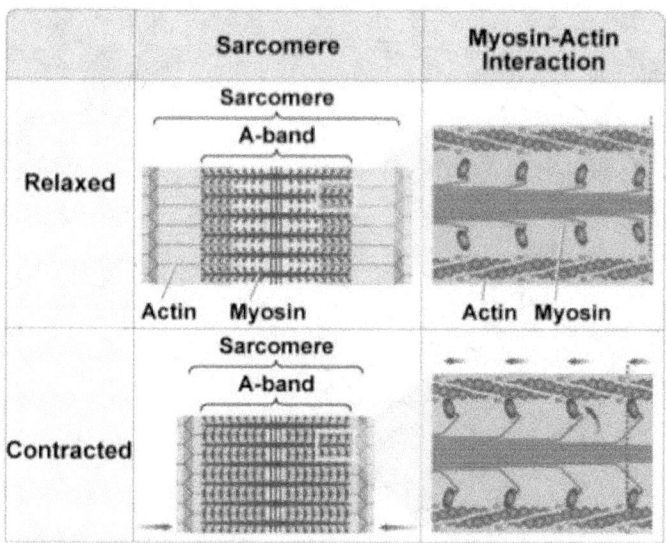

Sliding filament model: thick (myosin) and thin (actin) filaments slide past each other during muscle contraction, shortening the sarcomere

Calcium in sarcoplasmic reticulum for muscle contraction

Nerves stimulate muscle cells during muscle contraction. An action potential runs along the muscle cell membrane and deep into the cell via *T-tubules* to stimulate the *sarcoplasmic reticulum* (terminal cisternae) to release calcium ions.

Calcium causes muscles to contract via the *sliding filament* mechanism.

Extracellular calcium enters the cell by opening Ca^{2+} plasma membrane channels. The rate of Ca^{2+} removal is slower, resulting in a muscle twitch. Ca^{2+} concentrations in response to a single action potential are only sufficient to activate a proportion of the cross bridges.

Therefore, tension in smooth muscle can be graded by varying cytosolic Ca^{2+} concentrations. A low-level tension is maintained, even without external stimuli, as smooth muscle tone.

Cytosolic Ca^{2+} binds to calmodulin proteins. This newly formed calcium-calmodulin complex binds to the *myosin light-chain kinase* (MLCK) enzyme.

Activated kinase uses ATP to phosphorylate the myosin cross bridges. The phosphorylated cross-bridges bind to actin, resulting in muscle contraction. In response, myosin is dephosphorylated by the myosin light chain phosphatase (MLCP) enzyme, an antagonist to MLCK. This enzyme inhibits contraction, thus causing smooth muscle relaxation.

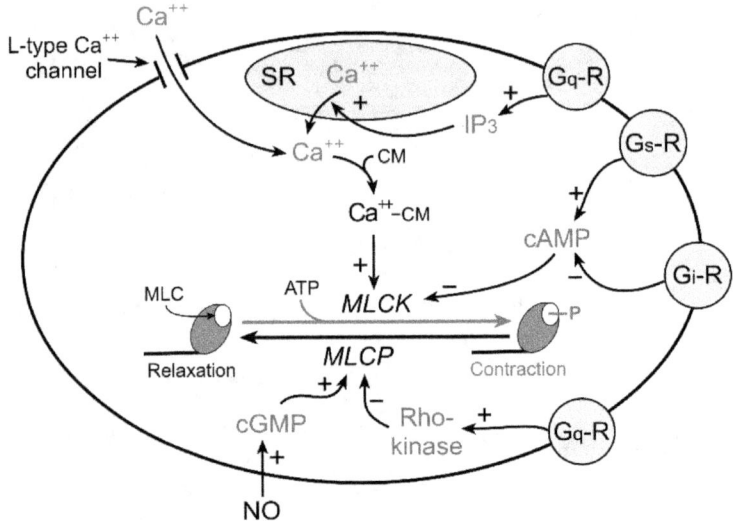

Smooth muscle stores Ca^{2+} in the sarcoplasmic reticulum and receives extracellular Ca^{2+} for muscle contractions. Overview of enzymatic cascade for Ca^{2+} and nitrous oxide.

Temporal and spatial response to force

Muscle spindles monitor muscle length changes and rates by stretch receptors in modified muscle fibers as *intrafusal fibers*. Other fibers responsible for skeletal movement are *extrafusal fibers*. Stretching muscle fires these spindles, while muscle *contraction slows* the firing.

Passive tension in a relaxed fiber increases with stretch due to the elongation of *titin filaments*. However, the maximum tension during contraction depends primarily on the overlap between the thick and thin filaments, depending on the *resting length* of the muscles.

Two factors allow for the highest maximum tension during contraction.

> *Increased resting length* increases maximum tension because it allows the thick and thin filaments room to slide, allowing more cross-bridge cycling.

> *Decreased resting length* can increase the maximum tension. Tension can arise due to increased overlap between thick and thin filaments, allowing greater interaction during contraction.

Maximum tension in a muscle is opposed by 1) increasing the resting length too much, which does not permit enough interaction between filaments, and 2) decreasing the resting length too much, which causes the thick filaments to hit the Z lines and stop the contraction.

Hence, an optimal resting length between the two extremes results in the greatest maximum tension during contraction.

Most fibers are near this length, l_0, and are relaxed.

When muscles contract (or shorten), they cannot inherently lengthen independently. Instead, skeletal muscles work in antagonistic pairs for skeletal muscles to return to their original length. One muscle of an antagonistic pair bends the joint and brings a limb toward the body. The other straightens the joint and extends the limb. In this mechanism, one muscle's shortening leads to another's lengthening.

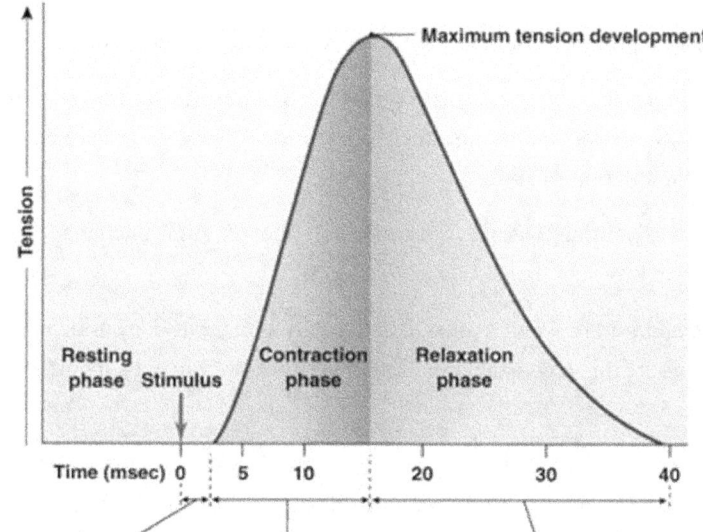

Muscle contraction with tension vs. time. Contraction phase produces a maximum tension force before the relaxation phase returns the muscle to the resting phase for a 40 msec twitch.

Muscle tension responds to force applied

Force exerted on an object by a contracting muscle is *muscle tension*, while force exerted on the muscle by the object (e.g., weight) is *load*.

Muscle tension and load are opposing forces, and whether the exertion of force leads to a change in fiber length depends on the *relative magnitudes* of the tension and the load.

Summation occurs when contractions combine and become stronger and more prolonged (i.e., an increase in muscle tension from successive action potentials).

Summation can be *temporal* (i.e., successive in time) or *spatial* (i.e., separate in location).

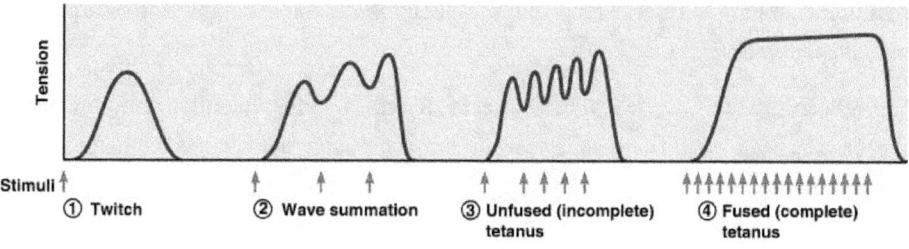

Muscle contraction types

Tetanus occurs when continuous contractions are sustained, and the muscle cannot relax.

In tetanus, the rate of muscle stimulation is so fast that twitches blur into one smooth, constant motion. If tetanus oscillates, it is *unfused* (or incomplete) tetanus, while tetanus without oscillations is *fused* (or complete) tetanus.

Tonus is a state of partial contraction. However, the muscle never wholly relaxes.

Twitch contraction refers to the mechanical response of a single muscle fiber to a single action potential. They are not tetanic because there is a period of relaxation between separate stimuli, preventing the summation of stimuli.

Two major types of contractions are *isometric* (i.e., fiber length is unchanged) and *isotonic* (i.e., fiber length shortens or lengthens).

Isometric contractions are when a muscle develops tension but does not change length when a muscle supports a load in a constant position or attempts to move a supported load greater than the tension.

During isometric contractions, the cross-bridges bound to actin do not move. The *latent period* is when the muscle receives stimulus and develops tension in the fiber.

Contraction time is required for the fiber to reach maximum tension.

Relaxation period releases the fiber's tension, and fibers rest until a new stimulus is received.

Isometric contractions *do not* move a load; they develop tension in a muscle fiber without changing fiber length. Therefore, the isometric contractions do not perform physical work, so they should be compared to isotonic twitches.

Isometric twitches have a *short latent period* and a *short contraction time*.

Isotonic contractions occur when the load remains constant while fiber length changes. If the fibers shorten, contraction is *concentric*, and cross-bridges are bound to actin move, shortening the fibers.

Before an isotonic shortening, there is a period of *isometric* contraction when the tension of the fiber increases to meet the load and move it.

In isotonic contractions, the *latent period* is between when the stimulus is received and when shortening occurs in the fiber. Time from the beginning of shortening to maximum shortening is the *contraction time*.

During relaxation, the fiber relaxes to a greater length. If fibers lengthen, isotonic contraction is an *eccentric contraction* when the load on a muscle is greater than the tension, forcing the muscle to lengthen.

Isometric and isotonic twitches are measured differently.

Isometric contractions do not change the muscle length, so plots show *tension vs. time.*

Isotonic contractions change muscle length, so plots show *distance shortened vs. time.*

Isometric contractions *do not* move a load; they only develop tension in muscle fiber without changing fiber length. Therefore, the isometric contractions do not perform physical work, and it is appropriate that they are compared to isotonic twitches. Isometric twitches have a *short latent period* and a *short contraction time.*

Isotonic twitches are compared at loads of different forces. With heavier loads, a longer time is required for the isometric component of the twitch to build tension to meet the load. Thus, increasing the load leads to a longer latent period. Heavier loads decrease the shortening distance that a single stimulus can provide.

Although the contraction time is slightly shorter with a heavier load, the decreased shortening distance leads to a slower velocity of contraction (or distance shortened) per unit time.

Relaxation phase depends on load as fibers return to their original length; increased loads have a shorter relaxation phase. Isotonic twitches *do move a load* and *involve a fiber length change.*

Compared to isometric twitches, isotonic twitches have a long latent and contraction period. Even though eccentric *isotonic contractions* involve muscle lengthening over time, they utilize *temporary* fiber shortening to control the load's movement.

For example, slowly lowering one's body from a pull-up requires eccentric muscle effort from the latissimus dorsi, whereas quickly dropping from a pull-up to a dead-hang position while gripping the bar would not involve isotonic contraction from the lats (and is painful).

Isometric twitches have a shorter contraction time but a more extended relaxation period and *overall duration* than isotonic twitches.

Isotonic twitches have shorter relaxation due to a load, bringing the muscle to its original length.

Notes for active learning

Muscle Regulation

Contractile velocity of different muscle types

Contractile velocity is the force that a muscle creates and depends on the muscle's length, volume, fiber type, and shortening velocity.

Muscle cross-sectional area (CSA) divides the volume by the length.

$$CSA = V / l$$

Physiological CSA $= m \cdot \cos \theta / l \cdot \rho$; where m is muscle mass, θ is the fiber angle, l is the length of the fiber, and ρ is muscle density.

Short fibers have a higher physiological muscle volume per unit of muscle mass. Greater force is produced, and it shortens at slower speeds.

Long fibers have a lower physiological muscle volume per unit of muscle mass, meaning there is a lower force production, and it shortens faster.

Type 1 fibers have a slow increase in force and low force production. They have a smaller diameter, which leads to *slower contractions*.

Type IIA fibers have *fast contractions* and a faster force production.

Type IIB fibers have a fast contraction, faster increase in force, and large force production.

Type IIB fibers are fatigued quickly, and maintaining that force is difficult.

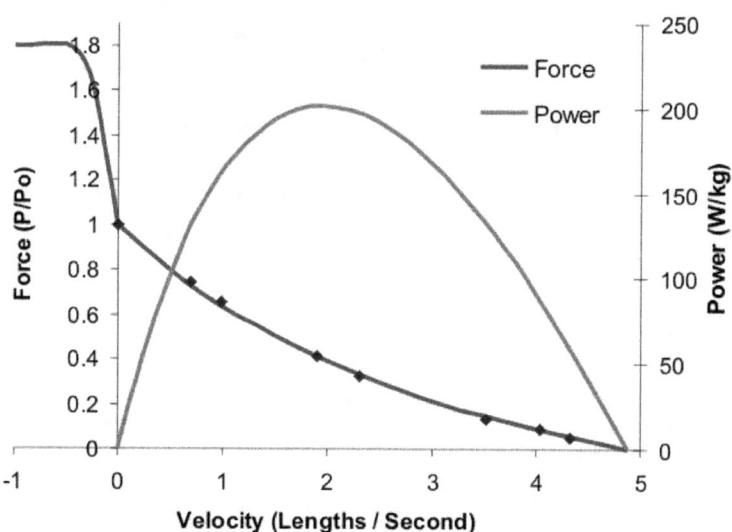

In the force-velocity relationship, changes in muscle lengths affect force generation. Force decreases with increasing contractile velocity.

Regulation of cardiac muscle contraction

Cardiomyocytes (i.e., cardiac muscle cells) coordinate contractions, regulated through *intercalated discs*, which spread action potentials to support the synchronized contraction of the myocardium.

Contraction in a cardiac muscle, as well as in smooth and skeletal muscles, occurs via *excitation-contraction coupling* (ECC).

ECC is where an electrical stimulus originating in neurons is converted into a mechanical response. In muscle cells, the electrical stimulus is the action potential, and the desired mechanical response is a contraction.

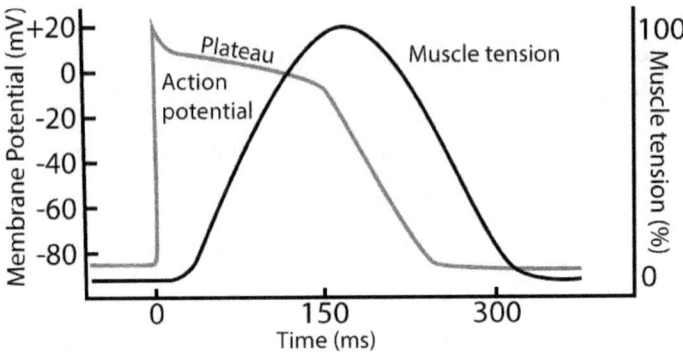

In particular cardiac muscle, ECC is dependent on calcium-induced calcium release. This involves conduction of calcium ions into the cell, triggering further release into the cytoplasm.

Like skeletal muscle, initiation and upshoot of the action potential in ventricular cardiac muscle cells are derived from the entry of *sodium ions* across the sarcolemma in a regenerative process.

In cardiac muscle, an inward flux of extracellular calcium ions through the calcium channels on the *T-tubules* sustains the depolarization of cardiac muscle cells for a *longer duration*.

Cardiac (like skeletal) muscle contraction occurs via the *sliding filament model*.

Cardiac muscle contraction pathways

Contraction pathway for cardiac muscle has five steps.

1. Action potential induced by pacemaker cells is conducted to contractile cardiomyocytes through intercalated discs (gap junctions).

2. As the action potential travels between sarcomeres, it activates the calcium channels in the T-tubules, resulting in an influx of calcium ions into the cell and releasing Ca^{2+} from the sarcoplasmic reticulum.

3. Calcium in the cytoplasm then binds to cardiac troponin-C, which moves the troponin complex from the actin-binding site. This movement of the troponin complex frees the myosin to bind actin and activates contraction.

4. Myosin head pulls the actin filament towards the center of the sarcomere, contracting the muscle.

5. Intracellular calcium is then removed by the sarcoplasmic reticulum, dropping the intracellular calcium concentration, returning the troponin complex to its inhibiting position on the actin, and effectively ending contraction.

Oxygen debt and muscle fatigue

Muscle fatigue is when there is a decline in muscle tension from previous contractile activity.

Fatigued muscle has *decreased shortening velocity* and a *slower rate of relaxation.*

Fatigue onset rate depends on the type of skeletal muscle and the duration of contractile activity. If a fatigued muscle is allowed to rest, it recovers. The recovery rate depends on the duration and intensity of the previous exercise.

Fatigue is not due to low ATP; a fatigued muscle still has a high ATP concentration but is an adaptation to prevent the rigor that results from a low ATP level.

High-frequency fatigue accompanies high-intensity, short-duration exercise due to failure in the T-tubule's action potential conduction. Recovery from fatigue is rapid.

Low-frequency fatigue (i.e., low-intensity, long-duration exercise) is due to *lactic acid* buildup, which changes muscle protein conformation (i.e., shape). Recovery from fatigue is slow.

Molecular mechanism underlying muscle fatigue is that the continuous *synaptic activity* causes depletion of the required *neurotransmitter*, leading to fatigue.

Notes for active learning

Neural Control of Muscular System

Motor and sensory neurons

Motor neurons are *efferent neurons* that send signals to muscles and organs.

Motor neurons have cell bodies in the CNS and contain large, myelinated axons that can propagate action potentials at high velocities.

Autonomic motor neurons control the sympathetic and parasympathetic branches of the nervous system, while *somatic motor neurons* control skeletal muscles.

Muscle fibers of a single muscle do not all contract at once.

A single motor neuron innervates multiple muscle fibers, collectively called a *motor unit*.

Motor units have varying amounts of muscle fibers. Usually, smaller motor units are activated; first, larger ones are activated as needed. This leads to smooth increases in force.

Fine movement only uses smaller motor units.

Total muscle tension depends on the tension in each fiber and the number of fibers contracting, which depends on fiber recruitment (or activation).

Sensory neurons, or *afferent neurons*, are the opposite of motor neurons.

Afferent fibers pathway

Afferent fibers from receptors have four pathways.

> Some fibers go directly to the same muscle's motor neurons without interposing any interneurons as *monosynaptic stretch reflex arcs*.
>
> Some fibers end on interneurons, inhibiting antagonistic muscles as *reciprocal innervation*.
>
> Some fibers activate motor neurons of synergistic muscles.
>
> Some fibers continue to the brainstem.

Motor program is the pattern of neural activities required to perform a movement. It is created and transmitted via neurons, organized hierarchically and is continuously updated. A skill is learned if the program is repeated frequently.

Local control of motor neurons is vital in keeping the motor program updated by gathering information from local levels through afferent nerve fibers.

Alpha and gamma motor neurons and reflex response

Alpha motor neurons are larger motor neurons that control *extrafusal fibers* responsible for skeletal movement.

Gamma motor neurons are smaller motor neurons that control *intrafusal fibers*. Neurons in these intrafusal fibers are excited or co-activated with the neurons in the extrafusal fibers to get continuous information about muscle length.

Withdrawal reflex activates flexor motor neurons and inhibits extensor motor neurons to move the body away from an external stimulus. The effect is *ipsilateral* (i.e., same side) of the body where the stimulus arose.

An opposite effect (i.e., *crossed extensor reflex*) may be produced on the contralateral side to compensate for any lost support due to the withdrawal.

Interneurons are synapses that integrate inputs from higher centers and peripheral receptors.

Afferent inputs to local interneurons bring information such as muscle tension or movement of joints, which influence movements.

Golgi tendon organs are receptors in tendons that monitor muscle tension.

Complex muscular activities (e.g., maintenance of posture and balance) require coordination from several muscles. *Afferent vestibular apparatus* pathways of the eyes and *somatic receptors* must first relay sensory information to brain centers. Information is compared with an internal representation of the body's geometry, and corrections to skeletal muscles are made through alpha motor neurons in the efferent pathways.

For example, walking coordinates multiple muscles. Extensor muscles are activated on one leg to support the body's weight. At the same time, contralateral extensors are inhibited through reciprocal inhibition, allowing flexors to swing the non-supporting leg forward.

Neuromuscular junctions and motor end plates

Muscles contract when stimulated by motor nerve fibers.

Before a signal crosses the neuromuscular junction, an action potential must reach the axon terminal of a motor neuron containing *acetylcholine* (ACh) vesicles.

Neurotransmitters are released into the synapse, where they travel across the gap and reach receptors on the motor end plate, a part of the sarcolemma (i.e., the sheath around skeletal muscle fibers) on the muscle cell.

A graded potential is created across this junction, and if the potential reaches a threshold, an action potential is created.

The action potential then travels down the sarcolemma and causes the muscle to contract. An action potential opens Ca^{2+} channels in the nerve plasma membrane, allowing Ca^{2+} to diffuse and enable neurotransmitter vesicles to fuse with the plasma membrane.

After vesicles fuse, they release ACh into the extracellular space. ACh opens ion channels in the motor end plate and produces depolarization as *endplate potential* (EPP).

Acetylcholinesterase enzyme on the motor end plate degrades ACh to close the ion channels and return the plate to resting potential.

Neuromuscular junction is the meeting of a nerve (motor end axon terminal) with a muscle at the motor end plate. *Motor end plate* is the sarcolemma that synapses with the motor neuron and has neurotransmitter receptors.

When nerve impulses travel down a motor neuron to the axon bulb, ACh-containing vesicles merge with the presynaptic membrane, releasing ACh into the synaptic cleft. ACh rapidly diffuses to and binds with receptors on the sarcolemma.

Sarcolemma generates impulses spreading along T-tubules into the *sarcoplasmic reticulum*, which triggers the release of Ca^{2+} ions from the sarcoplasmic reticulum. Ca^{2+} ions bind to *troponin* to initiate muscle contraction.

Sympathetic and parasympathetic innervation

Sympathetic and parasympathetic nerves have motor neurons innervating involuntary muscles.

Sympathetic nervous system controls "*fight or flight*" when heart rate and blood pressure increase, pupils dilate, less blood is directed to the digestive system, and more blood is directed to the muscles.

Parasympathetic nervous system controls "*rest and digest*" responses. Contrary to sympathetic responses, heart rate and blood pressure decrease, pupils constrict, and more blood is directed to the digestive system rather than muscles.

Voluntary and involuntary muscles

Voluntary muscles are consciously controlled muscles with cylindrical fibers.

Muscles are generally attached to bones (i.e., skeletal muscles), and the brain is involved in the movement of muscles. For example, a voluntary muscle is the biceps in the upper arm.

Involuntary muscles are spindle-shaped fibers associated with the autonomic nervous system and not consciously controlled. For example, smooth and cardiac muscles are involuntary.

Voluntary muscle contractions are rapid and forceful, while involuntary contractions are slow and rhythmic. Motor behaviors are a continuum of these two types of contractions, having varied voluntary and involuntary muscle components.

Muscle Cell

Muscle cell structure and function

Muscle consists of muscle cells bound by connective tissue. A single muscle fiber is a multinucleated cell formed from myoblasts during development. Muscle cells contain several parallel *myofibrils* composed of *myofilaments* (primarily actin and myosin).

Myofibrils contain *sarcomeres*, the basic units of contraction in the skeletal muscle. Myofibrils are packed within the multinucleated skeletal muscle cells.

Sarcolemma (i.e., plasma membrane) of muscle cells contain and pack myofibrils. The nuclei of the muscle fibers are at the edges of the diameter of the fiber, adjacent to the sarcolemma.

Sarcoplasm is the cytoplasm of muscle fibers and contains numerous mitochondria that produce ATP for muscle contraction.

Sarcoplasmic reticulum is like the smooth endoplasmic reticulum; it extends throughout the muscle cell's sarcoplasm and stores calcium ions in muscle contraction.

Muscles are attached to bones by collagen bundles of *tendons*. After infancy, new fibers are formed from undifferentiated satellite cells and generally do not undergo mitosis to create new muscle cells after development, which is called *hyperplasia*.

Muscle cells increase in size and overall volume, known as *hypertrophy*. In adulthood, any compensation for lost muscles occurs by an increase in the size of fibers.

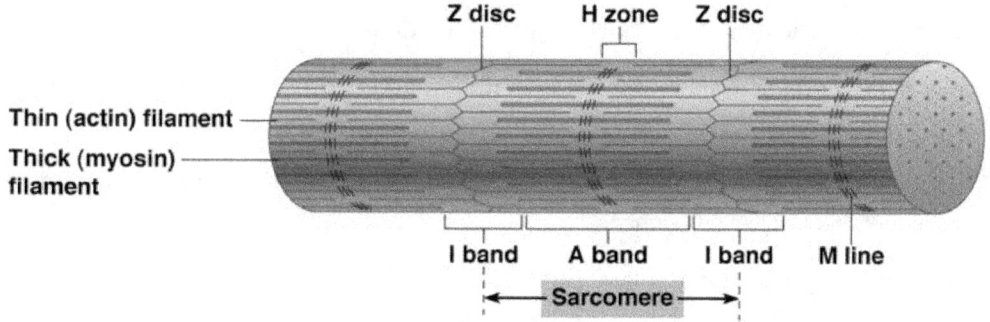

Sarcomere is the functional unit of muscle cells

Transverse tubules and calcium

Transverse tubules (*T-tubules*) are tunnel-like extensions of the sarcolemma that pass-through muscle cells from one side of the cell to another, forming a network around myofibrils. They are referred to as transverse because of the way they are oriented. The transverse tubules play a vital role in muscle contraction.

Muscle action potentials (i.e., electrical charge movement) travel along the transverse tubules and stimulate the release of *calcium ions* from the *sarcoplasmic reticulum*, allowing calcium ions to flood into the sarcoplasm and bind to troponin.

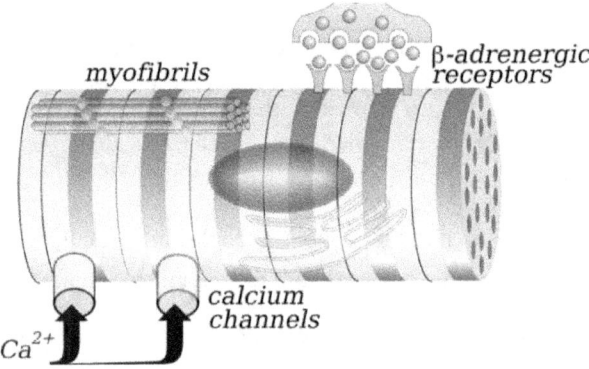

Calcium triggers the movement of various protein filaments (including *actin, myosin,* and *tropomyosin*) within the myofibrils, which results in muscle contraction. T-tubules' general function is to conduct impulses from the cell's surface to the sarcoplasmic reticulum, where Ca is released.

Sarcoplasmic reticulum stores calcium for contractions

Sarcoplasm in muscle cells is equivalent to the cytoplasm of other cells. The sarcoplasmic reticulum in muscle cells is homologous to the endoplasmic reticulum.

Unlike the endoplasmic reticulum, the sarcoplasmic reticulum stores and secretes Ca^+, the essential ion in muscle contraction.

Sarcoplasmic reticulum forms a sleeve around myofibrils, with enlarged *lateral sacs* that store Ca^{2+}. It is abundant in skeletal muscle cells and is related to myofibrils.

Sarcoplasmic reticulum membrane contains active pumps that move calcium into the sarcoplasmic reticulum from the sarcoplasm. The sarcoplasmic reticulum contains specialized gates for calcium.

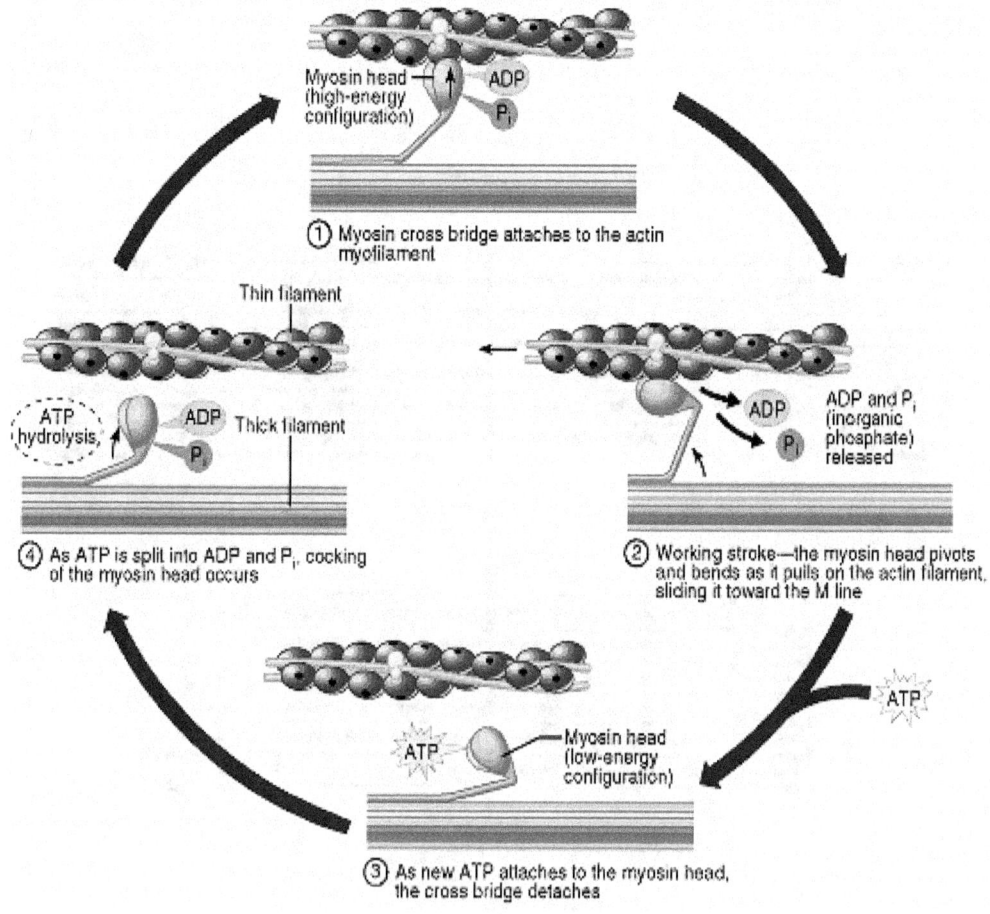

Calcium binds to troponin to cause a conformational change in tropomyosin and expose the myosin-binding sites on the actin myofilament (step 1)

Action potentials lead to depolarization of the sarcoplasmic reticulum membrane, leading to depolarization of the T-tubules. This opens the Ca^{2+} channels of the lateral sacs, causing the contraction to begin.

Contraction ends when Ca^{2+} is pumped into the lateral sacs by active transport proteins called plasma membrane Ca^{2+} ATPase (PMCA).

Sarcomere anatomy and function for muscle contractions

Sarcomeres with I and A bands, M and Z lines, and the H zone.

Skeletal muscle cells have longitudinal bundles of myofibrils.

Myofibrils consist of thin (i.e., actin) and thick (i.e., myosin) filaments, which repeat along the myofibril in units such as sarcomeres.

Organelles within the sarcomeres resemble the form and function of other eukaryotic cells.

H zones, the sarcomere's central region, have no overlap of thin and thick filaments.

In the center of the H zone, the M line links the center regions of thick filaments and divides the sarcomere vertically.

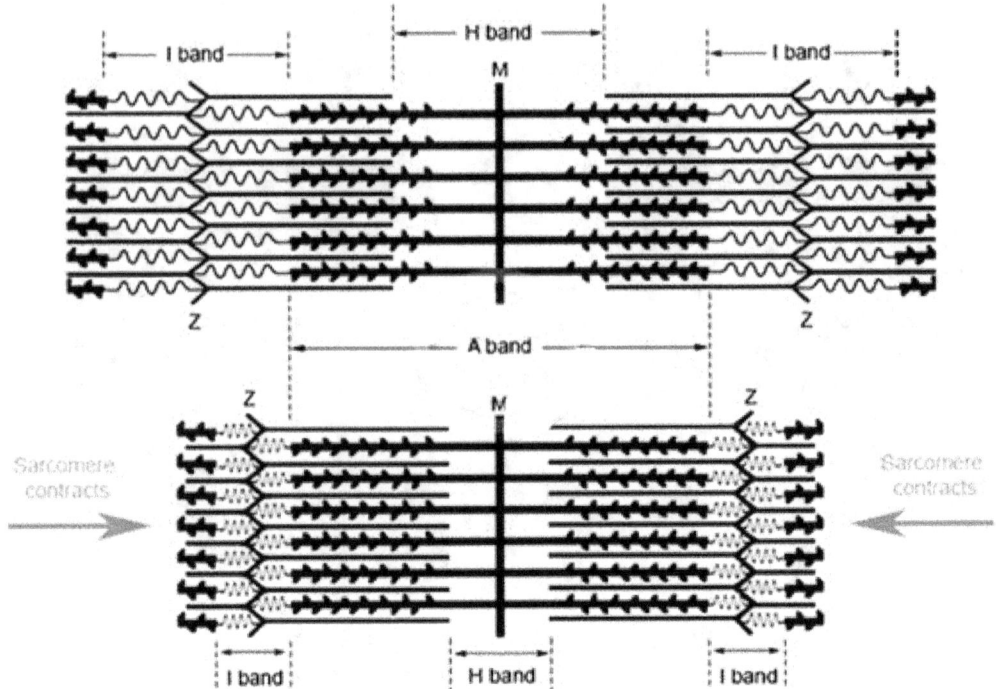

Sarcomere with associated banding regions

Each sarcomere has a band of thick filaments in the middle as the *A band*.

Sarcomeres are flanked on both sides by thin filaments.

Vertical borders between sarcomeres are *Z lines*, which anchor thin filaments.

I bands represent thin actin filaments, and *H bands* represent thick myosin filaments.

Titin protein fibers from the Z line are linked to the M line and thick filaments.

Due to the banded pattern provided by thin and thick filaments, *skeletal muscle* is *striated*.

Muscle fiber types and functions

Fibers within muscle tissue are organized into fast and slow fibers.

Fast fibers contain myosin with high ATPase activity and high shortening velocity.

Slow fibers contain myosin with low ATPase activity and low shortening velocity.

Fast fibers fatigue rapidly, while slow fibers fatigue gradually.

Oxidative fibers have many mitochondria and a high capacity for oxidative phosphorylation. ATP production is dependent on oxygen.

Oxidative fibers contain myoglobin, an oxygen-binding protein, which increases the rate of oxygen diffusion into fibers.

Myoglobin gives oxidative fibers a red color, like red muscle fibers.

Glycolytic fibers have few mitochondria but a high concentration of glycolytic enzymes and glycogen. Therefore, glycolysis, rather than oxidative phosphorylation, fuels the contractions.

These fibers are white muscle fibers due to their pale color.

Glycolytic fibers can develop more tension than oxidative fibers because they are larger and contain more thick and thin filaments. However, they get fatigued rapidly.

Myosin ATPase activity

Skeletal muscle fibers, determined by their myosin ATPase activity and energy source, are:

    1) slow oxidative,

    2) fast oxidative / glycolytic, and

    3) fast glycolytic.

Most muscles contain all three types of fiber.

Slow oxidative fibers are one of two skeletal muscle fibers with abundant mitochondria and myoglobin. They generate energy predominantly through aerobic conditions.

Slow muscle fibers have a lot of oxidative enzymes but are low in ATP activity. Slow oxidative fibers twitch at a slow rate and are resistant to fatigue, and the peak force exerted by these muscles is low.

Fast oxidative / glycolytic fibers can contract faster, producing a large peak force while resisting tiring even after several cycles.

These fibers have a large amount of ATP activity and are high in oxidative and glycolytic enzymes. They are used for anaerobic activities that must be sustained for a prolonged time.

Fast glycolytic fibers can exert a large force and contract fast. However, this comes at the expense of the fibers tiring quickly.

After a small amount of exertion, the muscle requires rest to recover. These fibers have low oxidative capacity, while ATP and glycolytic activity is high. These fibers are used during anaerobic activity for short durations of time.

Abundant mitochondria in red muscle cells as ATP source

Mitochondria are abundant in muscle cells because of the need for a quick energy source at any time. However, certain types of muscles have more mitochondria than others.

> *Type I muscle* (slow twitch or red muscle) contains more mitochondria than other types of muscle. Type I muscles are desirable for long-distance running, where muscles use mitochondria to produce ATP from oxygen *aerobically*.

> *Type IIB muscles* are common in weightlifters. These muscles require short bursts of energy and are less dependent on mitochondria. Type IIB muscles are mitochondria-poor and appear white. These muscles rely more on short bursts of glycolysis and, therefore, have greater glycogen stores. While they can generate greater force than type I muscles, type IIB muscles experience muscle fatigue much faster.

> *Type IIA muscles* are intermediate between types I and IIB. They have fewer mitochondria than type I but more than type IIB. Type IIA muscles fatigue less easily than type IIB but cannot replenish ATP as efficiently as type I. Type IIA muscles are often pink.

Muscle type properties

Red muscle (type I)	White muscle (type IIB)
High endurance but slow	*Fast, but fatigue easily*
• Predominantly aerobic respiration	• Anaerobic respiration (glycolysis)
• Many mitochondria because red muscles undergo aerobic respiration	• Few mitochondria because white muscles mainly undergo glycolysis
• Equipped to receive abundant oxygen supply: many capillaries and much myoglobin	• Equipped for short bursts of glycolysis: store high amounts of glycogen

Long-distance runners typically have a greater percentage of red fibers than white fibers.

Short-distance runners typically have a greater percentage of white than red fibers.

Many muscle cells rely on ATP to perform their function. Muscle cells contain myoglobin, which stores oxygen.

Cellular respiration does not immediately supply the ATP needed. Since ATP availability is essential, the body has adapted additional mechanisms other than glycolysis to generate it.

For example, when needing ATP, muscle fibers rely on *creatine phosphate* (phosphocreatine), a stored form of high-energy phosphate.

Creatine phosphate does not directly participate in muscle contraction; however, it contributes by regenerating ATP rapidly:

$$\text{Creatine-P} + \text{ADP} \rightarrow \text{ATP} + \text{Creatine}.$$

When all creatine phosphate is depleted, and O_2 is limited, fermentation produces a small amount of ATP to compensate. Over time, however, this results in a buildup of lactic acid, leading to muscle fatigue due to oxygen debt.

Lactic acid is transported to the liver, where 20% is broken down to CO_2 and H_2O via aerobic respiration. ATP gained from respiration is then used to convert 80% of the lactate to glucose.

For example, those who train for marathons increase the number of mitochondria, allowing aerobic respiration for longer periods. Rigor mortis, the stiffness seen in a recently deceased corpse, occurs because non-living organisms do not produce ATP.

Therefore, the mechanisms of muscle contraction cannot allow muscles to relax; muscles remain contracted until enzymatic breakdown of cross-linking of actin and myosin filaments occurs.

Increased amounts of contractile activity (exercise) increase muscle fibers' size (hypertrophy) and capacity for ATP production.

> *Low-intensity exercise* affects *oxidative fibers*, increasing the number of mitochondria and capillaries.
>
> *High-intensity exercise* affects *glycolytic fibers*, increasing their diameter by an increased synthesis of actin, myosin filaments, and glycolytic enzymes.

Muscle glycogen is the primary fuel in the *initial stages* of exercise.

After the initial stages, blood glucose and fatty acids are used. Muscle fiber generates ATP by one phosphorylation of ADP using *creatine phosphate*, which is the source of ATP during the initial phase of contraction. The slower pathways of second oxidative phosphorylation in mitochondria or glycolysis in the cytosol follow this.

At the end of muscle activity, *creatine phosphate* and glycogen levels are restored by energy-dependent processes, leading to a continued elevated level of oxygen consumption, called *oxygen debt*, even after exercise finishes.

Notes for active learning

Notes for active learning

CHAPTER 12

Skeletal System

Skeletal System Functions

Axial Skeleton Structures

Appendicular Skeleton Structures

Bone Characteristics

Cartilage and Joints

Bone Composition

Bone Growth and Remodeling

Endocrine Control of Skeletal System

Page intentionally left blank

Skeletal System Functions

Endoskeleton *vs.* exoskeleton

Humans possess an *internal endoskeleton that* contains both bone and cartilage. The endoskeleton does not limit the space for internal organs but supports greater weight. Soft tissues surround the endoskeleton to protect it because injuries to soft tissues are easier to repair. Usually, an endoskeleton has elements that protect vital internal organs.

Insects, crustaceans, and some other animals have external exoskeletons. Mollusks have exoskeletons that are predominantly calcium carbonate ($CaCO_3$). *Chitin*, present in insects and crustaceans, has jointed exoskeletons and a strong, flexible, nitrogenous polysaccharide. The exoskeleton protects against damage and keeps tissues from drying out.

Although stiffness supports muscles, the exoskeleton is less strong than an endoskeleton. The exoskeletons of clams and snails grow with the animals; their thick, non-mobile $CaCO_3$ shell is used for protection. The chitinous exoskeleton of arthropods is jointed and moveable.

Arthropods must molt when their exoskeleton becomes too small; a molting animal is vulnerable to predators. The jointed endoskeleton of vertebrates and exoskeleton of arthropods allows for flexibility. Exoskeletons made arthropods well-adapted for colonizing land because they protected against desiccation and allowed locomotion without water.

Structural rigidity and support

Bones provide a rigid framework for the body to move muscles anchored to them. For example, large leg bones support the body against gravity.

Leg and arm bones permit flexible body movement, pelvis bones support the trunk, and the atlas (i.e., 1st vertebra) support the skull.

Storage of calcium under hormonal influences

Bones store essential minerals needed to sustain life (e.g., calcium, phosphorus, and others).

Bones are critical in maintaining calcium homeostasis.

When blood calcium is low, parathyroid hormones (PTH) signal bone osteoclasts to break down the bone matrix and release calcium.

Most Ca^{2+} in the body is stored in the bone matrix as *hydroxyapatite*.

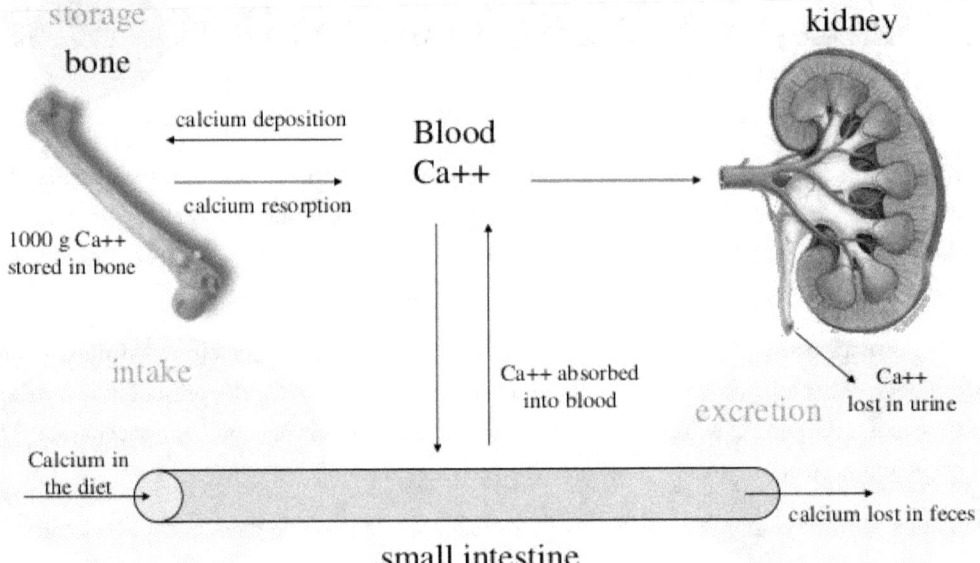

Calcium homeostasis with calcium stored in bone

Physical protection

One of the skeletal system's functions is to protect the internal organs.

The rib cage protects delicate internal organs, including the heart and the lungs.

The skull protects the brain, and the spine protects the spinal cord.

Many large bones shelter bone marrow, which contains stem cells needed to produce blood.

Skeletal tissues

Skeletal system has three main components:

      bone, cartilage, and joints.

Bone is a tough, rigid form of connective tissue that strengthens the human skeleton.

Cartilage is a form of connective tissue but is not rigid and tough compared to the bone.

Joints are where bones connect, allowing the skeletal system to be mobile.

Axial Skeleton Structures

Cranium bones

Human vertebrate skeletal system divides into the axial (midline) and appendicular skeletons.

Axial skeleton at the midline consists of the skull, vertebral column, sternum, and rib cage.

Cranium and the facial bones form the skull.

Newborns have membranous junctions as *fontanels* that usually close by age two.

Cranium bones contain *sinuses*, air spaces lined with mucous membranes that reduce the skull's weight. Sinuses give a resonant sound to the voice.

Two mastoid sinuses drain into the middle ear; *mastoiditis* is an inflammation of the sinuses that can lead to deafness.

Cranium has eight bones: one frontal, two parietal, one occipital, two temporal, one sphenoid, and one ethmoid bone.

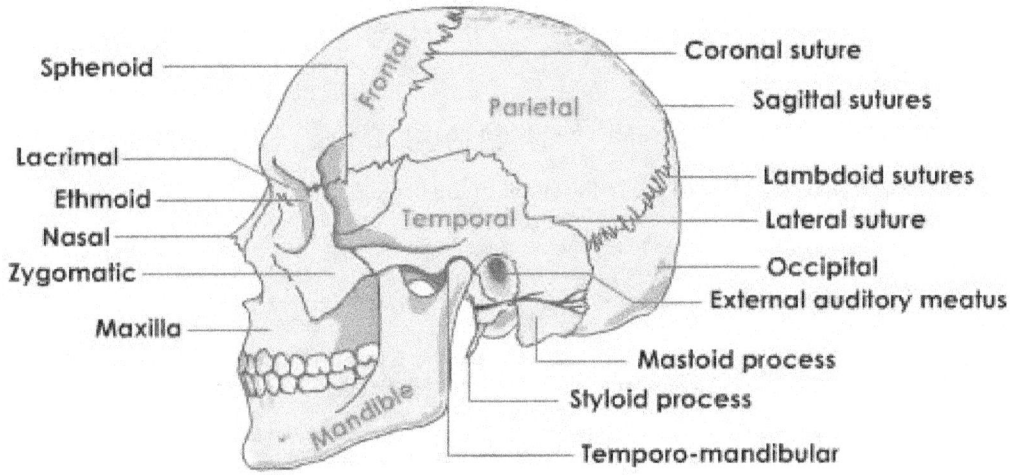

Human skull with bones and associated structure

Spinal cord passes through *foramen magnum*, an opening at the skull base in the *occipital bone*.

Temporal bones have an opening that leads to the middle ear.

Sphenoid bone completes the skull's sides and forms the floors and walls of the eye sockets.

Ethmoid bone, in front of the sphenoid, is part of the orbital wall and the nasal septum.

Facial bones

Fourteen facial bones include one mandible, two maxillae, two palatines, two zygomatic, two lacrimal, two nasal, and one vomer.

Mandible bone (lower jaw) is the movable portion of the skull; it contains tooth sockets.

Maxilla bone forms the upper jaw and the anterior of the hard palate; it contains tooth sockets.

Palatine bones comprise the posterior portion of the hard palate and the floor of the nasal cavity.

Zygomatic bone gives prominence to the cheekbones.

Nasal bones form the bridge of the nose. Other bones make up the nasal septum, which divides the nasal cavity into two regions.

Ears are elastic cartilage and lack bone, whereas the nose is a mixture of bone, cartilage, and fibrous connective tissue.

Vertebral column

Vertebral column supports the head and trunk and protects spinal cord and spinal nerve roots.

Vertebral column serves as an anchor for other skeletal bones.

Cervical vertebrae (7) in the neck.

Thoracic vertebrae (12) are in the thorax (or chest).

Lumbar vertebrae (5 or 6) are in the small of the back.

Sacrum is formed from five fused *sacral vertebrae*.

Coccyx is formed from four fused *coccygeal vertebrae*.

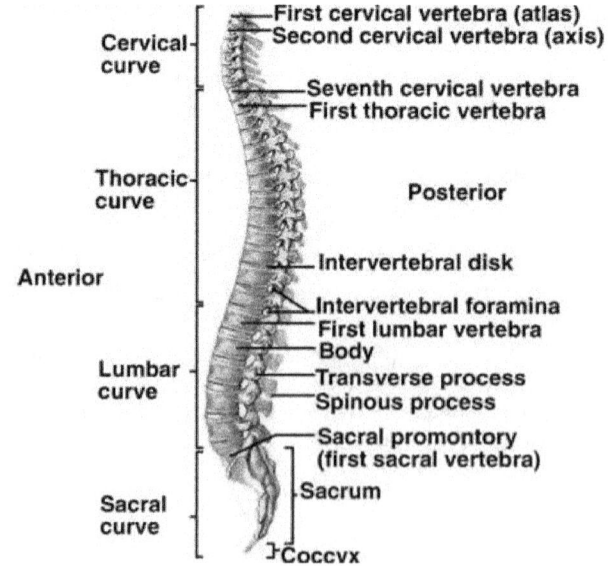

Spinal column has four normal curvatures that provide strength and resiliency in posture.

Scoliosis is a sideways curvature; *hunchback* and *swayback* are conditions of the spinal column.

Intervertebral discs between the vertebrae act as padding to prevent the vertebrae from grinding against each other and absorbing physical shock. Intervertebral discs weaken with age.

Vertebral discs allow movement between vertebrae, such as bending forward.

Rib cage protects the heart and lungs yet is flexible enough to allow breathing.

Twelve ribs connect to thoracic vertebrae in the back; seven pairs attach directly to the sternum.

Three pairs connect to the sternum indirectly via cartilage at the front of the sternum. '

There are two pairs of ribs (floating ribs) unattached to the sternum and attached to vertebrae.

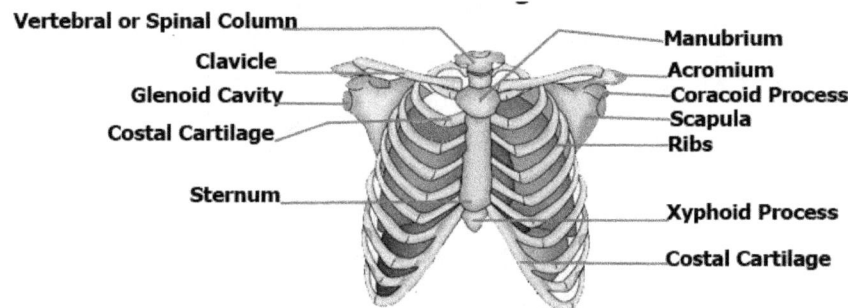

Rib cage with twelve pairs of ribs

Appendicular Skeleton Structures

Pectoral and pelvic girdles

Appendicular skeleton consists of the bones within the pectoral girdle, pelvic girdle, and upper and lower limbs.

Pectoral girdle is specialized for flexibility and built for strength. Ligaments loosely link the components of the pectoral girdle.

Clavicle (i.e., collarbone) connects with the *sternum* in the front and the *scapula* in the back. The scapula is held in place by muscles and can move freely.

Pelvic girdle consists of two heavy, large coxal (hip) bones.

Coxal bones are anchored to *sacrum*; together with the sacrum, they form a hollow cavity wider in females than males to transmit weight from the vertebral column via the sacrum to the legs.

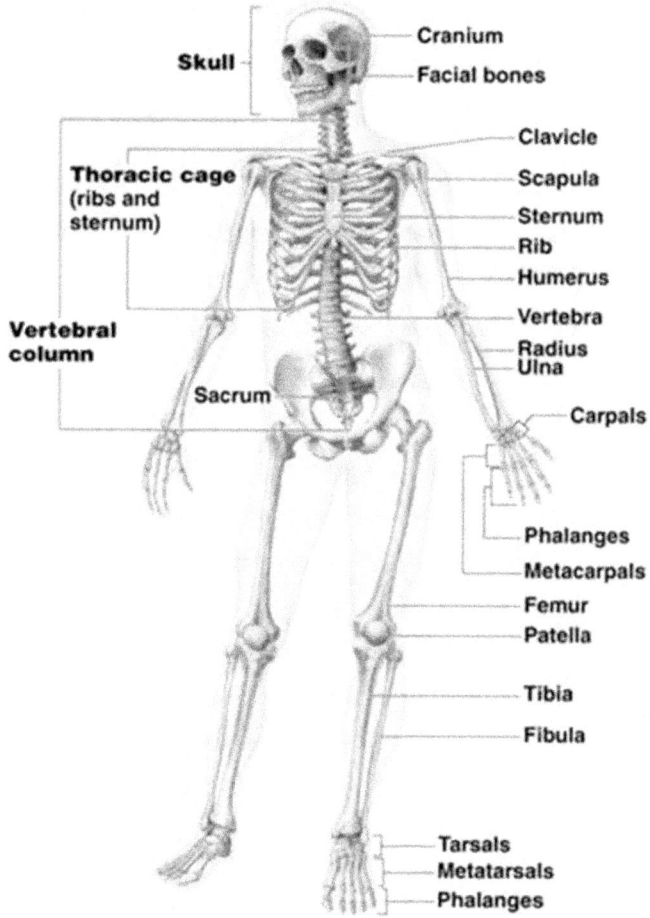

Human adult skeletal system (anterior view)

Upper limbs

Humerus is the long bone of the upper arm; its rounded head fits into a socket of the scapula.

Radius is lateral of bone in the lower arm (i.e., the forearm); it articulates with the humerus at the elbow joint (a hinge joint), and the radius crosses in front of the ulna for easy twisting.

Ulna (i.e., elbow bone) is the medial of the two bones in the lower arm. The larger end of the ulna joins with the humerus to make the elbow joint.

Hand flexibility is attributable to the presence of many bones.

Wrist has eight *carpal bones* that look like small pebbles.

Metacarpal bones (5) fan out to form the framework of the palm.

Phalanges are the bones of the fingers and thumb.

Lower limbs

Femur is the largest, longest, and strongest body bone; however, it is limited to support weight.

Patella is the kneecap and is a thick, roughly triangular bone that allows for knee extension.

Tibia has a ridge called the "shin;" its end forms the inside of the ankle. The shin bone is strong.

Fibula is the smaller of the two bones; its end forms the outside of the ankle.

Tarsal bones are in the ankle. For example, when standing or walking, tarsal bones receive the weight and pass it to the heel and ball of the foot.

Metatarsal bones form the foot's arch and provide a springy base.

Phalanges are the bones of the toes, which are stouter than those of the fingers.

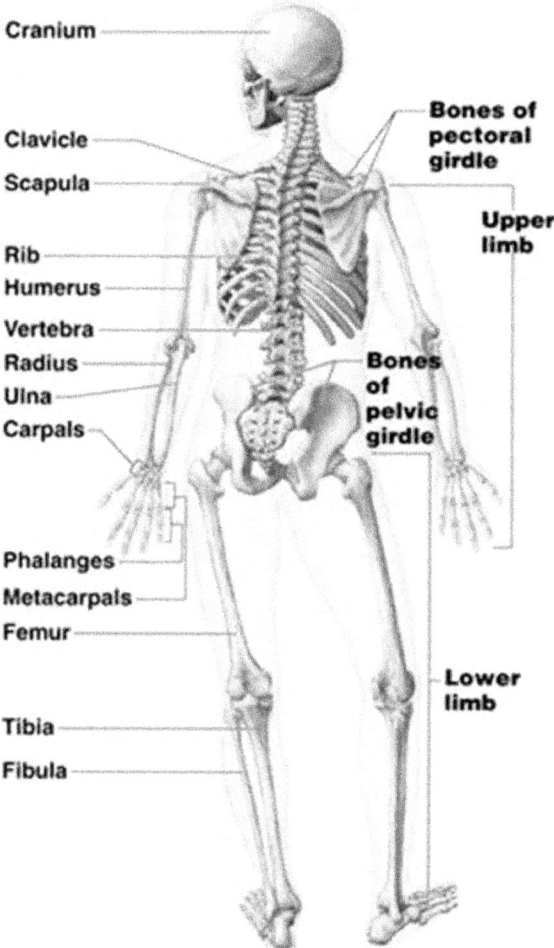

Human adult skeletal system (posterior view)

Notes for active learning

Bone Characteristics

Bone shapes

Bones are classified by their shape.

Long bones consist of a *diaphysis* (shaft) with two ends shaped like rods.

Examples include the thigh (*femur*), upper arm (*humerus*), and finger bones (*phalanges*).

Short bones are cube-like. The outer surface is a thin layer of compact bone and internally contains spongy bone. Short bones are in the hands and feet, with predominantly spongy bones. Short bones contain a tubular shaft and articular surfaces at the ends but are smaller than long bones. Articulations they join allow for increased flexibility and decreased mass. Bones provide stability and strength. Examples include wrists (i.e., carpals) and feet (i.e., tarsals) bones.

Flat bones are thin and usually curved, with an outer layer of a periosteum-covered compact bone surrounding an inner core of endosteum-covered spongy bone. Spongy bone is sandwiched between two layers of thin, compact bone.

Spongy bone within the epiphyses of flat and long bones contains hematopoietic tissue (i.e., red marrow). Their structure provides a flat and broad surface area for tendon attachment.

Strong bone structures offer protection to internal organs [e.g., most skull bones, breastbone (sternum), shoulder blades (scapulae), and ribs].

Irregular bones are not long, short, or flat. Their complicated shape is due to their specialized function of providing mechanical support for the body and protecting the spinal cord. Their structure consists of a thin layer of compact bone with an internal component of spongy bone (e.g., the vertebrae, hips, and auditory ossicles).

Sesamoid bones develop within a tendon; they hold the tendon away from the joint, causing the angle of the tendon to increase and the force of muscles to increase (e.g., patella and pisiform).

Wormian bones (sutural bones) are small bones that lie within the major skull bones.

Irregular isolated bones appear in addition to the usual centers of ossification of the cranium. They are predominantly in the lambdoid suture (posterior aspect of the skull), which is more tortuous than other sutures.

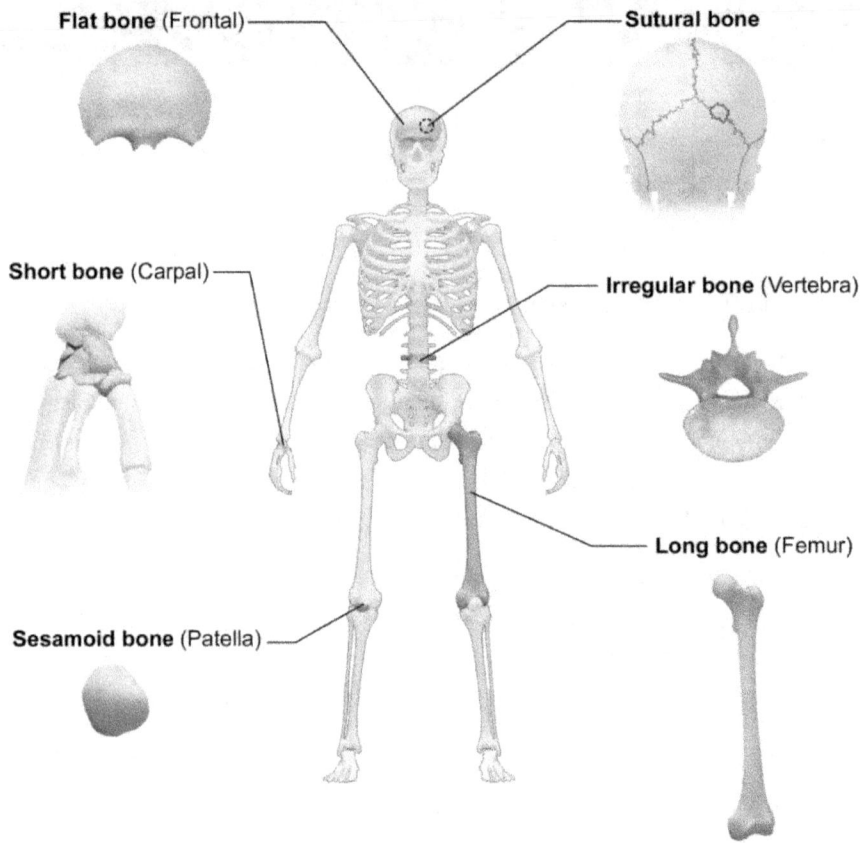

Bone classification by shape

Bone structure and function

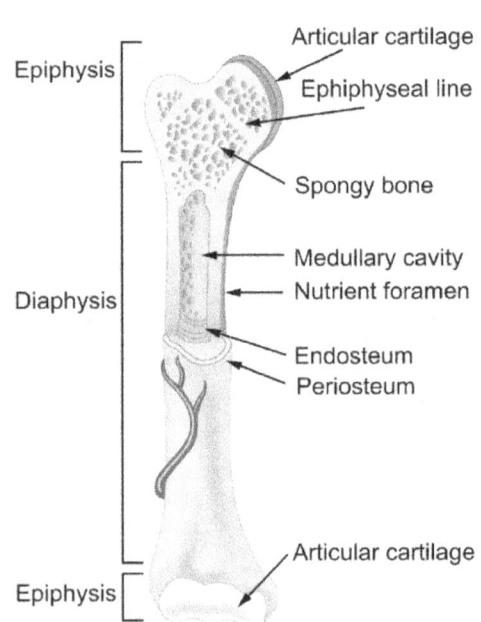

Diaphysis of the bone have a central medullary cavity filled with *fatty tissue* (i.e., yellow bone marrow) surrounded by a thick collar of compact bone. Yellow marrow in the shaft of long bones has fat molecules and is vital for energy reservoirs.

Epiphysis (i.e., the expanded end of the bone) consists mainly of spongy bone surrounded by a thin layer of compact bone.

Long bone with central diaphysis and terminal epiphysis

*Spongy bone*s have numerous plates separated by irregular spaces. It is lighter but designed for strength. Solid bones follow the lines of stress.

Bone spaces are often filled with *hematopoietic tissue* (i.e., red bone marrow), a specialized tissue that produces blood cells.

Epiphysis contains *articular cartilage*, which is a pad of hyaline cartilage. This is where long bones articulate (i.e., a joint) and function as a "*shock absorber*."

Epiphyseal line, or the remnant *epiphyseal disc* or *plate*, is cartilage at the diaphysis junction, and the epiphysis is the growth plate.

Periosteum (i.e., outer fibrous) protective diaphysis cover is richly supplied with blood vessels, lymph vessels, and nerves, which allows for the insertion of tendons and ligaments into bones.

Nutrient foramen is a perforating canal that allows blood vessels to travel in and out of the bone.

Osteons are the functional unit of *compact bones*. The bone cells are in small chambers of lacunae arranged in concentric circles around central canals.

Lacunae are separated by a matrix with protein fibers of collagen and mineral deposits.

Osteogenic layer contains *osteoblasts* (i.e., bone-forming cells) and *osteoclasts* (i.e., bone-destroying cells).

Endosteum layer is the inner lining of the medullary cavity and contains a layer of osteoblasts and osteoclasts.

Notes for active learning

Cartilage and Joints

Cartilage structure and function

Cartilage is an *avascular connective tissue* with a dense matrix of collagen and elastic fibers embedded in a rubbery ground substance.

Matrix is produced by *chondroblast* cells embedded in the matrix as *chondrocytes* (i.e., mature cartilage cells), individually or in groups within spaces of *lacunae* (sing. *lacuna*) in the matrix.

Three types of cartilage:

> hyaline cartilage, fibrocartilage, and elastic cartilage.

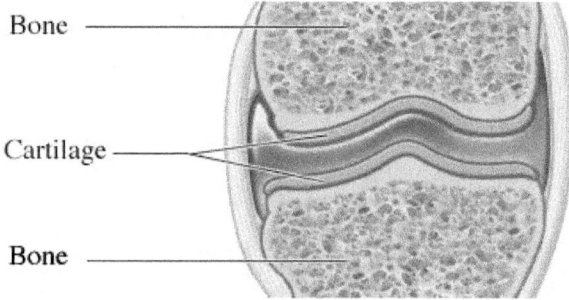

Cross section of a joint with cartilage cushioning the apposition of two bones

Cartilage cells secrete into the extracellular matrix, containing fiber meshwork that gives the cartilage its characteristic flexibility and resilience properties.

The surface of most cartilage in the body is surrounded by a membrane of dense, irregular connective tissue as *perichondrium*.

Unlike other connective tissues, cartilage contains no blood vessels or nerves.

Cartilage is softer and more flexible than *bone*. For example, the ear, nose, larynx, trachea, and joints are made of cartilage. Cartlidge possesses *compressibility* and *resilience* (i.e., the ability to resume its original shape after deformation), vital at the ends of bones in joints, knees, and between the vertebrae.

Hyaline cartilage is the most abundant of the three types. Hyaline cartilage consists of a bluish-white, shiny, ground elastic material with a chondroitin sulfate matrix into which fine collagen fibrils are embedded.

Mesenchyme tissue initiates the formation of chondrocytes, which produce collagen.

Collagen is present in tissue as a triple helix with hydroxyproline and hydroxylysine, ground substance, and elastin fibers.

Hyaline cartilage covers the surface of bones at joints (especially in osteoarthritis-prone areas vulnerable to damage due to wear), including the ends of long bones and the anterior ends of ribs. It facilitates smooth movements at joints, provides flexibility and support, reduces friction, and absorbs shock in joints.

Embryonic skeleton hyaline cartilage provides smooth surfaces, enabling tissues to move and slide easily over each other.

For example, hyaline cartilage is in the bronchi, bronchial tubes, costal cartilage, the larynx (i.e., *voice box*), the nose, and the trachea.

Fibrocartilage

Fibrocartilage (meniscus) is a tough form of cartilage that consists of chondrocytes scattered among clearly visible dense bundles of collagen fibers within the matrix.

Fibrocartilage lacks perichondrium. It provides support and rigidity to attached and surrounding structures and is the strongest of the three cartilage types.

A fibrocartilage is *calli*, the tissue formed between the end of bones at the healing fracture site.

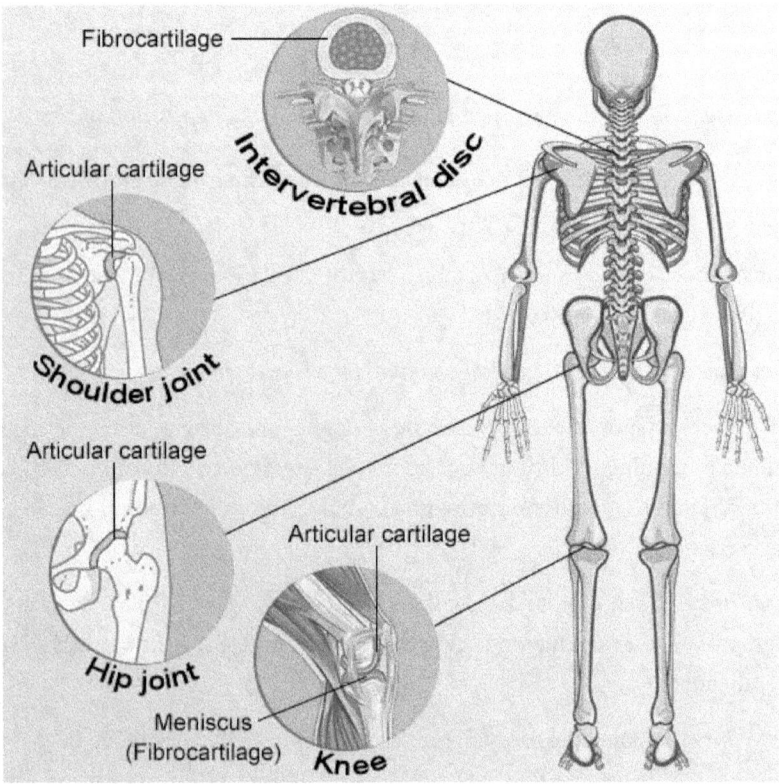

Fibrocartilage and articular cartilage

When blood clots, granulation tissue forms into cartilage and full-fledged bone.

Other examples include intervertebral discs (between the vertebrae of the spine), the menisci (cartilage pads of the knee joint), the pubic symphysis (hip bones join at the front of the body), and the portions of the tendons that insert into cartilage tissue, especially at the joints.

Knee bones are a capped crescent-shaped piece of *meniscus cartilage*.

Knee joints contain 13 fluid-filled sacs as *bursae*, easing friction between tendons, ligaments, and bones. Inflammation of the bursae (*bursitis*) is the cause of "*tennis elbow.*"

Elastic cartilage is yellowish, with cartilage cells (i.e., chondrocytes) in a threadlike network of elastic fibers within the cartilage matrix. A perichondrium is present.

Elastic cartilage supports surrounding structures and defines and maintains the shape of the area in which it is present (e.g., external ear). Other examples include the auditory (i.e., Eustachian) tubes, external ear (i.e., the auricle), and epiglottis (i.e., flap on the larynx).

Joint structure and function

*Joint*s are where bones meet. Joints connected to bones are synovial, fibrous, or cartilaginous.

Synovial joints (mobile joints) have a fluid-containing cavity that lubricates bone movement. They are usually involved with bones that move relative to each other.

Most joints are synovial, with two bones separated by a cavity (e.g., the carpals, wrist, elbow, humerus and ulna, shoulder, hip joints, and knee joints).

Synovial joints are subject to arthritis. In *osteoarthritis*, the cartilage at the ends of bones disintegrates, and the bones become rough and irregular from mechanical "wear and tear."

Rheumatoid arthritis is when the synovial membrane becomes inflamed and thickens. The joint degenerates and becomes immovable and painful. An autoimmune reaction likely causes this.

Synovial joint types include:

    ball and socket (e.g., shoulder and hip),

    hinge (e.g., fingers, elbow),

    gliding (e.g., scaphoid and lunate bones of the wrist), and

    immobile (e.g., plates of the skull and rib-to-sternum connection).

Ball and socket joints allow the most freedom of motion.

Fibrous joints (immovable) connect bone to bone with cartilage (or fiber). An example of an immovable joint is a suture, usually holding the bones of the skull; it includes the skull, pelvis, spinous process, and vertebrae.

Cartilaginous joints (i.e., slightly moveable) include joints between the vertebrae, spine, and ribs. For example, hipbones are slightly movable because they are ventrally joined by cartilage and respond to pregnancy hormones.

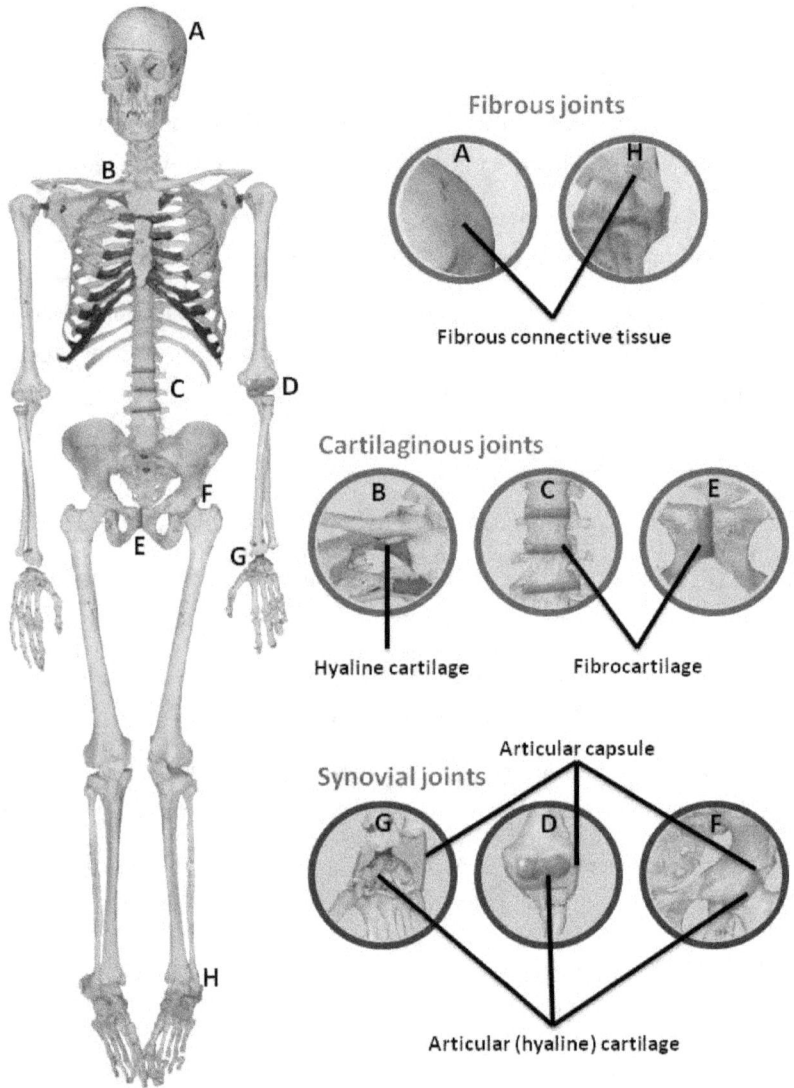

Three types of joints are synovial, fibrous, and cartilaginous, with cartilage and connective tissue examples. Note the reference to examples and locations in the body.

Hierarchical structure of ligaments and tendons

Ligaments and tendons are *soft collagenous tissues*.

Ligaments connect bone to bone, while *tendons* connect muscle to bone. Ligaments and tendons play a significant role in musculoskeletal biomechanics, and they represent an essential area of orthopedic treatment in which medical challenges remain.

A challenge is restoring the normal mechanical function of these tissues.

Ligaments and tendons have a hierarchical structure that affects their mechanical behavior. Ligaments and tendons adapt to mechanical changes due to injury, disease, or exercise.

Unlike bone, no quantitative structure-function relationships exist for ligaments and tendons.

1) Hierarchical structure of ligaments and tendons is more challenging to quantify than bone.

2) Ligaments and tendons exhibit nonlinear and viscoelastic behavior even under physiological loading, which is more difficult to analyze than bone's linear behavior.

Ligaments (or tendons) are the largest soft collagenous tissues that split into smaller *fascicles*.

Fascicle contains the basic *fibril* of the ligament (or tendon) and the *fibroblasts*, the biological cells of the ligament (or tendon). Structural characteristics are significant in the mechanics of ligaments (and tendons): the *crimp* of the fibril.

Crimp is the waviness of the fibril; this contributes significantly to the nonlinear stress-strain relationship for ligaments, tendons, and essentially all soft collagenous tissues.

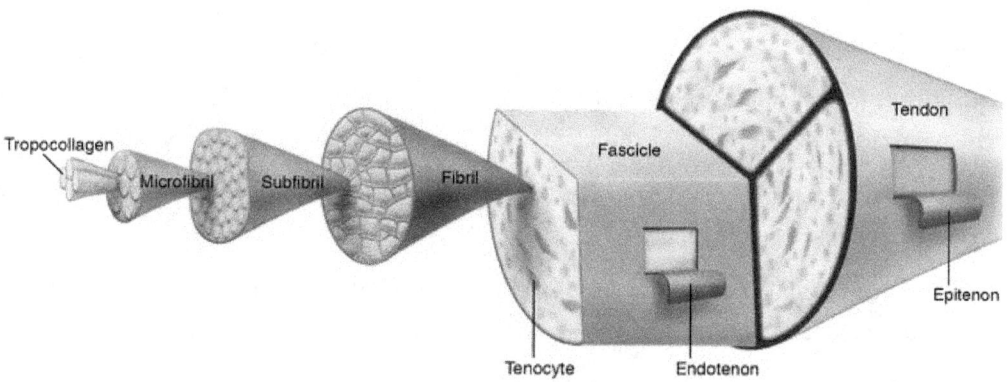

Ligaments and tendons have a hierarchical structure

Anatomy and functions of ligaments and tendons

Ligaments connect bones, forming a *joint capsule*, which stabilizes and strengthens the joints.

Joint capsules are lined with a synovial membrane that produces lubricating synovial fluid.

Ligaments are made of dense bundles of *connective tissue* made of collagenous fibers, surrounded and protected by *dense irregular connective sheaths*.

Blood is supplied to ligaments through microvascularity from insertion sites to supply the nutrition needed for growth, matrix synthesis, and repair.

Capsular ligaments are a part of the articular capsule that surrounds synovial joints. They act as mechanical reinforcements.

Extra-capsular ligaments join with other ligaments and provide joint stability.

Intra-capsular ligaments are uncommon and promote stability with a larger range of motion.

Cruciate ligaments occur in pairs of three.

Collagen fibrils in ligaments have slightly less volume and organization than tendons.

Ligaments have a higher percentage of *proteoglycan matrix* than *tendons*.

Fibroblasts are present in ligaments.

In "*double-jointed*" individuals, the ligaments are unusually loose, allowing them to stretch their ligaments more than average.

Tendon is a tough band of fibrous connective tissue that can withstand tension.

Tendons connect muscle to the bone at movable joints and anchor the muscle.

Tendons have *collagen fibrils* (Type I), a *proteoglycan matrix,* and parallel *fibroblasts*.

Type I collagen constitutes about 86% of dry tendon weight; glycine (~33%), proline (~15%), and hydroxyproline (~15%, to identify collagen because it is almost unique to it).

Tendons carry *tensile forces* from muscle to bone and *compressive forces* when wrapped around bone like a pulley.

Tendons procure blood through the vessels in the *perimysium*, a sheath of connective tissue that covers the tendon, through the periosteum, the membrane covering the bone's outer surface.

Origin is the point of attachment of the muscle to a stationary bone, and *insertion* is the point of attachment of the muscle to a bone that moves.

Mechanical properties of ligaments and tendons

Viscoelasticity is vital to ligaments and tendons with time-dependent mechanical behavior.

Stress and strain relationships are not constant but depends on displacement (or load).

Viscoelasticity has two significant types of characteristic behavior.

1) Creep is increasing deformation under constant load. This contrasts with elastic materials that do not exhibit increased deformation no matter how long the load is applied.

2) *Relaxation stress* is the second significant behavior, as the stress is reduced or relaxed under constant deformation.

Ligaments are viscoelastic as they gradually strain under tension and return to their original shape when the tension is released.

However, a joint cannot retain its original shape when extended past a certain point or extended for a prolonged period.

A joint becomes *dislocated* when this occurs, often due to trauma. Once a joint has become dislocated, it must be manually moved back to its original position as soon as possible. If the ligaments are lengthened for a prolonged period, the joint is weakened, making it susceptible to future dislocations.

Hysteresis (i.e., energy dissipation) is a characteristic of the viscoelastic material.

If a viscoelastic material is loaded and unloaded, the unloading curve differs from the loading curve. The difference between the curves represents the amount of energy dissipated (or lost) during loading.

Stress *vs.* strain for tendons and ligaments

Stress-strain curve has three regions:

1) toe region, 2) linear region, and 3) yield and failure region.

Most ligaments and tendons are in the toe and in a linear region during physiological activity. These constitute a *nonlinear stress-strain curve* since the slope of the toe region is different from the linear region.

Toe region represents "*un-crimping*" in the collagen fibrils for structure-function relationships. Since stretching out the collagen fibrils' crimp is easier, this part of the stress-strain curve shows a low stiffness.

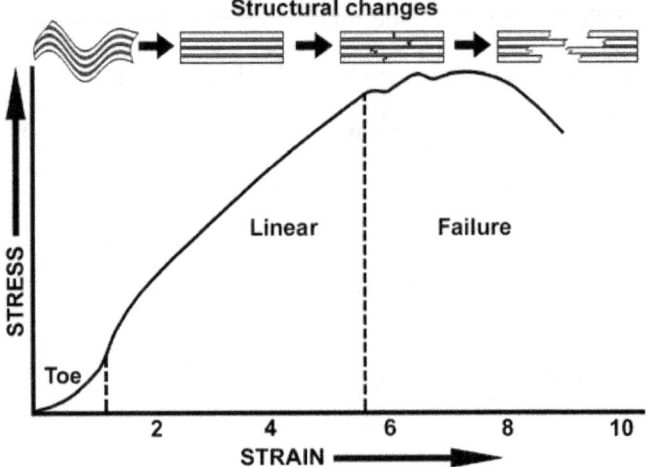

Nonlinear stress-strain curve with toe, linear, and failure regions noted

As the collagen fibrils become uncrimped, the collagen fibril backbone becomes stretched, giving rise to a stiffer material. As individual fibrils within the ligament or tendon begin to fail, damage accumulates, stiffness is reduced, and the ligaments and tendons begin to fail.

Thus, ligaments and tendons' overall behavior depends on the individual *crimp* structure and the *failure of collagen fibrils*.

Bone Composition

Chemical composition of bone

Bone's chemical composition is organic components (~25% by weight), inorganic components (~70% by weight), and water (~5% by weight). Bone is connective tissue and characteristically hard, strong, elastic, and lightweight.

Bones are made from a combination of compact and spongy bones.

Macroscopically, bone is a solid structure with internal canals where blood vessels run and holes where cells can reside. The structure is surrounded by membranes containing stem cells, including osteoblast (bone-building) and osteoclast (bone-degrading) cells.

Microscopically, bone is composed of cells, with the extracellular matrix arranged in cylinders as *osteons*, which contain blood vessels and nerves running through the middle.

Four types of bone matrix cells

Four types of cells make up the bone matrix.

Osteoprogenitor cells are derived from *mesenchyme* and may undergo mitosis and differentiate into *osteoblasts*.

Osteoblasts are *stem cells* that form the bone matrix by secreting collagen and organic compounds from which bone is formed. They *cannot* undergo mitosis.

As the collagenous matrix is released around them, they are enveloped by the matrix and differentiate into osteocytes. Osteoblasts secrete a matrix material of osteoid.

Osteoids are primarily made of collagen, which gives bone its high tensile strength. They contain *glycolipids* and *glycoproteins*.

Osteocytes are mature bone cells derived from *osteoblasts*. They are principal bone cells that *cannot* undergo mitosis. They maintain daily cellular activities to exchange nutrients and waste with blood.

Osteoclasts are multinucleated cells functioning in bone resorption, including the destruction of the bone matrix, and are essential in developing, growing, maintaining, and repairing bone. They develop from *monocytes*.

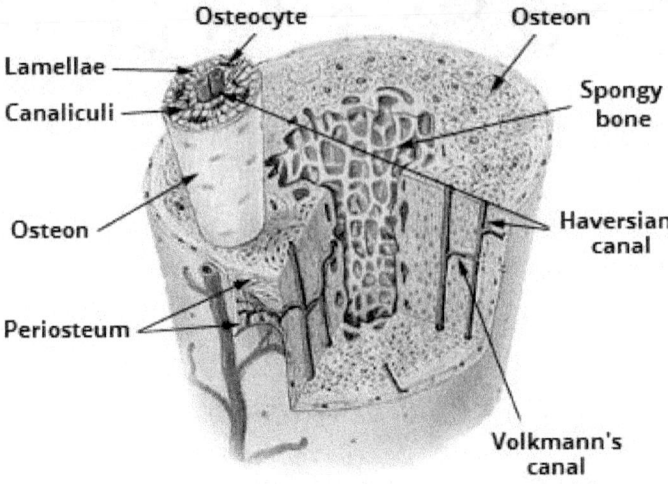

Bone cross-section with structure highlighted.

Compact and spongy bones

Compact bone is a highly organized, solid, smooth, dense bone with no external cavities. In compact bone, osteoclasts burrow tunnels, such as *Haversian canals*.

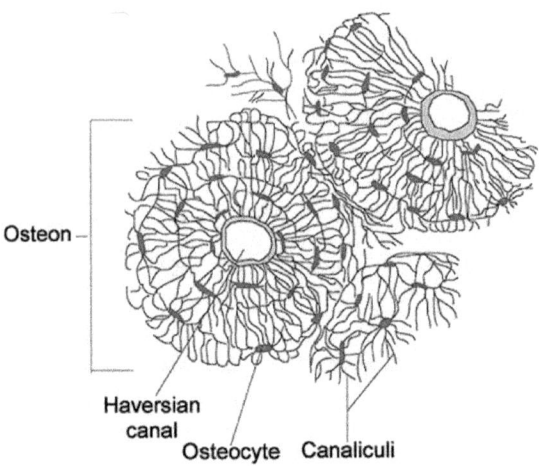

Compact bone from a transverse section of a long bone's cortex

Haversian system has osteocytes, the star-shaped bone cells in the *lacunae*.

Osteoblasts secrete the collagen and calcium salts matrix in concentric *lamellae* (i.e., layers) around the central Haversian canal, containing blood vessels and nerves. The elongated cylinders are bonded to form the long axis of a bone.

Canaliculi are a communication canal within the bone that connects the lacunae of the osteons.

Volkmann's canals, small channels that run perpendicular to the bone's surface, connect adjacent Haversian canals' blood and nerve supplies.

Spongy bone (i.e., cancellous) is less dense and consists of poorly organized *trabeculae*, small, needle-like pieces of bone with much open space between them. Spongy bone is nourished by diffusion from nearby Haversian canals.

Spongy bone supports soft tissue, protects internal organs, and assists in body movement, mineral storage, blood cell production, and energy storage as adipose (fat) cells in the marrow.

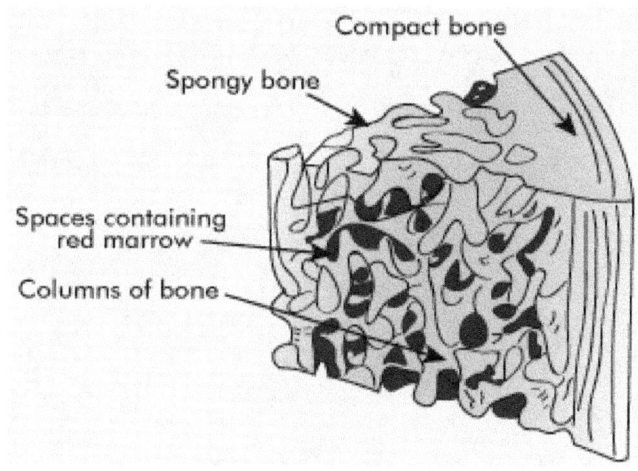

Bone with spongy bone in the medulla and compact bone along the cortex

Calcium–protein matrix of bones

Calcium is the most abundant mineral in bone and in the body. Calcium is an element that cannot be produced by any biological processes and must enter the body through diet.

Bones are storage sites for calcium. The extracellular matrix of bone consists of calcium salts, primarily calcium phosphate [$Ca_3(PO_4)_2(OH)_2$], which gives bone its hardness (or rigidity), collagen fibers, and ground substance (glue).

Calcium ions are vital for physiology and needed for bone mineralization, tooth health, regulation of the heart rate, blood coagulation, contractions of smooth and skeletal muscle cells, and regulation of nerve impulse conduction.

The calcium level in the blood is highly regulated at about 9-10 mg/dL. When the body cannot maintain this level, a person experiences hypocalcemia (or hypercalcemia), as described below.

Bones have a *mineral content* of roughly 50% by volume. The mineral content of the matrix consists primarily of *calcium phosphate* and *hydroxyapatite*, with minimal amounts of magnesium, carbonate, and acid phosphate.

Hydroxyapatite bone crystals are tiny and are soluble and vital in *mineral metabolism*.

The organic matrix of bone is composed of about 90% collagen protein. Collagen is formed through chains that resemble short threads twisted into triple helices (resembling strings). They line up and bind, forming fibrils arranged in layers and mineral crystals deposited between the layers.

Matrix maturation expresses *alkaline phosphatase* and *noncollagenous proteins* (i.e., *osteocalcin, osteopontin,* and *sialoprotein*).

Calcium and phosphate-binding proteins aid in the ordered deposition of minerals by regulating the amount and size of the hydroxyapatite crystals formed.

Matrix's *mineral* portion provides for the bone's *mechanical rigidity and strength*.

Matrix's *organic* portion contributes to the *bone's flexibility and elasticity*.

Bone Growth and Remodeling

Bone ossification, formation and growth

Human fetal skeleton is cartilaginous and serves as a bone construction scaffold.

Fetal skeleton is formed from mesenchyme and hyaline cartilage loosely shaped like bones. This "skeleton" provides supporting structures for ossification (hardening into bone).

At about 6-7 weeks' gestation, ossification begins and continues throughout adulthood. Cartilaginous structures are converted to bones when calcium salts are deposited in the matrix, first by *cartilaginous cells* and later by *bone-forming osteoblast cells*.

The main components of ossification are *cartilage cells* (i.e., chondrocytes), precursor cells (i.e., osteoprogenitor cells), bone deposition cells (i.e., osteoblasts), bone resorption cells (i.e., osteoclasts), and mature bone cells (i.e., osteocytes).

During ossification, blood vessels invade cartilage and transport osteoprogenitor cells to the center of ossification. Cartilage cells die at the center of ossification, forming *small cavities*.

Osteoblast cells form *progenitor cells,* depositing bone tissue outward from the center. Spongy textured calcaneus bone and smooth outer compact bone form from this process.

Endochondral ossification is the conversion of cartilaginous scaffolds to bones. Bones, such as facial bones, form without a cartilaginous scaffold and are *intramembranous ossification*.

Replacement of preexisting connective tissue with bone occurs through *intramembranous* and *endochondral ossification.*

Endochondral ossification occurs when a bone is formed from hyaline cartilage. Most bones in the skeleton are formed in this manner.

Primary ossification center is in the middle of a long bone; secondary centers later form at ends.

Primary ossification centers harden in a fetus and during infancy.

Secondary ossification centers develop in children and harden during adolescence and early adulthood. Cartilaginous growth plates form between primary and secondary ossification centers. As the growth plate remains between the two centers, bone growth continues.

Perichondrium becomes the *periosteum*, containing layers of undifferentiated cells, including *osteoprogenitor cells* that later develop into *osteoblasts*.

Appositional growth is when *osteoblasts secrete osteoid* against the cartilage scaffold shaft to support the new bone.

Hypertrophy occurs when chondrocytes in the primary ossification center begin to grow. They stop secreting collagen and proteoglycans and begin secreting alkaline phosphatase and other enzymes essential for mineral deposition.

After calcifying the matrix, hypertrophic chondrocytes die to form cavities within the bone.

Hypertrophic chondrocytes start to secrete *vascular endothelial cell growth factors* that induce the sprouting of blood vessels from the perichondrium.

Blood vessels in the periosteal bud invade the cavity left by the chondrocytes and branches in opposite directions along the shaft length. Blood vessels carry *hematopoietic, osteoprogenitor*, and other cells within the cavity. Hematopoietic cells eventually form *bone marrow*.

Osteoblasts, differentiated from the *osteoprogenitor cells* that enter the cavity via the *periosteal bud,* use the calcified matrix as a scaffold and secrete osteoid, forming bone *trabecula*. Osteoclasts formed from macrophages break down spongy bone to form the *medullary* (or bone marrow) cavity.

Hematopoiesis is blood cell formation. Blood cells are formed in the red marrow of certain bones. Flat bones of the skull, ribs, and breastbone (i.e., sternum) contain red bone marrow that manufactures blood cells.

During *intramembranous ossification,* bone forms on (or within) a fibrous connective tissue membrane, eventually forming the periosteum, made of fibers and granular cells in a matrix. The peripheral portion is predominantly fibrous, whereas the internal environment is predominantly osteoblasts. The tissue is heavily supplied with blood vessels.

As ontogenetic fibers move out of the periphery, they *calcify* and form fresh *bone spicules*.

A network of bones is formed from meshes containing blood vessels, and the delicate connective tissue is populated with osteoblasts.

Bony trabeculae are thickened by additional fresh layers of bone formed by the osteoblasts on its surface, and the meshes are simultaneously encroached upon.

Layers of bony tissue are continuously added under the periosteum and around large vascular channels that eventually become the *Haversian canals*, which thicken the bone.

During infancy and childhood, *longitudinal growth* occurs, where long bones lengthen entirely by growth at the *epiphyseal plates*.

Bones grow in *thickness by appositional growth*.

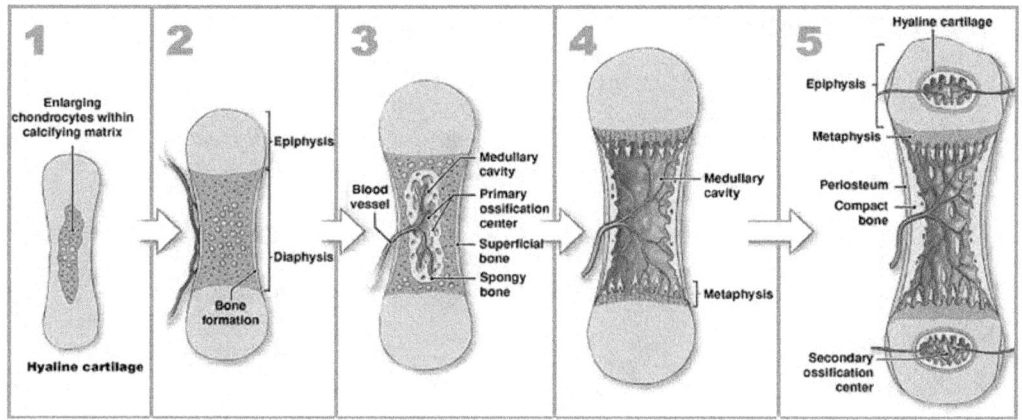

1) Enlargement of chondrocytes, 2) formation of a superficial layer of bone, 3) production of spongy bone at primary ossification center, 4) growth in length and diameter, 5) formation of secondary ossification centers

Epiphyseal plates contain four zones:

Zone of resting cartilage anchors the plate to the epiphysis.

Zone of proliferating cartilage is where chondrocytes divide to replace those that die at the diaphyseal surface of the epiphysis.

Zone of hypertrophic cartilage is the site of maturing cells.

Zone of calcified cartilage has dead cells in a calcified matrix.

Epiphyseal plates are replaced by bone in adulthood.

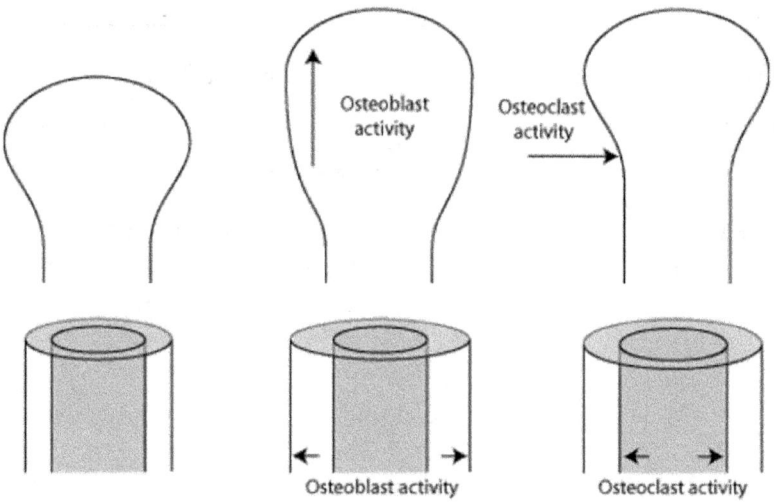

Bone growth and remodeling: longitudinal growth (top) and appositional growth (bottom)

Dynamic bone remodeling by osteoblasts and osteoclasts

Ossification of most bones is completed by age 25.

As a child grows, cartilage cells are produced by *mitosis* on the *epiphyseal side of the plate*. Epiphyseal plate's cartilage is destroyed and replaced by bone on diaphyseal side of the plate.

Thickness of the plate remains mostly constant while diaphyseal side bone increases in length.

Lengthwise, bone growth occurs at the *ends of long bones*, where *osteoblasts* add bone tissue at the bone ends.

Osteoblasts lengthen the knobs at bone ends, while *osteoclasts* remodel bone tissue by degrading (i.e., dissolving) the bone ends (i.e., knobs) until they are the right size and shape.

Along with the increase in *length*, bones increase in thickness (or diameter).

Appositional growth occurs in an osteogenic layer of the periosteum; *osteoblasts* lay down a matrix (i.e., compact bone) on the outer surface. This is accompanied by *osteoclasts* destroying the bone matrix at the *endosteal surface*.

> *Osteoblasts* add bone tissue to the outside of the bone for diameter growth.

> *Osteoclasts* remove bone tissue from the inside of hollow bones for diameter growth.

Without osteoclasts, diameter growth results in bones being too thick and too heavy. Even with osteoclasts, bones become thicker with age.

Age-related skeletal changes are apparent at the cellular and whole-body levels. For example, stature decreases incrementally at age 33, and bone loss gradually exceeds bone replacement.

Additionally, after menopause, females lose bone more rapidly than males.

By age 70, bone loss is similar in between the sexes and the likelihood of fractures increases as bones age.

Adults need more calcium than children to promote osteoblasts' work.

Remodeling rate varies. For example, the distal femur is replaced every four months, while the shift of the femur is not replaced during one's lifetime.

Endocrine Control of Skeletal System

Osteoblasts and osteoclasts

Hormones, including growth hormones and sex hormones, control the rate of bone growth. Eventually, the epiphysis plates become ossified, the bone stops growing, and a person reaches adult height.

In adults, bones are continually being remodeled (broken down and built up again). This involves osteoblasts, osteoclasts, calcitonin, and parathyroid hormone (PTH) hormones through the negative feedback mechanism, affecting blood calcium homeostasis.

Osteoclasts (i.e., bone-absorbing cells) break down bones, remove worn cells, and release Ca into the blood. Osteoclasts secrete lysosomal enzymes that digest the organic matrix by secreting acids that decompose calcium salts into Ca^{2+} and PO_4^- ions, which enter the blood.

Osteoclasts determine *blood calcium levels*, vital for muscle contraction and nerve conduction.

Osteoblasts (i.e., blood-forming cells) form new bones, taking calcium from the blood. They get incorporated into the bone matrix and become osteocytes in the lacunae of osteons.

This continual remodeling allows the bone to change in thickness gradually.

Minerals and vitamins for bone deposition and remodeling

Minerals needed for bone growth and remodeling include *calcium*, phosphorus (a component of the hydroxyapatite matrix), *magnesium* (regular osteoblast activity), *boron* (inhibiting calcium loss), and *manganese* (formation of new matrix).

Vitamins are needed for bone growth, remodeling, and repair.

For example, vitamin A is required for bone resorption and controls the activity, distribution, and coordination of osteoblasts and osteoclasts during development.

Vitamin B_{12} plays a role in osteoblast activity.

Vitamin C maintains bone matrix and collagen synthesis; deficiency of vitamin causes scurvy.

Vitamin D dramatically increases intestinal absorption of dietary calcium and slows urine loss. Vitamin D deficiency causes rickets in children and osteomalacia in adults.

Hormones of bone deposition and remodeling

Hormones stimulate the replacement of cartilage by bone in the epiphyseal plate.

Hormones needed for bone growth and remodeling include *human growth hormone* (HGH), *sex hormones*, *thyroid hormones*, *parathyroid hormone* (PTH), and *calcitonin*.

Pituitary gland secretes HGH for general tissue growth. HGH stimulates the reproduction of cartilage cells at the epiphyseal plate.

Sex hormones include *estrogen* and *androgens* (e.g., testosterone), which aid osteoblast activity by promoting new bone growth. Also, they degenerate cartilage cells in the epiphyseal plate by closing the plate.

Estrogen's effect is greater than androgen's effect.

Bone remodeling for calcium homeostasis

Thyroid hormones include *triiodothyronine* (T_3) and *thyroxine* (T_4).

Calcium homeostasis (blood Ca^{2+} level of 10 mg/dL) is critical for normal bodily functions.

Calcium homeostasis is controlled by PTH, vitamin D, calcitonin, and interactions of skeletal, endocrine, digestive, and urinary systems. Body systems maintain calcium levels in the blood.

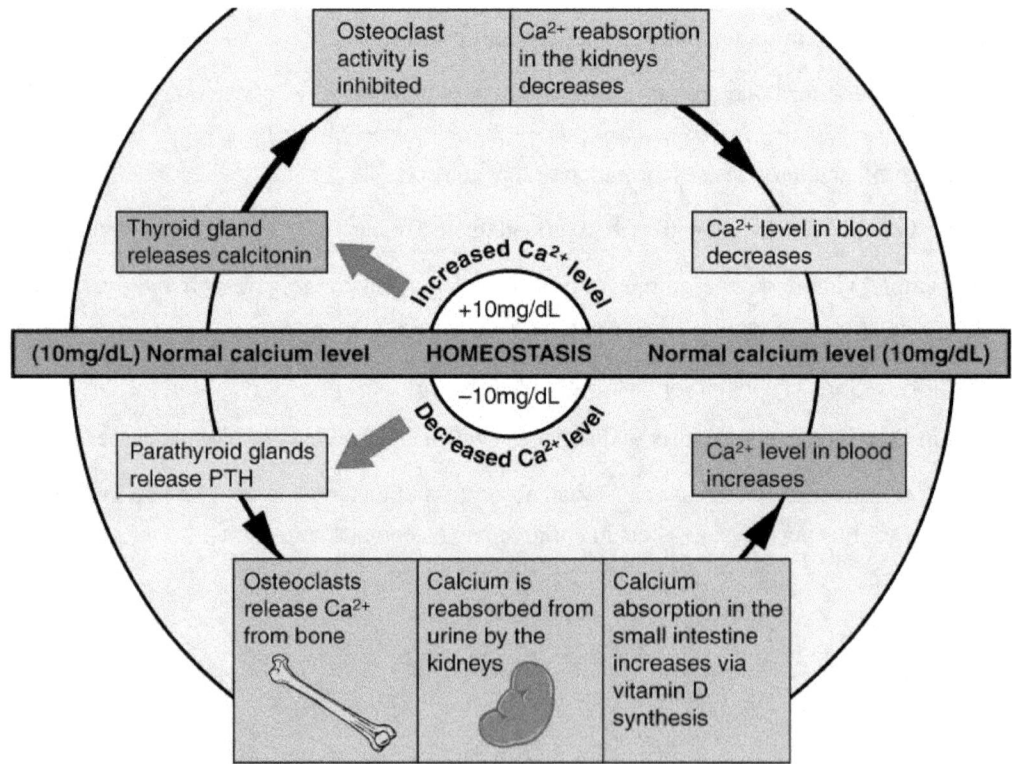

Calcium homeostasis includes bone formation and degradation.

PTH, vitamin D and calcitonin

Parathyroid glands secrete *parathyroid hormone* (PTH) if blood calcium levels are low. PTH stimulates *osteoclast proliferation* and bone *resorption* with demineralization, releasing calcium into the blood.

PTH causes kidney tubules to reabsorb Ca^{2+} into the blood. It causes intestinal mucosa to increase dietary absorption of Ca^{2+} and increase blood calcium levels (homeostasis).

PTH stimulates vitamin D synthesis, increasing Ca^{2+} absorption from food in the small intestine.

The body deposits calcium in the bones when blood levels are high and releases calcium when blood levels become low. PTH, vitamin D, and calcitonin regulate this.

When these processes return blood calcium levels to normal, there is Ca^{2+} to bind the receptors on the parathyroid gland surface cells, and this cycle of events is turned off.

Calcitonin is secreted by thyroid glands when blood calcium levels are high (hypercalcemia).

Calcitonin inhibits bone resorption and increases osteoblast activity (i.e., deposit bone matrix).

Calcitonin causes kidney tubules to secrete excess Ca^{2+} into the urine, decreasing blood calcium levels (homeostasis).

Parafollicular cells of thyroid glands secrete *calcitonin*, decreasing plasma calcium concentration by reducing bone resorption to lower blood calcium levels. When blood calcium levels return to normal, the thyroid gland stops secreting calcitonin.

Hypocalcemia is an abnormally low level of blood calcium.

Notes for active learning

CHAPTER 13

Skin System

Skin Structure and Functions

Thermoregulation Function of Skin

Physical Protection by Skin

Hair Structure

Skin Tissue Damage

Hormonal Influences

Page intentionally left blank

Skin Structure and Functions

Integument

Integument is an organ system that functions as an outer protective layer and consists of skin, glands, and accessory structures (e.g., hair, nails, blood vessels, and nerves).

Integument is a *cutaneous membrane* covering the body's outer surface. It is the largest organ by surface area and weight.

Average adults have skin surface area of approximately 2 square meters. Skin weighs about 5 kg or approximately 16% of body weight.

Thickness varies from 0.5 millimeters on the eyelids to 6 millimeters on the heels of the feet.

Humans lose almost a kilogram of skin epithelium annually, which becomes a significant part of household "*dust*."

Cutaneous glands are glands in the skin: *merocrine sweat glands*, *apocrine sweat glands*, *sebaceous glands*, *ceruminous glands*, and *mammary glands*.

Tissue types are well-represented in the integument organ system: 1) epithelium in the hair, skin, nails, and blood vessels; 2) muscle tissue surrounding blood vessels and attached to hair follicles; 3) nervous tissue in the lower layers of the skin and 4) connective tissue (including blood) throughout the entire organ system.

Dermatology is a branch of medicine studying integumentary system.

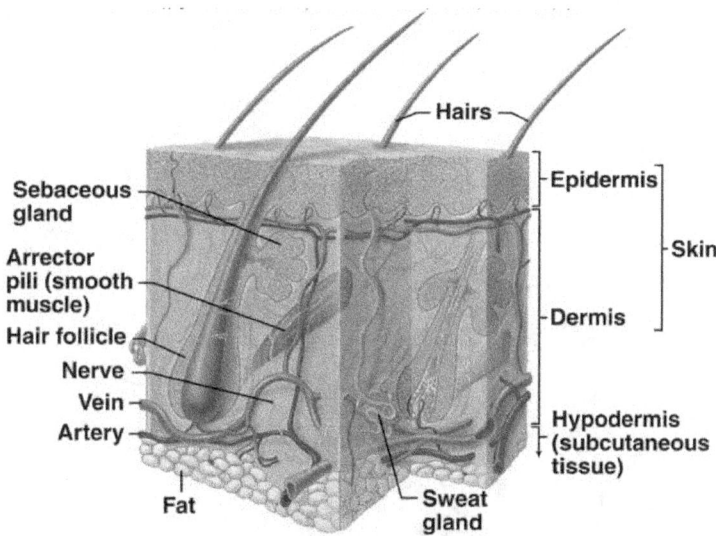

Skin with epidermis, dermis, fat cells, and accessory structures

Essential functions of skin

Integumentary system have several functions, including body temperature regulation, acting as a physical barrier, and protection against injury, dehydration, chemicals, UV radiation, and infectious agents.

Integument is a sensory organ that gathers information about temperature, pressure, and touch from the outside environment and transmits it to the central nervous system.

Integument has a storage function, keeping glucose and fat as energy stores and holding water and blood. Vessels in the dermis hold up to 10% of the blood in a resting adult.

Blood content of the skin and sweating are essential for *thermoregulation*. Sweating regulates the body's water content and excretes waste.

Skin synthesizes and *stores vitamin D*, which regulates blood Ca^{2+} levels and vital processes.

Layer differentiation, cell types, and tissue

Integument is stratified into three major layers.

Epidermis is the outer, thinner layer and consists of epithelial tissue. *Dermis* is the middle, thicker layer of epithelial, muscle, nervous, and connective tissue.

Subcutaneous (or *subQ layer*), known as *hypodermis*, below the dermis. Technically, it is not part of the skin as a supporting layer of loose connective tissue and fat that supplies blood to the dermis and attaches the skin to the underlying tissues and organs.

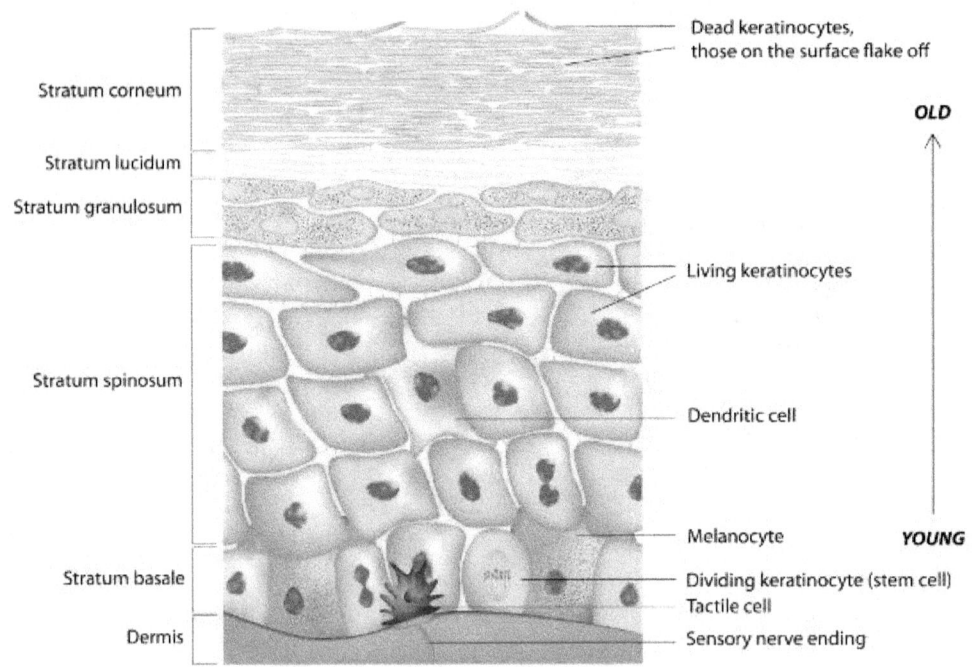

Most of the body is covered with thin skin, hair, and glands. *Volar surfaces*, which are on the palm and sole, are covered with thick skin.

Thick skin has an additional *epidermis stratification* level and lacks hair and sebaceous glands.

Epidermis is a superficial, stratified, *avascular* epithelial tissue needing the dermis for nutrients.

Oxygen enters the epidermis not from the dermal blood supply but from the atmosphere.

Epidermis comprises *keratinized stratified squamous epithelium*, an epithelial tissue with four major types of cells: keratinocytes, melanocytes, Langerhans (dendritic) cells, and Merkel cells.

Keratinocytes are most of the epidermal cells (nearly 90%) and produce *keratin*, a tough fibrous protein that provides protection.

Keratinocytes flatten as they die and migrate upward to the skin's surface, forming a tight layer of *dead keratinocytes* that give skin *waterproof quality*.

Keratinocytes are held by *desmosomes* (i.e., adhesion cell junctions) that resist stretching and tearing of the skin but still allow passage of materials between cells.

Epidermal layers' structure and function

Five layers of the epidermis include (from the superficial to the deepest):

> *stratum corneum, stratum lucidum, stratum granulosum, stratum spinosum*, and *stratum basale*.

Stratum corneum is the epidermal outermost layer with 25 to 30 layers of dead keratinocytes, called *corneocytes*. Keratin plates are sealed with lipids secreted by *lamellar granules*, organelles in living keratinocytes in the deeper layers of the epidermis.

Keratin packs in the *corneocytes,* and lipids seal gaps between cells, making skin impenetrable to many environmental agents and preventing water from entering or leaving.

Average keratinocyte flakes off the epidermal surface after one month, an *exfoliation process*.

Stratum lucidum is below the corneum and is in the thick skin at the fingertips, palms of the hands, and soles of the feet. It has 3 to 5 layers of dead keratinocytes, adding an extra layer of protection to the thick skin.

Stratum granulosum (i.e., granular layer) is an intermediate layer containing 3 to 5 layers of keratinocytes dying and migrating upward.

Keratinocytes in the stratum granulosum contain *lamellar bodies*, known as *membrane-coating vesicles,* which secrete lipids that seal the epidermis.

They are in the process of converting their cytoskeletal filaments into keratin so that they may become keratin-packed cells in the stratum corneum and/or stratum lucidum.

Stratum spinosum (spinous layer) lies under the stratum granulosum and provides strength and flexibility to the epidermis. It is made primarily of 8 to 10 layers of keratinocytes.

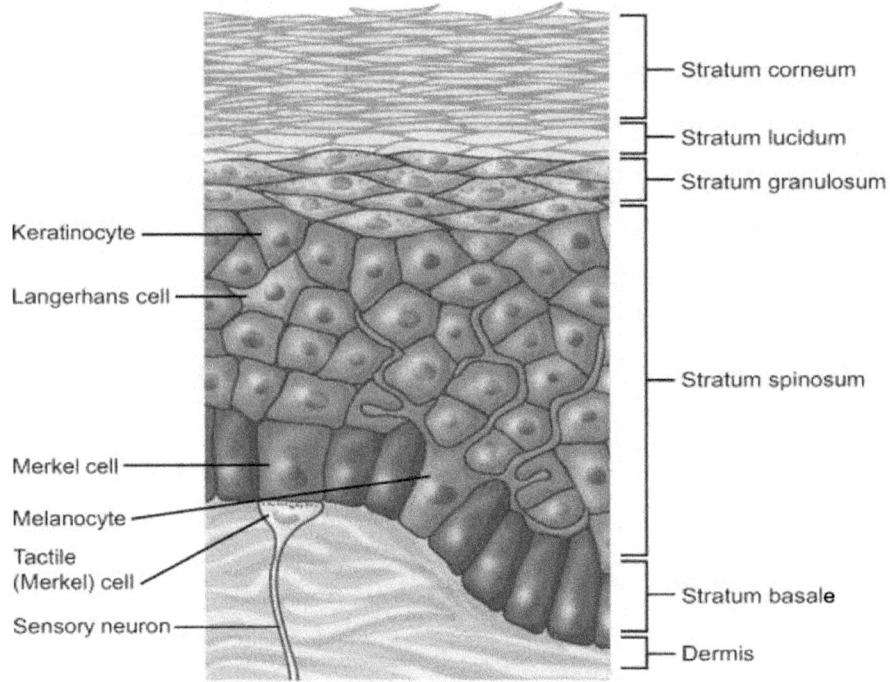

Skin layers are stratum corneum, stratum lucidum, stratum granulosum, stratum spinosum, and stratum basale

Langerhans cells are epidermis layers, but most predominantly in the *stratum spinosum*.

Langerhans cells are *macrophages* originating in the *red bone marrow* and are involved with immune responses. They interact with the *helper T-cells* of the immune system.

Stratum basale (basal layer) lies below the stratum spinosum and is the *stratum germinativum* or *germinal layer*. It is the deepest layer of the epidermis.

Continuous division of *stem cells* occurs in the stratum basale and supplies the upper layers.

Keratinocytes produced in the stratum basale are pushed to the top layer, losing their cytoplasm, nucleus, and organelles as they reach the stratum corneum before sloughing off.

Stratum basale contains *Merkel cells* associated with sensory neurons and touch sensation.

Melanocytes in the *stratum basale* produce *melanin* pigment, protecting against UV radiation.

Dermal layers' structure and function

Dermis is below the epidermis and is 0.2 to 4 millimeters thick and primarily connective tissue, mostly collagen, but includes elastic fibers, reticular fibers, fibroblasts, and other cell types.

Fibroblasts produce fibrous proteins for the extracellular matrix of connective tissue.

Dermis contains blood vessels, sweat glands, sebaceous glands, nerves, hair follicles, nail roots, and smooth muscle.

In most places, *dermal papillae* (upward projections of dermis) interlock with downward *epidermal ridges* to form a wavy boundary. Within the dermal papillae are the tiny *capillary loops* that supply blood. Papillae form *friction ridges* of fingertips and toes, increasing grip.

Papillary layer is the top 20% of the dermis. Papillary region lies below the epidermis and consists of *areolar connective tissue* with *thin collagen* and *elastic fibers*, *dermal papillae*, and *nerve endings*.

Papillary layer mobilizes *macrophages* for pathogens that breach the epidermis.

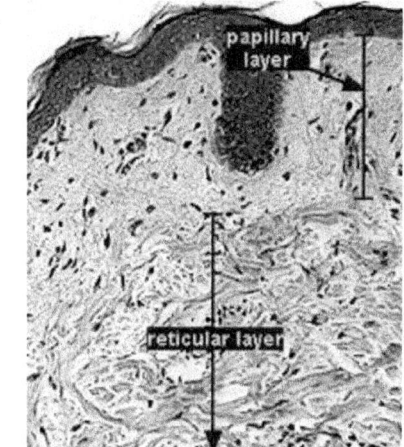

Reticular layer, deeper in the dermis, is a dense connective tissue (i.e., collagen and elastin fibers) packed with oil glands, nerves, sweat gland ducts, fat, and hair follicles.

Reticular layer provides strength and elasticity to the skin. Dermal tears cause stretch marks.

Cleavage lines (or *Langer lines*) are "*tension lines*" on the skin that indicate the predominant direction of collagen fibers in the dermis.

Skin receptor structure and functions

Dermis has *thermoreceptors* detecting temperature, especially in the skin of the ears and face.

Mechanoreceptors, which recognize sensations such as texture, pressure, and vibration, are in all layers of the integumentary system.

Merkel cells and *Meissner corpuscles* are sensitive on the top layer of the dermis and epidermis, usually on non-hairy parts of the body (e.g., lips, palms, soles of the feet, and tongue).

Merkel cells (or tactile epithelial cell) are mechanoreceptors essential for *light touch sensations*.

Mechanoreceptors include *Ruffini* and *Pacinian corpuscles*, both in *hypodermis*.

Ruffini corpuscles are mechanoreceptors that have a thermoreceptor-like function.

Pacinian corpuscles are low-threshold mechanoreceptors responsive to vibration or pressure in the skin and internal organs.

Nociceptors are in the dermis as receptors detecting stimuli that may cause damage to the skin or other parts of the body. They signal an individual experiencing pain to avoid the stimulus causing the pain.

Nociceptors cause dull pain in an area where injury has occurred to signal the individual not to use that appendage.

Subcutaneous layer (hypodermis) is not part of the skin. It is composed of areolar and adipose tissue in a larger quantity than the reticular layer of the dermis.

Subcutaneous layer securely attaches the dermis and epidermis to the body's deeper tissues.

Additionally, blood vessels and nerves in the hypodermis extend to the dermis.

Hypodermis stores fat in adipose tissue to absorb shock, provide insulation, and protect organs.

Hypodermis areas composed mainly of adipocytes are *subcutaneous fat*.

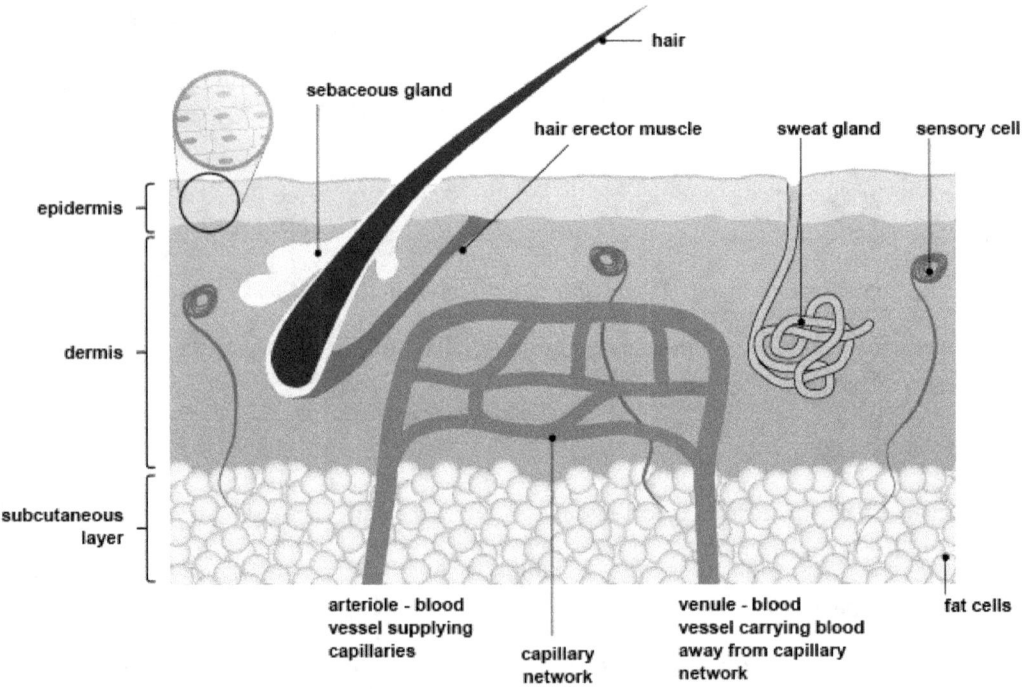

Skin and accessory structures

Skin pigmentation and melanocytes

Skin color is from skin pigments (e.g., eumelanin, pheomelanin, hemoglobin of the blood, white collagen of the dermis) and dietary carotene.

Pathological conditions include skin discoloration, such as cyanosis, erythema, pallor, albinism, jaundice, and hematomas.

Hair color is attributable to the relative amounts of eumelanin and pheomelanin.

Melanocytes are specialized skin cells that produce protective skin-darkening pigment *melanin*.

Melanocytes are *dendritic* (branched), and dendrites transfer pigment granules to adjacent cells.

Melanin is in the *stratum basale* of the epidermis and the *hair matrix*.

Skin markings include fingertip friction ridges, flexion lines of palms, wrists, and other places, and freckles, moles, and *hemangiomas* (i.e., bright red birthmarks).

Freckles are clusters of concentrated melanin triggered by sunlight exposure, and their amount is determined by genetics.

Nevi are chronic skin lesions and are, by definition, benign. A *melanocytic nevus* is a mole or birthmark. Some nevi can become cancerous; *malignant melanoma* is melanocyte cancer.

Melanin decreases typically as an individual ages and loses melanocytes, resulting in gray hair and atypical skin pigmentation. However, certain disorders cause melanin deficiency.

Vitiligo is a chronic disorder that causes depigmentation of skin patches. Pathogenesis (cause) is unknown but is likely a combination of genetics and an immune system disorder.

Albinism is a congenital condition characterized by the complete (or partial) absence of skin, hair, and eye pigments due to a defect of a melanin production enzyme.

Relative impermeability to water

Epidermal water barrier is created by keratinocytes and desmosomes linking them, 1) a lipid coating that fills the gaps between keratinocytes, and 2) a thick protein layer on the inner surface of the keratinocyte plasma membranes.

The water barrier reduces water loss from the body.

Keratin is water-insoluble; hydrophobic glycolipids seal dead keratin-packed cell spaces.

Sebum (i.e., oily substance) from sebaceous glands contributes partly to impermeability.

Sebum glands are absent from the palms and soles.

Notes for active learning

Regulatory Functions of Skin

Osmoregulation

Homeostasis is when the internal environment remains relatively constant despite changes in the external environment. Organisms usually strive for homeostasis, and the body's organ systems, including the integumentary system, are dedicated to maintaining homeostasis.

Integumentary systems have a crucial role in water homeostasis via *osmoregulation.*

Osmoregulation is the process by which the *osmotic pressure* of an organism's fluid is actively regulated to maintain the homeostasis of the body's water content.

Water homeostasis insulates the body against losing water to the outside (or taking it in).

Intercellular spaces of the epidermis are sealed with lipids and amino acids that counteract water and salt loss from the skin and the penetration of water-soluble materials into the skin.

Water loss from stratum corneum into the environment is *transepidermal water loss*, a normal process. The integumentary system ensures that excessive transepidermal water loss does not occur. However, it may occasionally promote water loss through the sweat glands to regulate body water content and temperature.

Perspiration excretes *salt* and *nitrogenous waste* (e.g., urea, uric acid, ammonia).

Increased sodium retention in the blood must offset sodium loss through perspiration.

Aldosterone is a steroid hormone that promotes sodium reabsorption in the kidneys with associated water retention and is a vital regulator for *osmoregulation.*

Thermoreceptors in skin

Homeothermy is the ability to maintain body temperatures within a normal range. Bodily heat content is the net difference between heat production and heat loss.

In a steady state, *heat production equals heat loss*.

Water loss through the skin, sweat, and respiratory tract contributes to heat loss. Body surfaces lose heat through radiation, conduction, convection, and evaporation.

Sensory information from *thermoreceptors* in the skin travels to the hypothalamus, integrating and responding to this information to maintain homeothermy.

Hypothalamus signals the body (e.g., sweat glands, skin arterioles) to initiate thermoregulation.

Two types of thermoreceptors detect changes in body temperature:

peripheral thermoreceptors (in the skin) and

central thermoreceptors (in the brain and spinal cord).

Central thermoreceptors provide the essential *negative feedback* for maintaining core body temperature, while peripheral thermoreceptors provide feedforward information.

Thermoreceptors are classified as *cold receptors* and *hot receptors*.

Cold receptors perceive a cold sensation when skin surface temperatures drop below 95 °F and are most stimulated when the skin's surface is at 77 °F. However, they are no longer stimulated when the temperature drops below 41 °F. This is why feet and hands go numb when submerged in ice-cold water for an extended period.

Hot receptors perceive hot sensations when the skin surface temperature rises above 86 °F; they are most stimulated at 113 °F.

Pain receptors take over above 113 °F to avoid damage to the skin and underlying tissues.

Hair and erectile musculature of skin

In animals, hairs insulate the body by trapping air. Typically, hair lies at an angle to the skin, with a bundle of the smooth muscle of the *arrector pili* or *piloerector* attached to the follicle.

When body temperature drops, the *piloerector contracts*, and the hair stands up.

In mammals, this erect position fluffs up the fur and traps a layer of air between fur and skin. This provides better insulation and thus increases body temperature. However, because humans are primarily hairless, this response is the *goosebumps* on the skin.

Adipose tissue layer for energy reserves and insulation

Adipose tissue in the hypodermis, which functions as protective padding and energy storage, acts as an insulator.

Fat is an ideal insulating tissue because heat travels poorly through this medium.

Two types of mammalian fat are brown fat and white fat.

Brown fat generates heat due to its mitochondria and is abundant in infants, the neck, and around the large blood vessels of adults. It can be in hibernating animals.

White fat is the primary insulator and energy storage in adults.

Fat layer thickness varies widely depending on location in the body. For example, the eyelids' fat layer is a fraction of an inch, while the fat layer on the buttocks can be several inches.

Merocrine and apocrine sweat glands

Human have two types of skin sweat glands. Both are simple, coiled tubular glands.

Sudoriferous glands produce sweat, cooling the body through evaporative cooling. Increased sweating is a corrective response to reduce the organism's temperature.

Merocrine (or *eccrine*) sweat glands are the body's major sweat glands; they are most numerous on the palms and soles of feet. These glands secrete a watery solution (600 ml per day) that cools the body and eliminates tiny amounts of waste like urea. Eccrine glands can release sweat in response to emotional stress (e.g., fear or embarrassment); this type of sweating is emotional or a "cold sweat."

Apocrine sweat glands are larger than eccrine glands and associated with hair follicles mainly on the skin of the axillae (i.e., armpit), groin, areolae, and bearded facial regions of adult males.

Apocrine sweat glands become active during puberty, have hair appearance in these regions, and secrete *pheromones* (or pheromone-like) substances. Sweat of apocrine glands is slightly viscous and usually odorous (unlike eccrine sweat). Much body odor is due to apocrine sweat.

Apocrine sweat gland's secretions are mainly in the hypodermis, with the excretory duct directing into hair follicles.

Myoepithelial cell contractions around the base of a follicle squeeze the secretion up the duct to the skin surface.

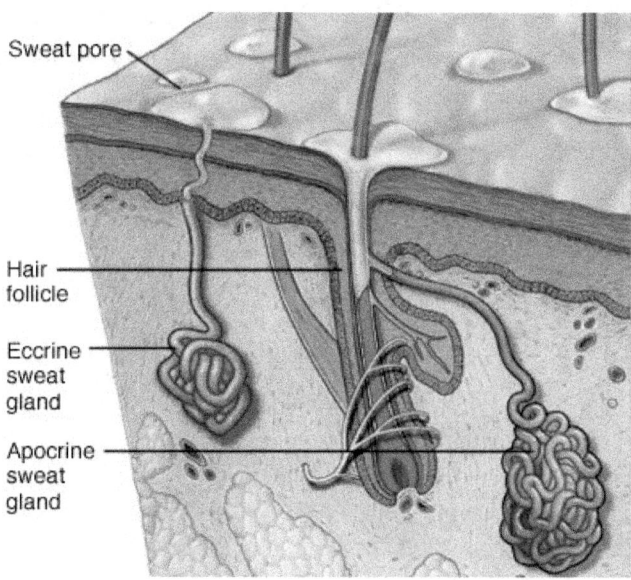

Eccrine (merocrine) gland, apocrine gland, hair follicles, and sweat pores

Notes for active learning

Vasoconstriction and vasodilation of surface capillaries

Skin's effectiveness as an insulator is under physiological control by changing skin blood flow. For example, blood vessels reduce the insulating capacity of the skin by shunting heat to the surface to be lost to the external environment (e.g., evaporation).

At low temperatures, the hypothalamus initiates *vasoconstriction*.

At elevated temperatures, the hypothalamus initiates *vasodilation*.

Vasodilation is the distention of blood vessels. It relaxes the smooth muscle around a blood vessel, increasing its diameter and promoting blood flow. For example, when the temperature is high, the hypothalamus initiates *vasodilation* of arterioles near the skin to increase blood supply to the skin's capillaries, leading to heat loss at the skin surface.

Vasoconstriction of arterioles causes blood to bypass the skin capillaries. It redirects blood to the veins, reducing blood supply to skin capillaries and reducing heat loss at the skin surface.

Regulation beyond the thermoneutral zone

Thermoneutral zone is the range of environmental temperatures over which the basal metabolic rate maintains body temperature and is adjusted by *vasoconstriction* or *vasodilation*.

When the temperature is below (or above) the thermoneutral zone, the body must use energy that exceeds the basal metabolic rate to alter heat production (and heat loss).

Heat production includes shivering and exercising in temperatures below the thermoneutral zone. Behavioral mechanisms include curling up when cold, reducing the surface area exposed to the environment, and decreasing heat loss by radiation and conduction.

Heat production decreases by lowering the metabolic rate at temperatures above the thermoneutral zone.

Heat loss is promoted by evaporative cooling via sweating.

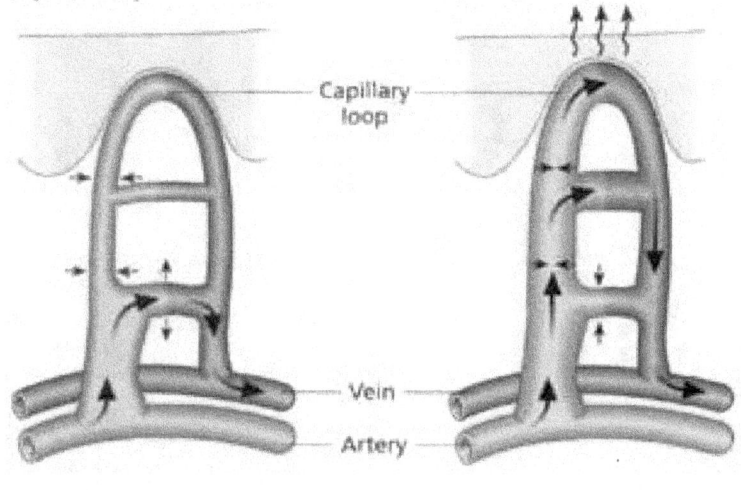

Vasoconstriction in cold environments and vasodilation in warm environments are physiological responses to regulate body temperature.

Notes for active learning

Physical Protection by Skin

Skin functions as the first barrier of defense

Skin is an excellent line of defense because it provides an almost impenetrable physical barrier protecting the internal environment. Multiple layers in the skin allow for specialization.

Epidermis is adapted to fast cell turnover, heals quickly, and resists damage. It offers waterproofing and protection from pathogens to underlying tissues.

Dermis provides temperature stability and reduces dehydration, but unlike the epidermis, it undergoes limited healing.

Nails and hair originate in the dermis and provide additional protection.

Protection against abrasion and pathogens

Keratinization replaces viable cells in the stratum basale with waxy, water-resistant keratin.

Constant friction stimulates this process as *callus*, a thick buildup of keratinocytes in the stratum corneum. They are responses to repeated physical stress that protect the dermis from this stress.

Excessive friction (or pressure) in a short time usually results in *blisters*.

Skin forms a physical barrier that prevents pathogens from entering the body. Besides its physical toughness, the skin has *chemical defenses*.

Sebaceous glands, associated with hair follicles, produce *sebum* (i.e., an oily secretion), which 1) prevents the dehydration of hair and skin and 2) inhibits the growth of certain bacteria.

Lactic acid and *fatty acids* in sebum create an *acidic environment* on the skin's surface that discourages the growth of pathogens. Sebum contains antibodies that fight infection.

Sebaceous glands are *holocrine glands* that break down to form secretions.

Ceruminous glands are modified sweat glands in the auditory canal that produce cerumen (i.e., a waxy secretion) along with nearby sebaceous glands.

Cerumen (or earwax) is a mixture of ceruminous gland secretion, sebum, and dead epidermal cells. It keeps the eardrum pliable, waterproofs the auditory canal, and kills bacteria.

Lymphocytes (i.e., immune cells) are abundant throughout the dermis and suppress infection.

Epidermis contains lymphocytes and other cells with immune function (e.g., *Langerhans cells*).

Mucous membranes are another barrier against pathogens. These are soft and moist areas of internal organs exposed to external environments (trachea) and specific skin areas (nose, ears, genitals).

Mucous membranes are not strong enough to create a physical barrier, but they produce mucus-containing antibodies, lysosomal enzymes, and other immune system agents.

Mucus in the respiratory tract traps pathogens and irritants expelled from the nose or trachea.

Senescence (or *cell aging*) of the integumentary system is marked by thinning and graying of the hair, dryness of the skin and hair due to atrophy of the sebaceous glands, and thinning loss of elasticity in the skin.

Subcutaneous fat loss reduces thermoregulation capacity.

UV radiation accelerates skin aging, promoting wrinkling, age spots, and skin cancer. Aged skin is more vulnerable to trauma and infection than younger skin and heals slowly.

Nail anatomy

Nails are hard, densely keratinized epidermal cells over dorsal surfaces at the ends of fingers and toes.

Nail structure has a free edge (i.e., a transparent nail body) with a whitish *lunula* at its base and a nail root embedded in the skin fold.

Skin underlying the nail is the nail bed; its epidermis is the *hyponychium*.

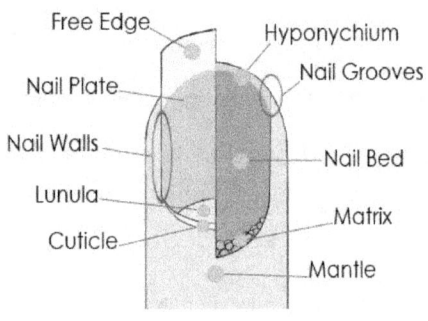

Nail anatomy

Nail matrix is a growth zone of the epidermal stratum basale at the nail bed's proximal end.

Hair Structure

Keratin structure

Nails and hair are formed of hard keratin and are tougher than the soft keratin in the skin.

Hard keratin is more compact and extensively cross-linked than soft epidermal keratin.

Pilus (hair) is a slender filament of dead, keratinized epidermal cells growing from an oblique tube, the *hair follicle,* composed of epidermal and dermal tissue.

Hair is on the skin's surfaces except for palms, fingers' anterior surfaces, and feet' soles.

Genetics determines hair color, thickness, and distribution. Hair functions vary by type and location, including thermal insulation, protection from sun and foreign objects, sensation, facial expression, signaling of sexual maturity, and pheromone dispersal.

Hair types and texture

Three hair types are: *lanugo hairs*, *vellus hairs*, and *terminal hairs.*

Lanugo hairs are fine, unpigmented, downy hairs that cover the fetus' body and are shed before or shortly after birth.

Vellus hairs are short, fine, pale hairs barely visible to the naked eye. They develop in childhood and are in all humans.

Terminal hairs are long, coarse, heavily pigmented hairs.

Deep in the follicle, hair begins with a dilated *bulb,* continues as a narrower *root* below the skin surface, and extends above the skin as the *shaft.*

Bulb contains a *dermal papilla* of vascularized connective tissue which nourishes hair.

Hair matrix above the papilla is the site of hair growth by dividing the matrix cells.

Hair has a thin *outer cuticle* in cross-section, a thicker layer of *keratinized cells* (forming the hair cortex), and a *medulla* core.

Hair follicles have an inner *epithelial root sheath* (i.e., an extension of the epidermis) and an outer *connective tissue root sheath* (i.e., condensed dermal tissue). It exhibits a *bulge,* a site of stem cells for follicle growth.

Hair follicles are associated with *hair receptors* (i.e., nerve endings) that detect hair movements.

Differences in hair texture are attributable to differences in cross-sectional shape: *straight hair* is round, *wavy hair* is slightly less round, and *curly hair* has oval or elliptical cross section.

Hair life cycle

Hair has a life cycle consisting of a growing *anagen* stage of 6 to 8 years, a shrinking *catagen* stage of 2 to 3 weeks, and a resting *telogen* stage of 1 to 3 months.

Hairs usually fall out during the *catagen* or *telogen stage*.

Catagen phase **begins with the end of the anagen phase and is characterized by a transition into quiescence**. During this phase, which lasts a few weeks, hair follicles undergo apoptosis-driven regression and lose about one-sixth of their standard diameter.

Telogen stage.is the resting stage when hair follicles are dormant and without growth.

Scalp hair typically lives 6 to 8 years and grows at a rate of 10 to 18 centimeters per year.

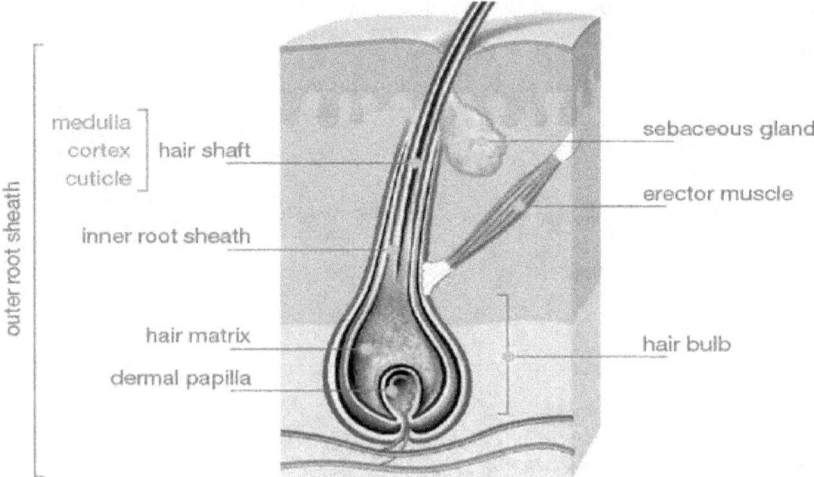

Hair anatomy with bulb, root, and shaft

Skin Tissue Damage

Tissue damage by burns

A burn is tissue damage caused by excessive heat, electricity, radioactivity, or corrosive chemicals *denaturing proteins* in skin cells.

Burns destroy skin's contributions to homeostasis (e.g., resistance to microbial invasion, protection against desiccation, and thermoregulation).

Burns are graded according to their severity; see the table below.

Burn Type	Layers affected	Sensation	Healing time	Prognosis
Superficial (1°)	Epidermis	Painful	5–10 days	Heals well; repeated sunburns increase the risk of skin cancer
Superficial partial thickness (2°)	Extends into superficial (papillary) dermis	Very painful	Less than 2–3 weeks	Local infection and cellulitis but no scarring
Deep partial thickness (2°)	Extends into deep (reticular) dermis	Pressure and discomfort	3–8 weeks	Scarring, contractures (may require excision and skin grafting)
Full thickness (3°)	Extends through the entire dermis	Painless	Prolonged (months) and incomplete	Scarring, amputation (early excision recommended)
Fourth degree (4°)	Extends through the entire skin and into underlying fat, muscle, and bone	Painless	Requires excision	Amputation, significant functional impairment, and death

First-degree burn involves only the epidermis and is characterized by mild pain and *erythema* (redness) but no blisters; the skin quickly regains function.

Second-degree burn destroys the epidermis and part of the dermis; some skin functions are lost. Indications of a second-degree burn include erythema, blister formation, edema, and pain.

Third-degree burn is a full-thickness burn, destroying the epidermis, dermis, and hypodermis. After a third-degree burn, most (if not all) skin functions are lost. The region becomes numb because sensory nerve endings have been destroyed.

According to the American Burn Association's classification of burn injury, a major burn includes third-degree burns over 10% of body surface area; second-degree burns over 25% of body surface area; or any third-degree burns on the face, hands, feet, or perineum (which includes the anal and urogenital regions).

Burns exceeding 70% of the body area result in death for more than half of the victims.

Wound healing

There are two wound-healing processes depending on the depth of the injury.

Epidermal wound healing follows superficial wounds that affect the epidermis. This healing serves to restore normal function.

Deep wound healing occurs when an injury extends to the dermis and subcutaneous layer. This process is serious and requires scar tissue formation (i.e., fibrosis), which reduces some function of the skin of the repaired wound.

Skin cancer classification

Skin cancer is classified by the cells of origin and the lesions' appearance:

> *basal cell carcinoma,*
>
> *squamous cell carcinoma,* and
>
> *malignant melanoma.*

Malignant melanomas are the least common form but are the most dangerous because they tend to quickly metastasize (i.e., move to other regions by circulatory or lymphatic systems).

Hormonal Influences

Hormone modulations of skin and fluid balance

Hormones are chemical messengers that relay information throughout the body, usually maintaining homeostasis.

Estrogen is the primary sex hormone in females but is present in males. Estrogen affects skin thickness, elasticity, and fluid balance. It increases glycosaminoglycans (GAGs) production, such as hyaluronic acid, which maintains the skin's structure and fluid balance.

Additionally, estrogen increases collagen production to maintain epidermal thickness and smooth the appearance of wrinkles.

Estrogen insufficiency, which occurs in menopausal women, can cause excessive perspiration.

Thyroid hormones affect body temperature and skin dryness. Excess thyroid hormone causes the skin to become warm, sweaty, and flushed. Conversely, thyroid hormone deficiency causes skin to become dry, coarse, and thick.

Serotonin affects mood, sleep, digestion, and memory; serotonin deficiency causes excessive perspiration.

Testosterone is present in both sexes but is the primary male sex hormone. Coarser hair, oily skin, and general skin aging are due to testosterone activity.

Females can experience increased oiliness and acne when their hormones are not balanced.

Hormones regulate blood flow during thermoregulation

Vasodilation and *vasoconstriction* control blood flow distribution and heat loss. They are influenced by chemicals (CO_2, H^+, and K^+), sympathetic nerves, and autonomic nerves.

Hormones play an essential role in regulating this system.

Vasodilation is the relaxation of smooth muscle around the blood vessels. Muscle relaxation depends on the intracellular concentration of Ca^{2+} related to myosin contractile protein's light chain phosphorylation.

Vasodilation is stimulated by decreased intracellular Ca^{2+} levels or dephosphorylated myosin. Hormones promote vasodilation through specific pathways by decreasing Ca^{2+} within cells.

Endogenous vasodilators include *epinephrine*, *histamine*, *prostacyclin*, and *prostaglandins*.

Vasoconstriction uses blood vessel constriction and increases intracellular calcium levels.

Vasoconstriction uses norepinephrine, dopamine, thromboxane, and vasopressin (ADH).

Epinephrine and norepinephrine have the same effect on the heart, but they have vastly different effects on blood vessels.

Epinephrine causes *vasodilation*, while norepinephrine causes *vasoconstriction*.

Heart contains *beta-2 receptors*, while blood vessels contain alpha and beta-2 receptors.

Epinephrine preferentially activates *beta-2 receptors*, so vasodilation occurs if there are sufficient beta-2 receptors.

Notes for active learning

Notes for active learning

CHAPTER 14

Reproductive System

Female Reproductive Structures and Functions

Male Reproductive Structures and Functions

Gametogenesis

Meiosis

Oogenesis

Spermatogenesis

Gametes' Structure and Functions

Sexual Development

Hormonal Control of Ovarian Cycle

Hormonal Control of Female Reproductive Cycle

Hormonal Control of Gestation and Birthing

Female Reproductive Structures and Functions

Genitalia of the reproductive system

Genitalia is the external genital organs of the reproductive system.

Female reproductive system includes the ovary, oviduct, uterus, and vagina.

The major difference between the male and female reproductive structures is that male structures are mostly external for the delivery of sperm.

Female structures are mainly internal to nurture a growing fetus.

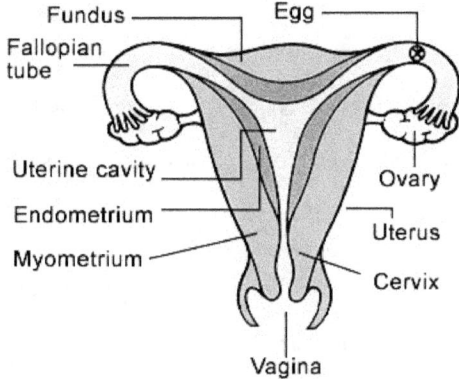

Female reproductive system with associated structures

Female genitalia

vulva is the collective external genitalia of females. The urethra opens into the vulva.

Vulva (pudendum or external genitalia) includes the *clitoris, mons pubis, labia majora,* and *labia minora*. The labia are on each side of the vaginal and urethral openings.

Clitoris is a short shaft of erectile tissue capped by a pea-shaped gland at the front juncture of the labia minora. This structure is homologous to the male penis.

Additionally, the vulva contains the vaginal orifice, *greater* and *lesser vestibular glands, paraurethral glands,* and *vestibular bulbs* (erectile tissues).

Vagina

Vagina is a tubular organ at a 45° angle with the small of the back.

Vagina is connected to uterus by the cervix, a cylinder-shaped neck of tissue 1 inch across.

Cervix is cartilage covered by smooth, moist tissue.

Vagina *tilts posteriorly* between the urethra and rectum.

It has no glands but is moistened by the transudation of serous fluid through the vaginal wall and mucus from glands in the cervical canal.

Stratified squamous epithelium with antigen-presenting *dendritic cells* line the vagina.

Vagina's mucosal lining lies in folds, extending as necessary in childbirth.

Vagina receives the penis during copulation.

Copulation is a sexual union that facilitates the reception of sperm by a female.

During birthing, the vagina is where the fetus passes out of the body (i.e., the birth canal).

Uterus

Uterus has upper *fundus,* middle *corpus* (body), and lower *cervix* (neck), meeting the vagina.

A narrow *cervical canal* connects the uterine lumen with the vaginal lumen.

Cervical glands in the canal secrete mucus, preventing vaginal microbes from spreading into the uterus.

Uterus is a hollow, thick-walled muscular organ superior to the urinary bladder; its size and shape are comparable to an inverted pear, where the fertilized ovum develops until birth.

Uterine wall has three layers:

> an outer serosa *perimetrium,*
>
> thick muscular *myometrium,* and
>
> an inner mucosa *endometrium.*

Endometrium contains tubular glands divided into two layers –

> thick superficial *stratum functionalis* (shed during menstrual periods) and
>
> thinner basal *stratum basalis* (retained from cycle to cycle).

The uterus is supported by a pair of lateral wing-like *broad ligaments* and cordlike *cardinal, uterosacral,* and *round ligaments.* It receives blood from a pair of *uterine arteries.*

Fallopian tubes

Fallopian tubes (or *oviducts*) are two tubes that branch from the uterus and provide a passage to the uterus for the ovum released by the ovary.

Fallopian tubes, uterine tubes, and salpinges (singular salpinx) are the expected fertilization sites. They are lined with ciliated epithelia.

After fertilization, the embryo is slowly moved by ciliary movement toward the uterus.

The flared distal end of the Fallopian tube, near the ovary, is the *infundibulum* and has feathery projections of *fimbriae* to receive the ovulated egg.

Its long midportion is the *ampulla,* and a short, constricted zone near the uterus is the *isthmus. Mesosalpinx* is a ligamentous sheet that supports the tube.

Gonad anatomy and functions

Female gonads are *ovaries* with immature eggs that mature one (or more) at a time (monthly).

Ovary is where ova (or eggs) are produced (ovaries produce a secondary oocyte each month) along with female sex hormones, *estrogen*, and *progesterone*, during the ovarian cycle.

Ovaries are in the *abdominal cavity*.

Females typically have two ovaries.

Oviduct (Fallopian or uterine tube) is a tube for egg movement from the ovary to the uterus.

Ovarian anatomy

Each ovary is associated with an *oviduct* and has the following:

    a central *medulla,*

    a surface *cortex,* and

    tunica albuginea as an outer fibrous capsule.

Fimbriae are finger-like projections that sweep over the ovaries and waft the egg into the Fallopian tubes when released from the ovary.

Generally, the ovaries alternate in producing one oocyte every month.

Ovary is supported by:

    medial *ovarian ligament*,

    lateral *suspensory ligament,* and

    anterior *mesovarium*.

Ovary receives blood from a branch of *uterine artery* medially and *ovarian artery* laterally.

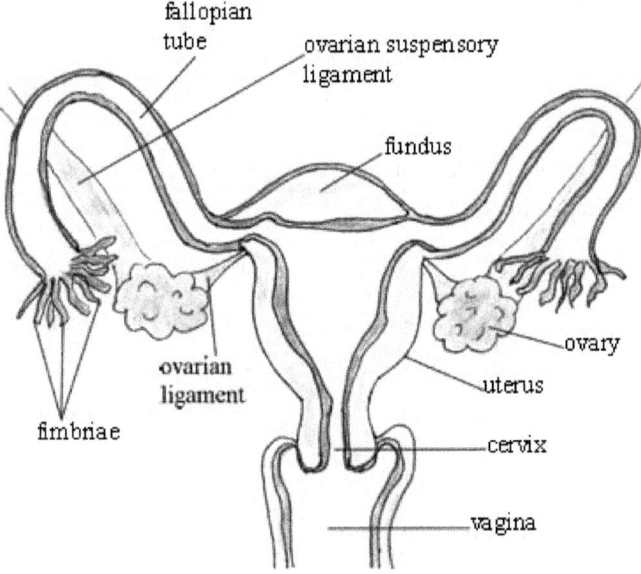

Female ovary with fallopian tube and ovarian ligament

Male Reproductive Structures and Functions

Male genitalia

Genitalia is the external genital organs of the reproductive system. External genitalia of men consists of the *penis*, *male urethra*, and *scrotum*.

Male reproductive system consists of the testes, epididymis, vas deferens, prostate gland, bulbourethral glands, and penis.

Males have one opening for urine and sperm, while females have one opening for urine and another for menstruation and sexual intercourse.

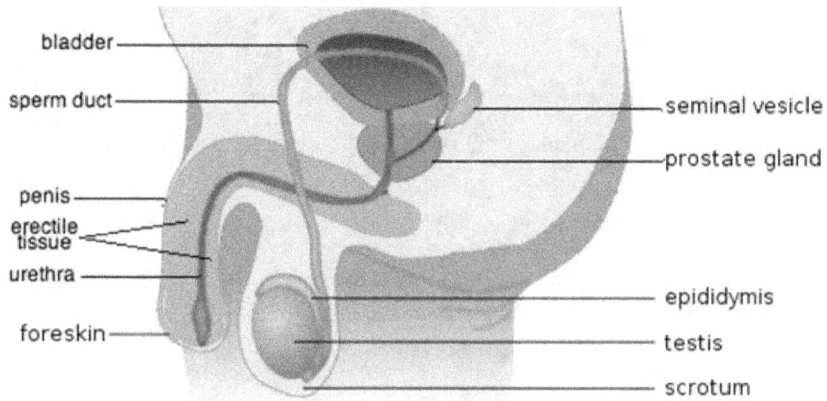

Male reproductive system with anatomy and glands

Penis

Penis is a cylindrical copulatory organ that introduces semen (a fluid containing spermatozoa) and secretions into the female vagina.

The penis is divided into an internal *root* and an external *shaft* and *glans*. It is covered with loose skin that extends over the glans as the *prepuce* (foreskin).

Internally, the penile shaft consists mainly of three spongy long *erectile tissues*:

> pair of dorsal *corpora cavernosa* (engorge with blood and effect of erection) and a
>
> single ventral *corpus spongiosum* (contains the urethra).

All three tissues have *lacunae* (or *blood sinuses*) separated by *trabeculae* composed of connective tissue and *trabecular muscle* (or *smooth muscle*).

At the proximal end of the penis, the *corpus spongiosum* dilates into a *bulb* that receives the urethra and ducts of the *bulbourethral glands*. *Corpora cavernosa* diverges into a pair of *crura,* anchoring the penis to the pubic arch and perineal membrane.

Blood supply

A pair of internal *pudendal arteries* supply the penis.

Pudendal arteries branch into a *dorsal artery*, travelling dorsally under the skin of the penis.

Deep artery travels through the corpus cavernosum and supplies blood to the lacunae.

Dorsal arteries supply most of the blood when the penis is flaccid, and the deep arteries supply blood during an erection.

Scrotum

Scrotum is part of the external male genitalia behind and underneath the penis. It is a pouch of skin surrounding and protecting the testicles.

The scrotum contains the testes and the *spermatic cord*, a bundle of *connective tissue*, *testicular blood vessels*, and *ductus deferens* (i.e., *sperm duct*).

Spermatic cord passes up the back of the scrotum and through the external inguinal ring into the inguinal canal.

Spermatic ducts

Spermatic ducts carry sperm from the *testes* to the *urethra*.

Spermatic ducts include:

> *efferent ductules* (leaving the testes);
>
> *duct of epididymis* (highly coiled structure adhering to the posterior side of testes);
>
> muscular *ductus deferens* (travels through the spermatic cord and inguinal canal into the pelvic cavity); and a
>
> short *ejaculatory duct* (carries sperm and seminal vesicle secretions towards the last 2 cm to the urethra).

Urethra completes the path of the sperm to the outside of the body.

Urethra is the duct by which *urine* is conveyed out of the body from the *bladder* and by which *male vertebrates convey semen*.

Gonads

Male gonads are the *testes* that produce sperm and testosterone.

Paired testes are suspended in the scrotal sacs of the scrotum.

Shortly before birth, the fetal testes descend through the inguinal canal into the scrotum.

Low temperature in the scrotum is vital to normal sperm production.

If testes do not descend, surgery or hormonal therapy is required; otherwise, sterility results.

Testis consists of *seminiferous tubules* to produce sperm and *interstitial cells* (Leydig cells) to produce testosterone.

Seminiferous tubule epithelium consists of *germ cells* and *sustentacular cells*.

Germ cells develop into sperm.

Sustentacular cells support and nourish germ cells by forming a *blood-testis barrier* between them and the nearest blood supply.

Like the ovary, the testis has a fibrous capsule of the *tunica albuginea*.

Fibrous septa extend from the *tunica* and divide the interior of the testis into 250–300 compartments of *lobules*.

Lobules contain one to three sperm-producing seminiferous tubules.

Testosterone-secreting interstitial cells lie in clusters in between the tubules.

Gonad anatomy and function

A long, slender *testicular artery* supplies each testis and is drained by pampiniform plexus veins, which converge to form the *testicular vein*.

Testis is supplied with *testicular nerves* and lymphatic vessels.

Epididymis is a coiled tube attached to each testicle for *maturation and storage of sperm*.

Vas deferens and *epididymis* store sperm until ejaculation.

Sperm is *non-motile* while stored in the *vas deferens* and *epididymis*. During the passage through the epididymis, they are concentrated by fluid absorption.

When a male is sexually aroused, the sperm enters the urethra, extending through the penis.

Sperm travels the *vas deferens* into the *ejaculatory duct*, which leads to the *urethra* and *penis*.

Urethra transports urine from the *bladder* during urination.

Blood supply and innervation

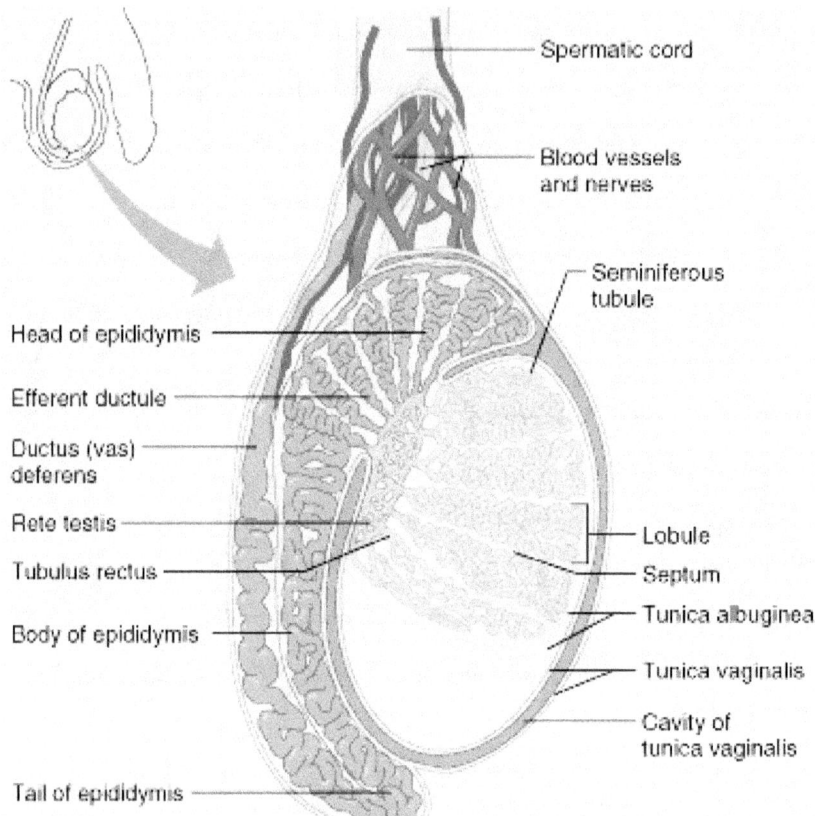

Male reproductive system with blood vessels, ducts and tissue shown

Accessory glands

Males have *three sets* of accessory glands:

    a pair of *seminal vesicles* posterior to the urinary bladder,

    a pair of small *bulbourethral glands* secreting into the proximal end of penile urethra.

    a single *prostate gland* inferior to the bladder (enclosing the prostatic urethra) and

Seminal vesicles lie at the urinary bladder base, which contains two glands that join the *vas deferens* (pl. *vasa deferentia*) to form an ejaculatory duct that enters the urethra.

A thick fluid containing nutrients, including mucus (liquid for the sperm), fructose (for ATP), and prostaglandins, is secreted into the ejaculatory duct.

Bulbourethral glands are below the prostate gland and on either side of the urethra; they release mucous secretions that provide lubrication.

Bulbourethral glands produce a small amount of clear, slippery fluid that lubricates the urethra and neutralizes its pH.

Prostate gland is below the urinary bladder and surrounds the upper portion of the urethra.

Prostate secretes a milky, slightly alkaline solution that promotes sperm motility and viability. This fluid neutralizes urine acidity in the urethra and neutralizes vaginal acidity.

Prostaglandin secretions neutralize seminal fluid, acidic from the metabolic waste of sperm.

Semen

Semen (seminal fluid) is a thick, whitish fluid containing about:

    10% sperm,

    30% glandular secretions from the prostate vesicles, and

    60% secretions from the seminal vesicles and bulbourethral glands.

Semen contains about 50–120 million sperm/mL and *seminogelin* (seminal vesicle protein), a serine protease (prostate-specific antigen), fructose, prostaglandins, and other substances.

The seminal vesicles and prostate secrete most of the semen.

Accessory muscles

Sperm cannot develop at the core body temperature of 37 °C.

Testis is about 2 °C cooler than average body temperature by three structures in the scrotum:

    cremaster muscle of the spermatic cord,

    dartos muscle in the scrotal wall, and the

    pampiniform plexus of veins in the spermatic cord.

Cremaster muscle relaxes when warm and contracts when cool, lowering or raising the scrotum and testes.

Dartos muscle contracts and tautens the scrotum when it is cool.

Pampiniform plexus is a countercurrent heat exchanger cooling blood on its way to the testes.

Sperm pathway

Mnemonic for the path of sperm:

"Seven Up" (Seminiferous tubules, Epididymis, Vas deferens, Ejaculatory duct, nothing, Urethra, Penis).

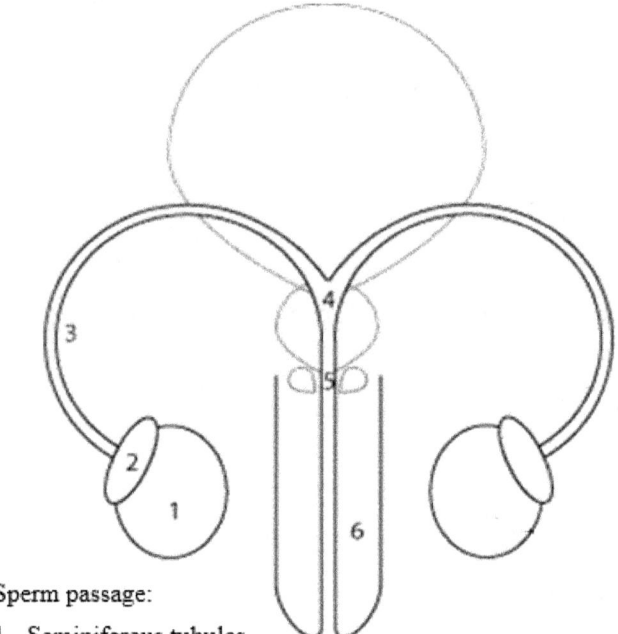

Sperm passage:
1. Seminiferous tubules
2. Epididymis
3. Vas deferens
4. Ejaculatory duct
5. Urethra
6. Penis

Path of sperm from the seminiferous tubules and through the penis as "Seven Up"

Gametogenesis

Gonads produce gametes

Gonads are *primary sex organs* specialized to produce *gametes* (haploid egg and sperm).

Two types of gonads:

      testes, which produce spermatozoa (sperm), and

      ovaries, which produce ova (singular ovum or egg).

Gamete formation

Gametogenesis is the meiotic cell division that produces eggs (oogenesis) and sperm (spermatogenesis).

Meiosis is a nuclear division that is broken into two broad stages (meiosis I and meiosis II), which reduces the chromosome number from *diploid* (2N) to *haploid* (N).

The haploid number is half of the diploid number of chromosomes.

Meiosis of one diploid cell produces four haploid cells.

These daughter cells, containing half the genetic information, are *gametes*.

Before fertilization, the building blocks to create that cell must be available so that the initial *fertilized cell* (i.e., zygote) can develop into an embryo, fetus, and adult.

Gamete development

Developing gametes (egg and sperm) are *germ cells*.

The first stage in their development is the proliferation of primordial germ cells by mitosis (replication via cell division); *daughter cells* receive a *complete set* of chromosomes identical to the original cell.

In females, germ cells' mitosis activity occurs during *embryonic development*, while in males, it begins at *puberty and continues throughout life*.

For years, females were believed to contain all their egg cells at birth. However, recent findings of mitotic activity in female gonads and the idea that females do not produce new eggs during their lifetime are actively researched.

Meiosis

The next stage of development is meiosis; each daughter cell receives half the chromosomes of the original cell.

During meiosis, chromosomes stay in their homologous pairs.

For example, instead of 46 individual human chromosomes, there are 23 chromosome pairs.

Gamete production via meiosis occurs in sexually reproducing eukaryotes, including animals, plants, and fungi.

Sexual reproduction forms gametes.

Human males produce tiny, motile sperm in the testes, and human females produce a large, immobile, nutrient-laden egg or ovum in the ovarian follicles.

Gametes fuse to form a *zygote* with the full or diploid (2N) number of chromosomes.

If gametes contained the same number of chromosomes as somatic (body) cells, the zygote would have twice the correct number of chromosomes.

Diploid zygote

When 1N gametes fuse, the chromosomes from both parents combine in the 2N zygote.

Each fertilized egg (i.e., zygote) cell has a pair of homologous chromosomes, one 1N homolog from the mother (*egg*) and one 1N homolog from the father (*sperm*).

Chromosomes align within the daughter cells in many combinations during meiosis. $(2^{23})^2$ or about 70 trillion combinations are possible without crossing over.

This allows for genetic variability in sexually reproducing organisms.

Crossing over occurs during meiosis I, where homologous chromosomes are paired (synapsis) and exchange some genetic material to form genetically unique (recombinant) chromosomes.

If crossing over occurs once, $(4^{23})^2$ or 70 trillion squared genetically unique zygotes are possible for one couple.

Crossing over is unique to prophase I of meiosis.

Meiosis

Two stages of meiosis

There are two divisions in meiosis: meiosis I and meiosis II.

During meiosis I, homologous chromosomes separate, resulting in two haploid daughter cells with one half the number of chromosomes as the parent cell.

In meiosis II, sister chromatids separate within each haploid cell, producing four haploid daughter cells with the number of chromosomes equal to that of starting cells, essentially acting like a mitotic division of haploid cells

Phases of meiosis I

Meiosis I and meiosis II have four phases: prophase, metaphase, anaphase, and telophase.

Before meiosis I, DNA replication occurs in the S phase of interphase, and each chromosome has a pair of *sister chromatids*.

Sister chromatids are attached at the centromere (like mitosis for somatic cells).

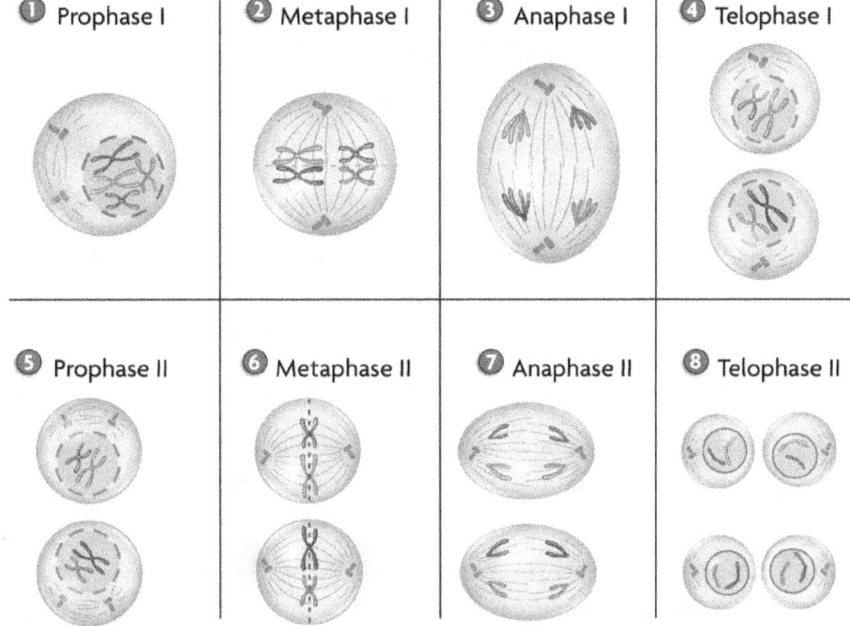

Meiosis I is a reduction stage (2N → 1N), meiosis II separates sister chromatids at the centromere

Meiosis I: reduction phase from diploid to haploid

During meiosis I, homologous chromosomes line up at the synapsis.

Two sets of paired chromosomes (1 from mother and 1 from father) are together as bivalents (tetrads) held by a chiasma complex.

Prophase I

1. Nuclear division occurs: nucleolus disappears, nuclear envelope fragments, centrosomes migrate away from each other, and spindle fibers assemble.

2. Homologous chromosomes undergo synapsis, forming bivalents; crossing over may occur as sister chromatids exchange genetic material by recombination.

3. Chromatin condenses, and chromosomes are microscopically visible.

Metaphase I

1. During prometaphase I, bivalents held by chiasmata move toward the metaphase plate at the equator of the cell.

2. The fully formed spindle aligns the bivalents at the metaphase plate.

3. Kinetochores are proteins associated with centromeres; they attach to *kinetochore spindle fibers* anchored to centrioles at each pole of the cell.

4. Homologous chromosomes independently align at the metaphase plate.

5. Maternal and paternal homologs may be oriented toward either pole.

Anaphase I

1. The homologs separate and move toward opposite poles.

2. Each chromosome is attached with a centromere and two sister chromatids (replicated previously during the S phase).

Telophase I

1. In animals, this occurs at the end of meiosis I.

2. The nuclear envelope reforms and nucleoli reappears.

3. This phase may or may not be accompanied by cytokinesis for portioning the two nuclei with separate plasma membranes (i.e., two daughter cells).

Interkinesis

1. Between meiosis I and meiosis II is like interphase in mitotic divisions.
2. However, no DNA replication (as in S phase of mitosis) occurs; the chromosomes are 1N (each chromosome has a sister chromatid).

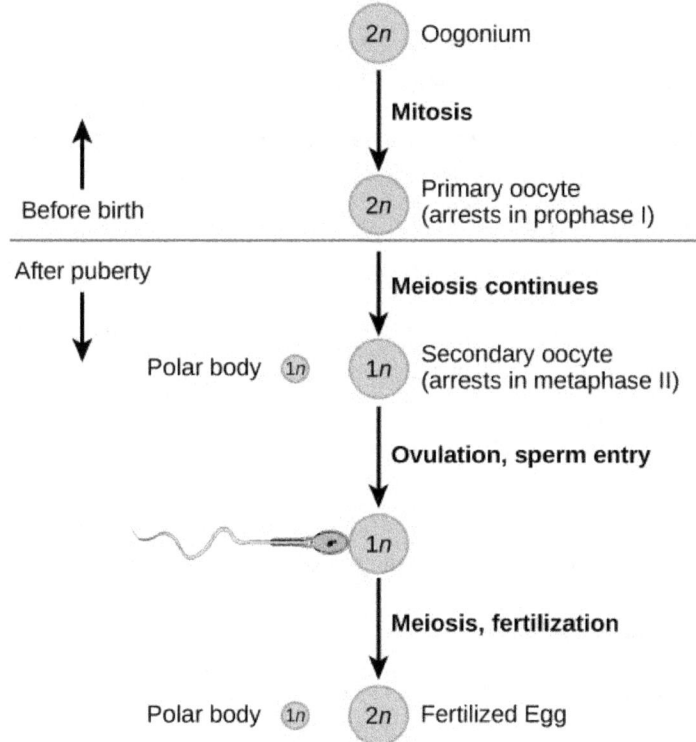

Meiosis generates 4 unique haploid cells, while mitosis generates two identical diploid cells

Meiosis II: 1N → 1N

Before meiosis II, DNA does *not* replicate, and centromere still attaches to sister chromatids.

During meiosis II, the centromeres split, and the sister chromatids separate.

Chromosomes in the four daughter cells contain one chromatid.

Counting the number of centromeres verifies the number of chromosomes.

Fertilization restores diploid number

Fertilization restores the diploid number (2N) in the zygote and somatic cells originating from a zygote.

1. During metaphase II, haploid chromosomes (with sister chromatids) align at the metaphase plate.

2. During anaphase II, sister chromatids separate at the centromeres, and the two daughter chromosomes move toward the poles.

3. Due to crossing over in prophase I, each gamete contains chromosomes with gene combinations, unlike either parent.

4. At the end of telophase II and cytokinesis, there are four haploid cells (1 sperm for males and 1 egg, and 3 polar bodies for females).

5. In animals, the haploid cells mature and develop into gametes, which may fuse into a zygote (2N) from a 1N sperm and 1N egg.

6. In plants, the daughter cells become spores and divide to produce a haploid adult generation.

7. In some fungi and algae, a zygote results from gamete fusion and immediately undergoes meiosis; therefore, the adult is haploid.

Haploid gametes fuse during fertilization

DNA is replicated once before mitosis and meiosis I and II;

> in mitosis, there is *one nuclear division*,
>
> in meiosis, there are *two nuclei divisions* between syntheses of DNA.

In humans, meiosis occurs in reproductive organs to produce gametes, while mitosis occurs in somatic cells (not germline cells) for growth and repair.

Meiosis *vs.* mitosis summary

- During **prophase I** of meiosis, homologous chromosomes pair for crossing over, increasing genetic variation.

    Crossing over does *not* occur during mitosis.

- During **metaphase I** of meiosis, *homologous chromosomes* align at the metaphase plate.

    In mitosis, individual chromosomes align.

- During **anaphase I** of meiosis, homologous chromosomes, with centromeres intact, separate and move to opposite poles.

    In mitosis, *sister chromatids separate* and move to opposite poles.

- During **meiosis II** of meiosis, the stages are the same as mitosis.

- Nuclei contain the *haploid* (1N) number of chromosomes in meiosis.

    Cell contains the *diploid* (2N) number of chromosomes in mitosis.

- Meiosis produces *four* genetically unique *haploid daughter cells* (4 sperm or 1 egg and 3 polar bodies).

    Mitosis produces *two* genetically identical *diploid daughter cells*.

Oogenesis

Ovarian cycle

Oogenesis produces a *single ovum* from a *single primary oocyte*.

Unlike spermatogenesis, the *ovarian cycle* occurs monthly and usually produces one gamete (egg) per month.

Each egg develops in its bubble-like *follicle*, located primarily in the cortex.

Each month, about 20 to 25 *primordial follicles* resume their development.

The single layer of squamous follicular cells around the oocyte thickens into cuboidal cells.

The follicle is a *primary follicle*.

As the egg enlarges, the follicular cells multiply and aggregate into multiple strata; the follicle is a *secondary follicle*, and the follicular cells are *granulosa cells*.

Oogenesis *vs.* spermatogenesis

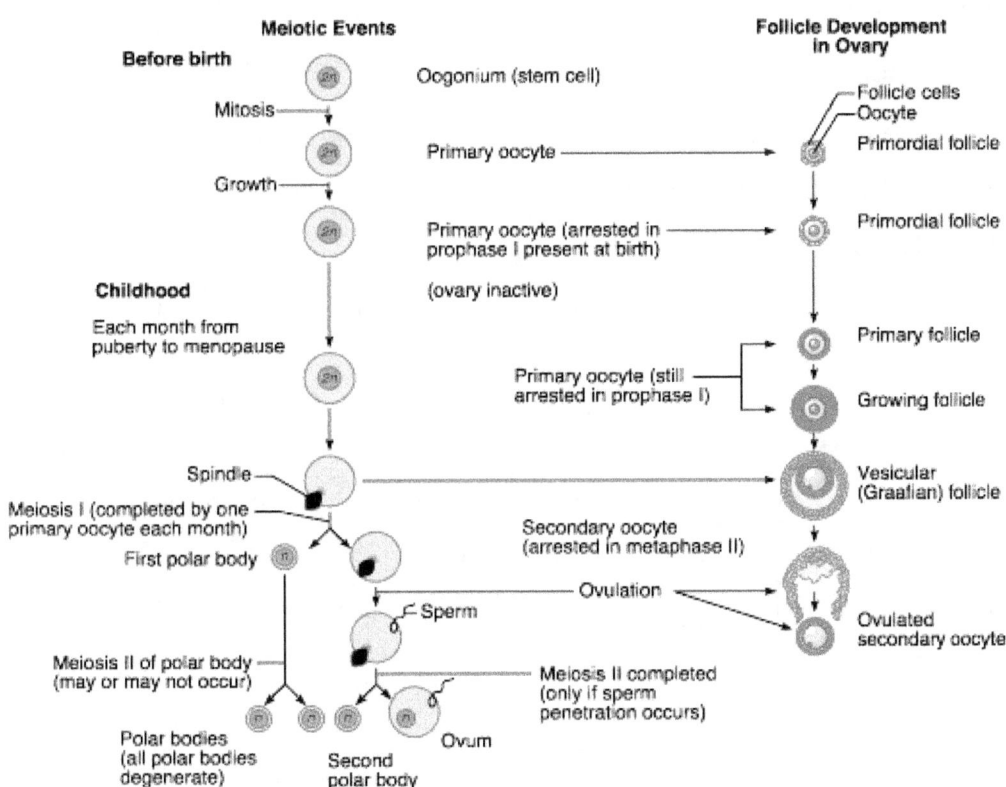

Oocytes

Oogonia are primitive germ cells that undergo mitosis and develop into *primary oocytes* (with 46 chromosomes), the initial cells in oogenesis.

Primary oocytes remain in meiotic arrest (i.e., begin first meiotic development but not completed).

The germ cells in a female are believed to be at this developmental stage at birth.

However, this is an area currently under investigation by researchers.

Primary oocytes are in the ovaries of the female reproductive system.

Oogenesis occurs monthly, beginning at puberty and ending at menopause.

At puberty, primary oocytes are destined for ovulation and complete meiosis, and each daughter cell receives 23 chromosomes.

Although some primary oocytes undergo *atresia* (immature and degraded) during childhood, there are about 300,000 to 400,000 oocytes at puberty.

When the primary oocyte divides, one of the two daughter cells, the *secondary oocyte*, retains most cytoplasm.

Polar bodies

First polar body is the nonfunctional daughter cell and (often) does not proceed to meiosis II.

The secondary oocyte proceeds to metaphase II of meiosis and suspends.

Meiosis II resumes if fertilization occurs.

Completing meiosis II allows the secondary oocyte to become a fertilized egg (2N zygote when fused with the sperm).

Meiotic division produces two *second polar bodies* that disintegrate because they receive insufficient cytoplasm.

The body absorbs second polar bodies and retains most of the egg's cytoplasm.

The cytoplasm serves as a source of nutrients for the developing embryo.

This is different from spermatogenesis, in which four functional, mature sperm are produced from a single spermatogonium.

Ovum development

An oocyte is a *developing egg*.

Oocytes undergo two separate *meiotic cell divisions* before becoming a mature *ovum*.

Oocytes differentiate into a mature egg (or ovum) by meiosis when germ cells complete two final, highly specialized divisions.

A single ovum is produced per month.

Ovulation

Typically, one tertiary follicle becomes a fully mature *vesicular* (Graafian) or *tertiary follicle* destined to ovulate.

Ovulation occurs around day 14 of a typical cycle.

Follicle swells and bursts, releasing the egg and *cumulus oophorus* (a mass of follicular cells surrounding the ovum in the vesicular ovarian follicle) into the opening of the uterine tube.

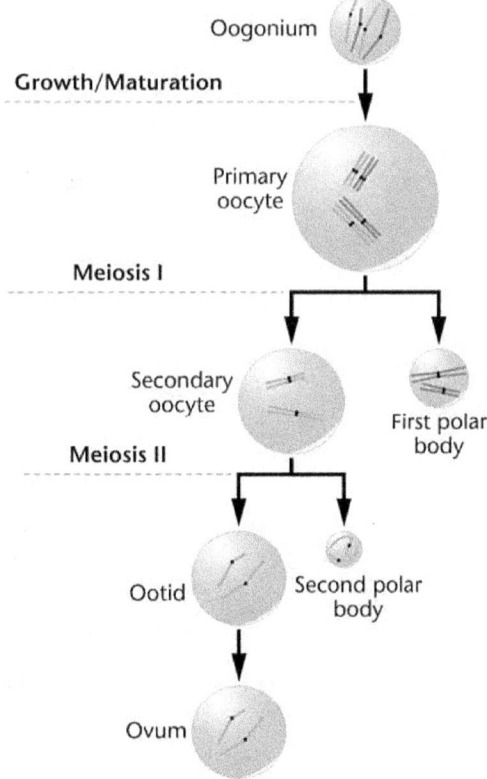

Female oogenesis with 1 ovum and (up to) 3 polar bodies

Notes for active learning

Spermatogenesis

Sperm formation

In human males, meiosis is part of *spermatogenesis*, producing sperm in the testes.

In human females, meiosis is in *oogenesis*, the production of egg cells occurring in ovaries.

Spermatogenesis occurs in the *seminiferous tubules* in the testes and produces *sperm* from *primary spermatocytes*.

Primary and secondary spermatocytes

Spermatogonia are undifferentiated germ cells that divide by mitosis and differentiate into *primary spermatocytes*.

Primary spermatocytes grow and undergo the *first meiotic division* to form *secondary spermatocytes*.

Spermatid formation

In secondary spermatocyte stage, cells undergo a *second meiotic division* to form *spermatids*.

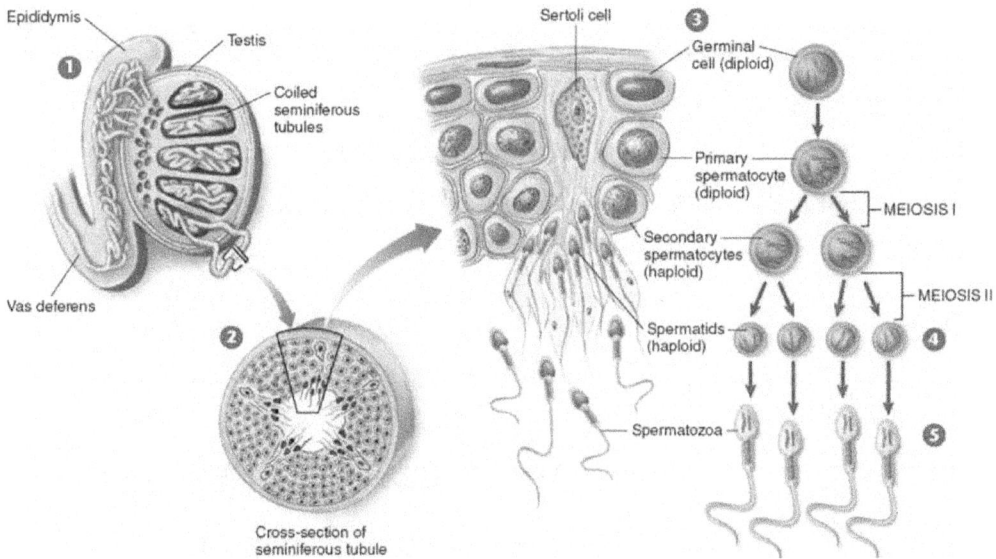

Testis and spermatogenesis. Mitosis (2N) is followed by meiosis I (1N) and meiosis II (1N)

Spermatogonium

Spermatogonium replicates all its chromosomes during interphase.

Spermatogonium has 46 primary spermatocyte chromosomes, and each chromosome is two sister chromatids joined by a centromere.

Cells undergo prophase I, where homologous chromosomes line up on spindles at the equator.

Cells undergo anaphase I (reduction phase of meiosis), but the centromeres do not divide; the *homologous chromosome pairs* separate.

During telophase I, two cells are formed.

Each cell is a secondary spermatocyte that contains 23 chromosomes (i.e., haploid cells), and each chromosome has *two chromatids* joined by a centromere.

Meiosis II

Haploid cells undergo meiosis II:

> prophase II, metaphase II, anaphase II, and telophase II.

This second set of divisions *does* resemble mitosis.

Chromosomes condense (but do not pair up) during prophase II.

Chromosomes align by spindle fibers during metaphase II, and the centromeres divide during anaphase II. The cells finish dividing during telophase II.

At end of meiosis II, there are *four haploid cells* with 23 chromosomes.

Spermatids, formed from the division of the secondary spermatocytes, develop into mature *spermatozoa* (or *sperm*).

Sertoli cells

Sertoli cells are stimulated by follicle-stimulating hormone (FSH) in the seminiferous tubules and surround and nourish spermatids during differentiation.

Spermatids complete maturation (e.g., a gain of motility) in the *epididymis*.

Sertoli cells secrete peptide hormones:

> *inhibin* (acts on the pituitary gland to inhibit FSH release) and
>
> *androgen-binding protein* (binds testosterone and is an intermediary between germ cells and hormones).

Sertoli cells divide the tubules into compartments with different environments where stages of spermatogenesis continue.

Leydig cells and epididymides

Leydig cells between tubules produce testosterone in presence of luteinizing hormone (LH).

Sperm produced in the testes mature within the *epididymides*.

Epididymides are tightly coiled tubules outside of the testes.

Maturation time in the epididymis is required for sperm to develop the ability to swim.

Once sperm matures, they are propelled into the *vasa deferentia* by muscular contractions.

Sperm is stored in the epididymides and the vasa deferentia.

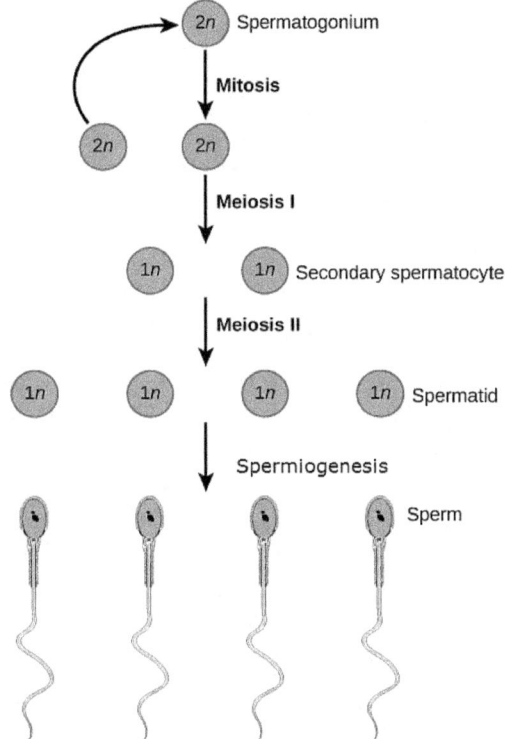

Male spermatogenesis with haploid secondary spermatocytes (1N) and spermatids (1N)

Notes for active learning

Gametes' Structure and Functions

Female *vs.* male gametes

Ovum (or unfertilized egg cell) is the female gamete.

Unlike sperm, the egg is not capable of active movement.

The egg is much larger than the sperm (visible to the naked eye).

Human sperm is about 55 micrometers (μm) long (head is 5 μm, and flagellum is 50 μm).

A mature ovum is between 120-150 μm in diameter.

Therefore, the ratio of the length of the sperm to the diameter of the egg is about 1:3.

Male	Female	Difference
Spermatogonium (2N)	Oogonium (2N)	Spermatogonium renews its population by mitosis throughout life. Oogonium stops renewing its population before birth
Primary spermatocyte (1 N)	Primary oocyte (1N)	Primary oocyte arrests at prophase I
Secondary spermatocyte (1N)	Secondary oocyte (1N)	Secondary oocyte arrests at metaphase II
Sperm (1N)	Ovum (1N)	Between the secondary spermatocyte and sperm is the spermatid

Egg morphology

Compared with the width of a sperm cell (~3 μm) to an egg's diameter, the ratio is about 1:50. Eggs are non-motile and filled with cytoplasm.

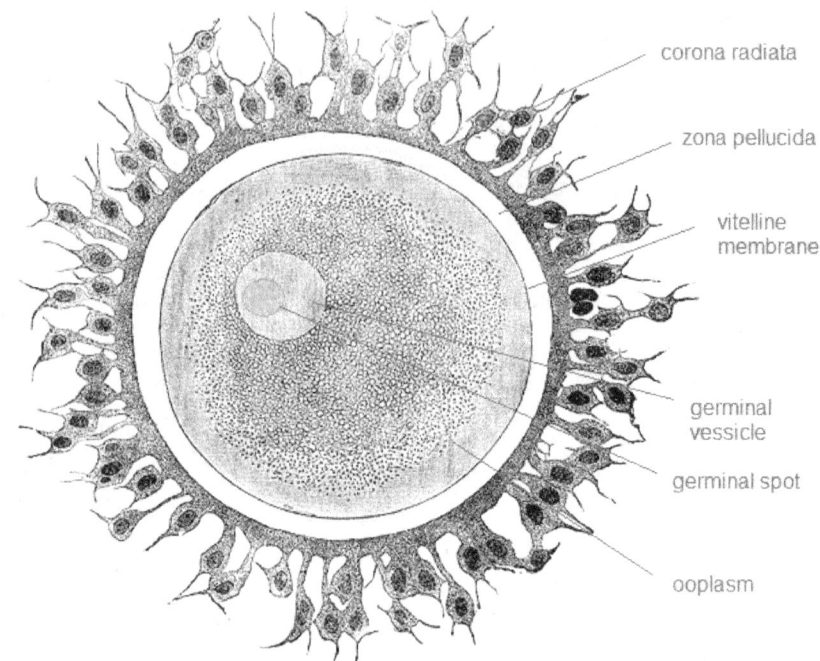

Human ovum with the protective glycoprotein layer of zona pellucida and inner vitelline membrane enclosing the ooplasm

Granulosa cell

Granulosa cells produce a glycoprotein gel layer as the *zona pellucida* around the egg; the connective tissue around the granulosa cells condenses into a tough fibrous *theca folliculi*.

Granulosa cells secrete *follicular fluid*, which forms small pools.

The follicle is *tertiary* with continued proliferation of granulosa and theca cells, increased thecal vascularization, and further oocyte enlargement.

Ovary functions as an endocrine organ when transitioning from secondary to tertiary follicles.

Fluid pools eventually coalesce to form a single cavity, the *antrum*.

The egg is held against one side of the antrum by a mound of cumulus oophorus cells; the innermost layer of these cells is the *corona radiata*.

Sperm morphology and mechanisms

Sperm is compact cells of haploid male DNA with flagella that provide motility.

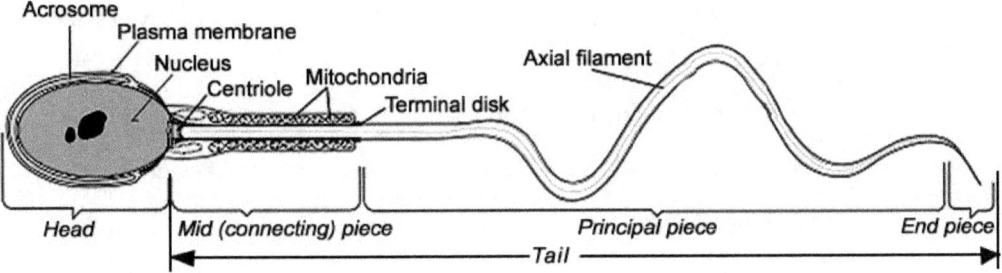

Human spermatozoon with head, midpiece, and tail with mitochondria for motility

Spermatozoa

Spermatozoa (i.e., mature sperm) have the following.

Sperm head (haploid with 23 chromosomes) has a nucleus and DNA covered by an acrosome.

Acrosome is a cap-like covering over the anterior end of the nucleus that stores enzymes to help sperm penetrate the several layers of cells and thick membrane enclosing the egg.

Middle piece contains multiple mitochondria wrapped around microtubules of the flagellum in a 9 + 2 microtubule array for energy.

Tail has microtubules as a flagellum for its whip-like movement, propelling sperm.

Ejaculate of a human male contains several hundred million sperm.

Fewer than 100 reach the vicinity of an egg, and usually, only one sperm enters an egg.

Egg and sperm contributions during fertilization

Sexual reproduction produces offspring that combine genes from each parent.

It is the union of two gametes (i.e., *ovum* and *sperm*) to form a zygote (i.e., *fertilized egg*).

Gametes contain half the genetic information needed to produce the 2N progeny.

Sperm contributes chromosomal DNA, as the egg actively destroys *sperm mitochondria*.

Egg contributes chromosomal DNA and mitochondria, organelles, and biomolecules within the ooplasm within the large volume of the cytoplasm.

Cytoplasmic volume requirements drive the partitions of gametes into 1 large egg and 3 small, non-functional *polar bodies*.

Cytoplasmic nutrients and biomolecules

Egg contains *cytoplasm nutrients* and *biomolecules* needed by a developing embryo.

A diploid zygote (haploid sperm and haploid egg) represents the first stage in developing a genetically unique organism.

Zygote contains essential components for development with genes on chromosomes.

Zygote genes are not activated to produce proteins until after several cleavage divisions.

During cleavage, the large zygote subdivides into cells of conventional size via mitosis.

After preliminary cleavage, blastomeres are the initial cells of an organism's development.

Sexual Development

Male and female sexual maturity

Ovaries produce *estradiol* and *progesterone*. Estradiol is the female hormone estrogen.

Testes produce *testosterone*, which is the main sex hormone in males. Testosterone is an androgen, which has masculinizing effects.

Androgens are not unique to males, and estrogens are not unique to females.

Many male and female reproductive system organs develop from the same embryonic organs.

Organs with the same embryonic precursor are *homologous*.

For example, the scrotum and labia majora are homologous because each develops from the labioscrotal folds.

Secondary sex organs are anatomical structures needed to produce offspring, such as the male glands, ducts, penis, female uterine tubes, uterus, and vagina.

Secondary sex characteristics are not essential to reproduction but help attract mates by indicating sexual maturity (e.g., breasts).

Secondary sex characteristics comprise the *external differences* between males and females.

Reproductive organs mature during puberty

Puberty is when reproductive organs mature, and reproduction becomes possible.

Puberty is initiated by the secretion of *gonadotropin-releasing hormone.*

(GnRH) by the hypothalamus. GnRH stimulates the release of *follicle-stimulating hormone* (FSH) and *luteinizing hormone* (LH) by the anterior pituitary.

FSH and LH act upon gonads to stimulate the development of sperm and ova and the secretion of sex hormones.

Sex hormones exert negative feedback on the secretion of GnRH, FSH, and LH.

Visible changes at puberty are from hormones (e.g., testosterone, estrogens, growth hormone).

After puberty, the individual attains fertility.

Adolescence continues until full adult height is attained.

Secondary male characteristics

The earliest visible sign of male puberty is an enlargement of the testes and scrotum; the ejaculation of motile sperm marks the completion of puberty.

Testosterone has three prominent roles:

1) stimulating the development of prenatal genitalia,

2) stimulating the development of male secondary sexual characteristics, such as the growth of skeletal muscle (longer legs and broader shoulders), development of pubic hair, facial hair, and chest hair, and

3) maintaining sex drive during adulthood. It stimulates the secretion of oil and sweat glands (i.e., attributed to body odor and acne).

Testosterone prompts the *larynx* and *vocal cords* to enlarge, resulting in a deeper voice.

Testosterone triggers baldness if "baldness genes" are present and regulates testosterone synthesis by acting on Leydig cells to stimulate testosterone secretion.

Secondary female characteristics

Female puberty is marked by:

thelarche (e.g., the onset of breast development),

pubarche (e.g., the appearance of pubic and axillary hair), and

menarche (i.e., the onset of menstruation).

Regular ovulation and fertility are attained about a year after menarche.

Estrogens maintain the development of related organs and female secondary sex characteristics.

Females have less body and facial hair and more fat beneath skin (i.e., a rounded appearance).

In females, the pelvic girdle enlarges, and the pelvic cavity is larger for wider hips.

Female breast development

Estrogen and progesterone are required for breast development.

Female breast has a conical or *pendulous body* and a narrower *axillary tail* extending toward the armpit. *Breast* contains 15–24 lobules, each with a mammary duct.

Nipple is at the apex and is surrounded by a zone of darker skin as the *areola*.

Areola has small *areolar glands* that may appear as bumps around the nipple. They produce a secretion that prevents chafing and cracking of the skin in a nursing mother.

Mammary duct begins at the nipple and divides into ducts that end in alveoli (blind sacs).

Prolactin hormone is for *lactation* (milk production) to begin.

The feedback inhibition suppresses the prolactin production of estrogens and progesterone in the anterior pituitary during pregnancy.

Therefore, it takes a couple of days after delivering a baby for milk production to begin.

Before this, the breasts produce a watery, yellowish-white fluid (*colostrum*) similar to milk but containing more protein and less fat, rich in IgA antibodies that provide immunity to a newborn.

Female hormone fluctuations

Breast cancer is a common cancer in females; women should have regular breast exams and mammograms as recommended.

At midlife, sexes go through a period of hormonal and physical changes of *climacteric*. This is marked by a decline in testosterone or estrogen secretion and a rise in FSH and LH secretion.

Female climacteric is accompanied by *menopause*, cessation of ovarian function and fertility.

Menopause is the age-related cessation of menstrual periods a decrease in the *number* of ovarian follicles and their *hypo-responsiveness to gonadotropins*.

Plasma estrogen levels decrease, resulting in high gonadotropin secretion.

A decrease in bone mass of osteoporosis occurs, hot flashes or the sudden dilation of arterioles, which increases body temperature and sweating.

Male reproductive cycle

Hypothalamus controls the testes' sexual function through the secretion of GnRH.

GnRH stimulates the pituitary to produce the gonadotropic hormones FSH and LH in the anterior pituitary gland.

FSH promotes male spermatogenesis by stimulating primary spermatocytes to undergo meiosis I (forming secondary spermatocytes).

FSH enhances Sertoli cells (nurse cell that helps develop sperm) by causing them to bind to androgens effectively.

In males, LH is an *interstitial cell-stimulating hormone* (ICSH).

LH acts on Leydig's cells and stimulates testosterone production and secretion.

Sperm production rate

Sustentacular cells of the seminiferous tubules release the hormone *inhibin*, which regulates the rate of sperm production and produces an androgen-binding protein, making the testes responsive to testosterone.

Hypothalamus-pituitary-testis system uses a *negative feedback* relationship that maintains a relatively *constant* production of sperm and testosterone.

Although hormone and gamete production is constant in males, this is not true for females.

Neural control of sexual arousal

The penis contains vascular compartments and arteries.

Typically, these vessels are constricted with little blood, causing the penis to remain flaccid.

During sexual arousal, nervous reflexes cause an increase in the arterial blood flow to the penis.

Nerves of the penis converge on a pair of *dorsal nerves*, which lead via the *internal pudendal nerves* to the sacral plexus and then the spinal cord.

Penis receives *sympathetic*, *parasympathetic*, and *somatic motor nerve fibers*.

Sexual excitation

Sexual excitation in higher brain centers, stimulation of mechanoreceptors in the penis, *inhibition of sympathetic fibers*, and release of *nitric oxide* contribute to arteriole dilation.

Dilation causes these compartments to engorge with blood at high pressure.

Erection results from increased blood flow fills and distends the erectile tissue, making the penis elongated and rigid.

Erectile dysfunction is the inability to achieve an erection due to physiological or psychological causes.

Viagra and related products release *nitrous oxide* (NO) and block the breakdown of cGMP, a messenger involved in the relaxation of the arterial smooth muscle, promoting erection.

Ejaculation

Stimulation of sympathetic nerves contracts the smooth muscles lining the ducts and discharges semen through the urethra.

Sphincter at base of the urinary bladder is closed so sperm cannot enter the bladder, and urine is not expelled.

Ejaculation is the expulsion of semen and is achieved at the peak of sexual arousal.

Emission is the *first phase of ejaculation.*

Nerve impulses from the spine trigger the epididymides and vasa deferentia to contract.

Subsequent motility causes the sperm to enter the ejaculatory duct.

Secretions are released from seminal vesicles, the prostate gland, and the bulbourethral glands.

A small amount of secretion from the bulbourethral glands may leak from the end of the penis to clean the urethra of acid, but it may contain sperm.

Expulsion is the *second phase of ejaculation.*

Rhythmical contractions at *penis base* and within the *urethral wall* expel the semen in spurts.

Rhythmical contractions are *myotonia* (muscle tenseness) release, a crucial sexual response.

Ejaculation lasts for a limited time, and the penis returns to a flaccid state following ejaculation.

Refractory period follows when stimulation does not result in an erection.

Orgasm

Orgasm is a physiological and psychological sensation at the climax of sexual stimulation.

During orgasm, heart rate and blood pressure increase, and skeletal muscles contract.

Clitoris in females contains many sensory receptors as a sexually sensitive organ.

Female orgasm releases neuromuscular tension in the genital area, vagina, and uterus muscles.

Notes for active learning

Hormonal Control of Ovarian Cycle

Female ovarian cycle

In longitudinal cross-section, an ovary has *cellular follicles*, each with an *oocyte* (egg).

A female is born with up to two million follicles.

The number is reduced to 300,000–400,000 by puberty, and a small number of follicles (about 400) fully mature.

As a follicle matures, it develops from a *primary* to a *secondary follicle* to a vesicular follicle (Graafian).

As oogenesis occurs, a secondary follicle contains a secondary oocyte pushed to one side of the fluid-filled cavity.

The vesicular follicle fills with fluid until the follicle wall balloons out on the surface and bursts, releasing a secondary oocyte surrounded by a *zona pellucida* and *follicular cells*.

During the *follicular phase*, FSH and LH stimulate primary follicles (containing primary oocytes) to grow and stimulate *theca cells*, expressing receptors for LH to produce androstenedione (androgen).

Menstrual cycle

Endometrium undergoes cyclic histological changes are the *menstrual cycle*, governed by the shifting hormonal secretions of the ovaries.

FSH, LH, estrogen, and progesterone are in a complex interaction to regulate menstruation.

An average 28-day uterine cycle is divided into four phases.

Proliferative phase is the mitotic rebuilding of tissue lost in the previous menstrual period and is primarily regulated by estrogens.

Secretory phase is regulated primarily by progesterone and consists of a thickening of the endometrium by secretions (not mitosis).

Premenstrual phase is ischemia and necrosis of the endometrium.

Menstrual phase

Menstrual phase begins when endometrial tissue and blood are first discharged from the vagina and mark day 1 of a new cycle.

Decline in ovarian secretions of progesterone and estrogen triggers the menstrual phase.

Menstrual cycle begins on day 1, with *menstruation* (sloughing of endometrium with bleeding).

During days 1 to 5, low levels of estrogen and progesterone cause menstruation.

Menstruation is the periodic shedding of tissue and blood from the endometrium; this lining disintegrates, and the blood vessels rupture.

Menses

Menses is the flow of blood and tissues discharged from the vagina.

FSH from the anterior pituitary stimulates the growth of a follicle in the ovary (the follicular phase), which secretes estrogen as it grows.

After day 5, the rising estrogen levels stimulate the uterus to grow a new inner lining.

Between days 6 and 13, increased production of estrogens by an ovarian follicle causes the endometrium to thicken and become vascular and glandular (proliferative phase).

By day 14, the endometrial lining is thick.

LH surge

LH surge from anterior pituitary releases oocytes and some ovarian follicular cells (ovulation).

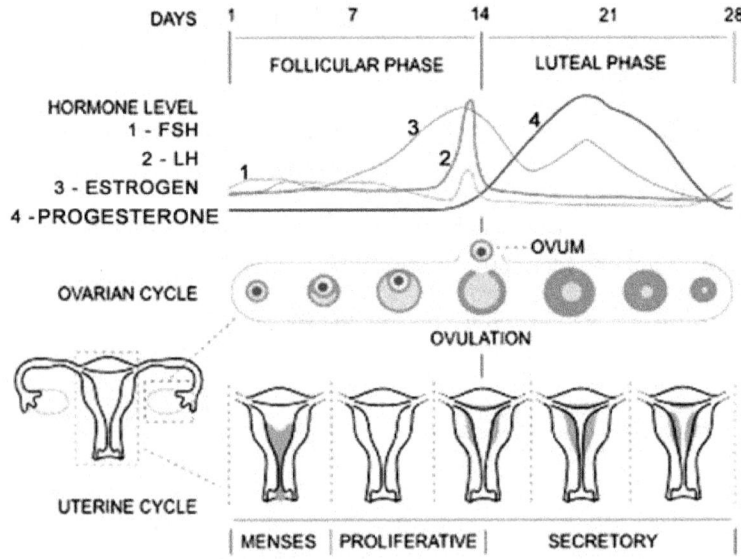

Female ovarian and uterine cycles with associated hormone levels

Endometrium formation

As a response to LH, androgens are converted into estrogen by follicle-stimulating (FSH-induced) hormone by granulosa cells.

Estrogen leads to the thickening of the endometrium (uterine epithelium).

As estrogen levels rise, it exerts feedback control over the anterior pituitary secretion of FSH, causing the follicular phase to end.

As FSH decreases, the follicles cannot be maintained, and all but one follicle degenerates.

One dominant follicle (*Graafian follicle*) survives because it is:

      1) hyperresponsive to FSH and can maintain itself under low FSH, and

      2) sensitive to LH.

Estrogen levels rise, causing hypothalamus to secrete GnRH, causing a surge in LH secretion.

LH does not drop but shoots up (LH surge) because increased estrogen exerts *positive feedback* on the pituitary's LH-releasing mechanism.

LH spike triggers *ovulation,* while the remaining follicular cells become the *corpus luteum.*

Notes for active learning

Hormonal Control of Female Reproductive Cycle

Ovulation

Ovulation is the rupture of *vesicular follicle* discharging a 2° oocyte into the pelvic cavity.

Ovulation usually occurs on day 14 of the 28-day cycle.

Secondary oocyte completes a second meiotic cell division when fertilization occurs. Meanwhile, the follicle develops into the *corpus luteum* (promoted by LH), which secretes progesterone.

Days 15 through 28 have increased progesterone production by the corpus luteum, causing the endometrium to double in thickness.

Uterine glands mature, producing a thick mucoid secretion (secretory phase).

Endometrium is now prepared to receive an embryo.

Progesterone is the hormone responsible for maintaining the endometrium.

Pregnancy maintains endometrium

Progesterone and estrogen levels decline *without pregnancy,* causing the lining to degrade and shed, initiating the next cycle.

With low levels of progesterone, the uterine lining begins to degenerate.

If pregnancy does not occur, the corpus luteum degenerates in about 14 days, and estrogen and progesterone levels recede.

Lack of estrogen and progesterone collapses vascular endometrium, leading to menstruation.

During menstruation, the anterior pituitary increases FSH production; a follicle begins maturation.

Ovarian cycle controls the *uterine cycle*.

Hormonal response to fertilization

Ovarian cycle is under the control of gonadotropic hormones FSH and LH in females.

Gonadotropic hormones are not constant but are secreted at varying rates during the cycle.

Luteal phase in the ovary (corresponding to the uterus's secretory phase) is the second half of the ovarian cycle following ovulation.

Progesterone and estrogen from the corpus luteum inhibit the normal functioning of GnRH, which slows the production of FSH and LH.

Progesterone converts the endometrium into a secretory tissue full of glycogen and blood vessels, ready to receive a fertilized egg.

As progesterone levels in the blood rise, negative feedback decreases the anterior pituitary's secretion of LH, and the corpus luteum degenerates.

If fertilization does occur, the corpus luteum persists for about three months.

For example, postcoital contraceptives (e.g., Plan B) include progesterone antagonists that prevent progesterone from binding to receptors, leading to erosion of the endometrium.

When oral contraceptives (i.e., birth control pills) are used, synthetic progesterone and estrogen inhibit pituitary gonadotropin release, thereby preventing ovulation.

Female and male infertility

Infertility is a condition where conception is difficult, but the individual *can conceive*.

Sterility means a person *cannot conceive*, regardless of medical or surgical interventions.

Major causes of female infertility:

    1) blocked oviducts

    2) failure to ovulate due to low body weight (<10-15%)

    3) *endometriosis*, the spread of uterine tissue beyond the uterus

    4) atypical hormone levels

Major causes of male sterility and infertility:

    1) low sperm count

    2) abnormal sperm from disease, radiation, chemical mutagens, or excessive heat near the testes

    3) atypical hormone levels

Viviparity

Mammals, including humans, are *viviparous*; the embryo develops in the female's body.

There are many forms of viviparity, but the most developed form is *placental viviparity*, where the mother constantly supplies the nutrients needed for development (e.g., placenta).

Human pregnancies are typically about *40 weeks* from the *first day* of the *last menstrual period*.

When the fetal brain matures, the hypothalamus causes the pituitary to stimulate the adrenal cortex to release androgens.

Hormonal Control of Gestation and Birthing

Pregnancy

Placental cells produce *human chorionic gonadotropin* (hCG), which maintains corpus luteum.

Human chorionic gonadotropin hormone is detected about 11 days after conception. Home pregnancy tests rely on the presence of HCG to confirm pregnancy.

In general, the level of HCG

> doubles every 48 hours during the first four weeks of pregnancy,
>
> doubles every 72 hours by 7-8 weeks, and
>
> peaks at 11-12 weeks of pregnancy.

Corpus luteum

Corpus luteum produces *progesterone* and *estrogen*, maintaining uterus during first trimester.

HCG maintains the corpus luteum until the placenta produces its progesterone and estrogen, as the corpus luteum regresses.

Progesterone and *estrogen* have two effects at this stage:

> inhibit anterior pituitary, so no new follicles mature,
>
> maintain uterus lining, so the corpus luteum is not needed, eliminating menstrual cycles during pregnancy.

Parturition

Childbirth (or *parturition*) is the completion of pregnancy and includes *labor* and *delivery*.

Placenta uses androgen precursors for estrogens stimulating prostaglandin and oxytocin.

Estrogen, prostaglandin, and oxytocin cause uterus to contract rhythmically and expel the fetus.

Labor

Labor is a series of strong uterine contractions and has three stages:

> 1) cervix thins and dilates; amniotic sac ruptures and releases fluids;
>
> 2) rapid uterine contractions, followed by the birth of a newborn;
>
> 3) uterus contracts and expels the umbilical cord and placenta.

The cervix dilates, and the newborn moves through the vagina.

Delivery

Delivery is the process of giving birth from the uterus or womb.

Following birth:

- oxygen is now supplied by breathing with functional lungs;
- switch from fetal circulation, which bypasses lungs and liver, to normal circulation (closing ducts and openings);
- nutrients now come from suckling rather than from the mother's blood.

Breast development during pregnancy

Outside of pregnancy or lactation, the breast is primarily adipose and fibrous tissue with small traces of mammary glands.

Estrogen and progesterone secretion at the onset of puberty leads to breast enlargement due to the development of the duct system.

During pregnancy, the ducts grow, and branch and secretory *acini* (cell clusters) develop at the ends of the smallest branches.

During pregnancy, estrogen stimulates the secretion of prolactin and placental lactogen, stimulating the development of the glands (the alveoli) in breasts.

During pregnancy, milk secretion is *inhibited* by estrogen and progesterone.

The inhibitory effect stops after childbirth once the placenta is removed.

Lactation

Lactation is the *secretion of milk* by the mammary glands.

Milk secretion is maintained by releasing prolactin from afferent input from nipple receptors to the hypothalamus during suckling.

Dopamine (inhibiting prolactin) secretion regulates *milk secretion*.

Milk ejection from the alveoli to ducts is stimulated by oxytocin, released by the suckling reflex.

Suckling inhibits hypothalamic-pituitary-ovarian (HPO) axis hormones, which, in effect, blocks ovulation.

Breast is internally divided into lobes, each with a *lactiferous duct* conveying milk to the nipple.

Each duct expands into a *lactiferous sinus* just beneath the skin of the nipple.

Acini have contractile *myoepithelial cells* responding to oxytocin, causing milk flow in ducts.

Notes for active learning

Notes for active learning

APPENDIX

Glossary of Anatomy & Physiology Terms

Abdominopelvic cavity – the division of the anterior (or *ventral*) cavity that contains the abdominal and pelvic viscera.

Anabolism – assembly of more complex molecules from simpler molecules.

Anatomical position – standard reference position used for describing locations and directions on the human body. Refers to the positioning of the body when it is standing upright and facing forward with each arm hanging on either side of the body and the palms facing forward. The legs are parallel, with feet flat on the floor and facing forward.

Anatomy – studies the form and composition of the body's structures.

Anterior (or *ventral*) – describes the front or direction toward the front of the body.

Anterior cavity (or *ventral cavity*) – larger body cavity located anterior to the posterior (dorsal) body cavity; includes the serous membrane-lined pleural cavities for the lungs, pericardial cavity for the heart, and peritoneal cavity for the abdominal and pelvic organs.

Catabolism – breaking down more complex molecules into simpler molecules.

Caudal (or *inferior*) – describes a position below or lower than another body part proper, near or toward the tail (in humans, the coccyx, or the lowest part of the spinal column).

Cell – smallest independently functioning unit of all organisms; in animals, a cell contains cytoplasm, composed of fluid and organelles.

Computed tomography (CT) – medical imaging technique in which a computer-enhanced cross-sectional X-ray image is obtained.

Control center – compares values to normal range; deviations cause activation of an effector.

Cranial (or *superior*) – describes a position above or higher than another body part proper.

Cranial cavity – the division of the posterior (dorsal) cavity that encloses the brain.

CT (computed tomography) – medical imaging technique in which a computer-enhanced cross-sectional X-ray image is obtained.

Deep – describes a position farther from the surface of the body.

Development – changes an organism goes through during its life.

Differentiation – a process by which unspecialized cells become specialized in structure and function.

Distal – describes a position farther from the point of attachment or the body trunk.

Dorsal (or *posterior*) – describes the back or direction toward the back of the body.

Dorsal cavity (or *posterior body cavity*) – encloses the brain and spinal cord.

Effector – an organ that causes a change in a value.

Frontal plane – a two-dimensional, vertical plane dividing the body or organ into anterior and posterior portions.

Gross anatomy (or *macroscopic anatomy*) – the study of the larger structures of the body, typically with the unaided eye.

Growth – the process of increasing in size.

Homeostasis – steady-state of body systems that living organisms maintain.

Inferior (or *caudal*) – describes a position below or lower than another part of the body proper, near or toward the tail (in humans, the coccyx or lowest part of the spinal column).

Lateral – describes the side or direction toward the side of the body.

Macroscopic anatomy (or *gross anatomy*) – the study of the larger structures of the body, typically with the unaided eye.

Magnetic resonance imaging (MRI) – a medical imaging technique in which a device generates a magnetic field to obtain detailed sectional images of the body's internal structures.

Medial – describes the middle or direction toward the middle of the body.

Metabolism – the sum of all the body's chemical reactions.

Microscopic anatomy – the study of tiny body structures using magnification.

MRI (magnetic resonance imaging) – a medical imaging technique in which a device generates a magnetic field to obtain detailed sectional images of the body's internal structures.

Negative feedback – the homeostatic mechanism that tends to stabilize an upset in the body's physiological condition by preventing an excessive response to a stimulus, typically as the stimulus is removed.

Normal range – the value of values around the set point that does not cause a reaction by the control center.

Nutrient – chemical obtained from foods and beverages critical to human survival.

Organ system – a group of organs that coordinate to perform a particular function.

Organism – a living being with a cellular structure that can independently perform all physiologic functions necessary for life.

Organ – a functionally distinct structure composed of two or more types of tissues.

Pericardium – the sac that encloses the heart.

Peritoneum – a serous membrane that lines the abdominopelvic cavity and covers the organs found there.

PET (positron emission tomography) – medical imaging technique in which radiopharmaceuticals are traced to reveal metabolic and physiological functions in tissues.

Physiology – studies the chemistry, biochemistry, and physics of the body's functions.

Plane – the imaginary two-dimensional surface that passes through the body.

Pleura – a serous membrane that lines the pleural cavity and covers the lungs.

Positive feedback – the mechanism that intensifies a change in the body's physiological condition in response to a stimulus.

Positron emission tomography (PET) – medical imaging technique in which radiopharmaceuticals are traced to reveal metabolic and physiological functions in tissues.

Posterior cavity (or *dorsal cavity*) – houses the brain and spinal cord.

Posterior (or *dorsal*) – describes the back or direction toward the back of the body.

Pressure – the force exerted by a substance in contact with another substance.

Prone – face down.

Proximal – describes a position nearer to the point of attachment or the trunk of the body.

Receptor (or *sensor*) – reports a monitored physiological value to the control center.

Regional anatomy – the study of the structures that contribute to specific body regions.

Renewal – the process by which worn-out cells are replaced.

Reproduction – the process by which new organisms are generated.

Responsiveness – the ability of an organism or a system to adjust to changes in conditions.

Sagittal plane – two-dimensional, vertical plane that divides the body or organ into right and left sides.

Section (in anatomy) – a single flat surface of a three-dimensional structure cut through.

Sensor (or r*eceptor*) – reports a monitored physiological value to the control center.

Serosa (or *serous membrane*) – a membrane that covers organs and reduces friction.

Serous membrane (or *serosa*) – a membrane that covers organs and reduces friction.

Setpoint – ideal value for a physiological parameter; the level or small range within which a physiological parameter such as blood pressure is stable and optimally healthful within its homeostasis parameters.

Spinal cavity (or *vertebral cavity*) – a division of the dorsal cavity containing the spinal cord.

Superficial – describes a position nearer to the surface of the body.

Superior (or *cranial*) – a position above or higher than another body part.

Supine – face up.

Systemic anatomy – the study of the structures that contribute to specific body systems.

Thoracic cavity – a division of the anterior (or *ventral*) cavity that houses the heart, lungs, esophagus, and trachea.

Tissue – a group of similar or closely related cells that perform a specific function.

Transverse plane – a two-dimensional, horizontal plane dividing the body (or organ) into superior and inferior portions.

Ultrasonography – ultrasonic waves to visualize subcutaneous body structures such as tendons and organs.

Ventral (or *anterior*) – describes the front or direction toward the front of the body.

Ventral cavity (or *anterior body cavity*) – larger body cavity located anterior to the posterior (dorsal) body cavity; includes the serous membrane-lined pleural cavities for the lungs, pericardial cavity for the heart, and peritoneal cavity for the abdominal and pelvic organs.

Vertebral cavity (or *spinal cavity*) – a division of the dorsal cavity containing the spinal cord.

X-ray – a form of high-energy electromagnetic radiation with a short wavelength capable of penetrating solids and ionizing gases. It is used in medicine as a diagnostic aid to visualize body structures such as bones.

Frank J. Addivinola, Ph.D.

This study guide's lead author and chief editor is Dr. Frank Addivinola. With his outstanding education, laboratory research, and decades of university science teaching, Dr. Addivinola lent his expertise to oversee the development of this series.

During his extensive career, Dr. Addivinola held faculty positions at colleges and universities, including Harvard University, Johns Hopkins University, University of Maryland, and Northeastern University, and taught undergraduate and graduate-level courses in biology, biochemistry, organic chemistry, inorganic chemistry, physics, anatomy and physiology, medical terminology, nutrition, and medical ethics. He received several awards for his research and presentations.

Dr. Frank Addivinola conducted original research in developmental biology as a doctoral candidate and pre-IRTA fellow in Molecular and Cell Biology at the National Institutes of Health (NIH). His dissertation advisor was Nobel laureate Marshall W. Nirenberg, Chief of the Biochemical Genetics Laboratory at the National Heart, Lung, and Blood Institute (NHLBI). Before NIH, Dr. Addivinola researched prostate cancer in the Cell Growth and Regulation Laboratory of Dr. Arthur Pardee at the Dana Farber Cancer Institute of Harvard Medical School.

Dr. Addivinola holds an undergraduate degree in biology from Williams College. He completed his Masters at Harvard University, Masters in Biotechnology at Johns Hopkins University, and five other graduate degrees at the University of Maryland University College, Suffolk University, and Northeastern University.

Everything You Always Wanted to Know About…

- Chemistry
- Physics
- Cell & Molecular Biology
- Organismal Biology
- Human Anatomy & Physiology
- American History
- American Law
- American Government & Politics
- Comparative Government & Politics
- World History
- European History
- Psychology
- Sociology
- Environmental Science
- Human Geography

Visit our Amazon store

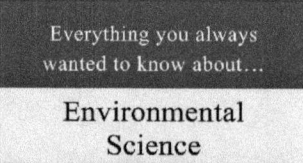

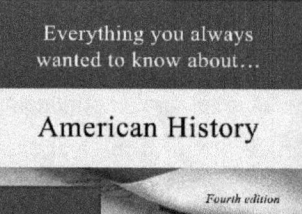

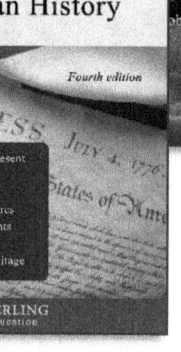